The Amazing Liver and Gallbladder Flush

Also by Andreas Moritz
==================

Timeless Secrets of Health and Rejuvenation

Cancer Is Not a Disease – It's a Healing Mechanism

Lifting the Veil of Duality

Vaccine-Nation

It's Time to Come Alive

Feel Great, Lose Weight

Simple Steps to Total Health

Heart Disease - No More!

Diabetes - No More!

Alzheimer's - No More!

Ending the AIDS Myth

Heal Yourself With Sunlight!

Hear the Whispers, Live Your Dream

Art of Self Healing

All of the above are available at www.ener-chi.com, www.amazon.com, and other online or physical bookstores

The Amazing Liver and Gallbladder Flush

*A Powerful Do-It-Yourself Approach to Optimize Your
Health and Wellbeing . . .
and Much More!*

Andreas Moritz

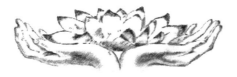

Your Health is in Your Hands

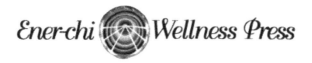

For Reasons of Legality

ISBN-13: 978-0-9845954-4-0

Published by Ener-Chi Wellness Press—Ener-chi.com, USA

First edition, *The Amazing Liver Cleanse*, 1998
Second edition, *The Amazing Liver Cleanse*, 1999 (revised)
Third edition, *The Amazing Liver Cleanse*, USA, 2002 (revised)
Fourth edition, *The Amazing Liver and Gallbladder Flush*, USA, 2005 (extended and revised)
Fifth edition, *same title* USA, Feb. 2007 (improved and reedited)
Sixth edition, *same title* USA, October 2012 (expanded and updated)
Cover Design/Artwork (Ener-Chi Art for the Liver): By Andreas Moritz

Clinical success is the final test.
This book is transforming our current medical model.

Be prepared to be WELL.

"This is more than a book—this is a powerful self-healing tool. At a time when we have given up on our body's own innate wisdom, Andreas Moritz offers a simple, self-directed remedy allowing for one's own self-empowered healing. It is simple, inexpensive, and easy to perform. The healing that occurred for my patients and myself has been life altering."
—**Gene L. Pascucci, BS, DDS** (dentist, metaphysician and mystic living in Reno, Nevada)

"I was intrigued to learn about the liver flush from a friend, although I put off doing it for a good few months. Having suffered from severe health problems for several years, I eventually took the plunge, but not really expecting any great results. Much to my amazement, the next day I excreted about six hundred gallstones of varying sizes and colors, and the relief was instantaneous. I was calmer, felt much less irritable, and had greater clarity of thought. I have now completed five flushes and am nearly back to normal functioning. Whilst I have used other treatment modalities in addition to this cleansing technique, I consider that the liver flush has had a major impact upon my recovery. I shall certainly be adding it to my health maintenance program for the rest of my life."
—**Dr. Diane Phillips, MB, BS, BSc (UK)**

Dedication

To all those who wish to take responsibility for their own health and
who care about
the health and well-being of their
fellow human beings.

TABLE OF CONTENTS

INTRODUCTION

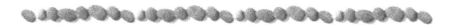

Most people believe that gallstones can be found only in the gallbladder. This is a common, yet false assumption. Most gallstones are actually formed in the liver, and comparatively few occur in the gallbladder. You can easily verify this by giving yourself a liver flush. It matters little whether you are a layperson, a medical doctor, a scientist, or someone whose gallbladder was removed and, therefore, is believed to be stone-free.

The results of the liver flush[1] speak for themselves. No amount of scientific proof or medical explanation can make such a cleanse any more valuable than it already is. Once you see hundreds of green, beige-colored, brown, or black gallstones in the toilet bowl during your first liver flush, you will intuitively know that you are on to something extremely important in your life.

To satisfy your possibly curious mind, you may decide to take the expelled stones to a laboratory for chemical analysis or ask your doctor what she thinks about all that. Your doctor may either support you in your initiative to heal yourself, or tell you this is just ridiculous and warn you against it. Regardless of what others may say to you, what is most significant in this experience is that you have taken active responsibility for your own health, perhaps for the first time in your life.

An estimated 20 percent of the world's population will develop gallstones in their gallbladder at some stage in their lives; many of them will opt for surgical removal of this important organ. Although gallbladder surgery is rarely necessary and can have long-term devastating consequences[2], most patients succumb to the pressure by their doctor and loved ones to have it removed. Some doctors even tell their patient that cutting out their gallbladder is inconsequential. If you no longer have a gallbladder, please read on. Purging your liver of stones is even more important for you than for those who still have a gallbladder.

There are far more people who have gallstones in the *liver* than people who have gallstones in the *gallbladder*. During some 35 years of working in the field of natural medicine and seeing thousands of people suffering

---

[1] When I refer to the liver flush, it includes flushing of the gallbladder as well
[2] Complications after Gallbladder Surgery, steadyhealth.com

from all types of chronic diseases, I can attest to the fact that each one of them, without exception, has had considerable amounts of gallstones in their liver. Surprisingly, relatively few of them reported to have had a history of gallstones in their gallbladder. Gallstones in the liver are, as you will understand from reading this book, the main impediment to acquiring and maintaining good health, youthfulness, and vitality. Gallstones in the liver are, indeed, one of the major reasons people become ill and have difficulty recuperating from illness.

The failure to recognize and accept the incidence of gallstone formation in the liver as an extremely common phenomenon may very well be the most unfortunate oversight that has ever been made in the field of medicine, both orthodox and holistic.

Relying so heavily on blood tests for diagnostic purposes, as conventional medicine does, may actually be a great disadvantage with regard to assessing liver health. Most people who have a physical complaint of one kind or another may show to have perfectly normal liver enzyme levels in the blood, despite suffering from chronic liver bile duct congestion.

Congestion in the liver bile ducts is among the leading health problems, yet conventional medicine rarely refers to it, nor do doctors have a reliable way to detect and diagnose such a condition. Standard liver tests involve measuring liver enzyme counts in the blood. Liver enzymes are only elevated when there is advanced liver cell destruction, as is the case, for example, in liver inflammation, hepatitis, and cirrhosis. It usually takes many years of chronic liver bile duct congestion before liver damage becomes apparent.

Standard clinical tests almost *never* reveal the occurrence of gallstones in the liver. So when a doctor sees the handful of stones that his patient has just released during a liver cleanse, she may just shake her head and proclaim, "These are not gallstones!" In fact, most doctors don't even know that gallstones grow inside the liver, in spite of the fact that medical literature is replete with studies that describe them in great detail.

That said, most of the relevant research was conducted before digital archiving was available (between 1920s and 1960s), and today's health practitioners simply don't have the time to study the research that was done over 50 years ago, not to mention the research published during the past 2-3 years. Now that digital scanning technology provides us with easy access to such historic medical information, we have a better understanding of what these scientists have referred to as *intrahepatic stones* or *intrahepatic gallstones*.

In a more recent publication titled "Intrahepatic Stones - A Clinical Study", a team of researchers describes the results of examining patients afflicted with stones congesting the liver bile ducts. This research, which was published in the Annals of Surgery in February 1972[3], clearly distinguishes between gallstones in the gallbladder and gallstones in the liver. The authors state that "For centuries, both surgeons and pathologists have noticed another type of stone in the intrahepatic biliary ducts. The location, consistency, number, and behavior of such stones were found to be entirely different from choledocholithiasis (stone formation) of gallbladder origin. Liver stones or intrahepatic stones were the names designated for this condition."

Some of the more advanced research universities, such as the prestigious Johns Hopkins University, have begun to describe and illustrate these liver stones in their literature or on their websites. Regardless of the overwhelming scientific evidence of the existence of liver stones, it is remarkable that trained medical professionals still vehemently deny that stones could possibly occur in the liver. They insist that the stones released during liver flushes are merely *olive oil soap stones* that are somehow produced from the ingredients used for the liver cleansing procedure. (I will address this subject later in Chapter 7)

I have frequently argued that intrahepatic gallstones are a relatively new occurrence among populations in the Western Hemisphere. The subjects in this study were mostly people who were undernourished and must have lost weight, and not have had enough fats in their diet to keep bile production stimulated and the bile flora balanced. Weight loss is a well-known, leading cause of intrahepatic gallstones.

In the West, food was a lot more plentiful (except during times of war), organically grown, free of contamination and pesticides, and unprocessed. Most foods eaten consisted of homegrown fresh produce or natural foods purchased from local farmers. No chemical preservatives were used. With the onset of food factories and lab-made foods (now over 44,000), mass vaccination campaigns, toxic cosmetic products, water fluoridation, environmental toxins, chemtrail spraying, and the consumption of medical drugs filled with toxic ingredients, etc., the human liver started mass-producing intrahepatic stones. Today, it's almost impossible not to make

---

[3]Intrahepatic Stones – A Clinical Study: Ann Surg. 1972 February; 175(2): 166–177

them, unless you know how to avoid them. Still, most people, including doctors, are completely unaware of them.

By understanding how gallstones in the liver contribute to the occurrence or deterioration of nearly every kind of illness, and by taking the simple steps to remove them, you will put yourself in charge of restoring your own health and vitality, permanently. The implications of applying the liver flush for yourself (or if you are a health practitioner, for your patients) are immensely rewarding. To have a clean liver equals having a new lease on life.

Although there are numerous factors than can impact your health in one way or another, most of them affect the liver. While it is very important to take care of these other disease-causing factors, leaving the liver out of the equation would be unwise and may actually render any other healing approaches ineffective.

The liver has direct control over the growth and functioning of every cell in the body. Any kind of malfunction, deficiency, or abnormal growth pattern of the cell is largely due to poor liver performance. Even when it has lost up to 60 percent of its original efficiency, the liver's extraordinary design and resourcefulness may still allow it to perform *normally*, as indicated by *in the proper range* blood values. As unbelievable as this may sound to the patient and his doctor, the origin of most diseases can easily be traced to the liver. The first chapter of this book is dedicated to this vitally important connection.

All diseases or symptoms of ill health are caused by an obstruction of some sort. For example, a blood capillary that is blocked can no longer deliver vital oxygen and nutrients to a group of cells it is in charge of supplying to. To survive, these cells will need to enforce specific survival measures. Of course, many of the afflicted cells will not live through the *famine* and will simply die off. Yet other, more resilient cells will adjust to this adverse situation through the process of cell mutation and learn to utilize trapped metabolic waste products, such as lactic acid, to cover their energy needs. These cells may be compared to a man in the desert who, for lack of water, relies on drinking his own urine in order to live a little longer than he would otherwise.

Cell mutation leading to cancer is merely the body's final attempt to help prevent its demise through an overload of toxins and a damaged organ structure. Although common practice, it is farfetched to call the body's predictable response to the accumulation of toxic waste matter and decomposing cell material a *disease*. Unfortunately, ignorance of the body's true nature has caused many to believe that this instinct-driven survival mechanism is an *autoimmune disease*. The word autoimmune suggests that the body attempts to attack itself and practically tries to commit suicide. Nothing could be further from the truth. Among other reasons, cancerous tumors result from major congestion in the connective tissues, blood vessel walls, and lymphatic ducts, all of which prevent healthy cells from receiving enough oxygen and other vital nutrients.

All cancer cells are oxygen-starved. To initiate healing and undo or repair the damage in the affected organ, the body builds new blood vessels to sustain the cancer cells and prevent complete organ failure, at least for as long as possible[4].

Other, more apparent obstructions in the body can also seriously affect your well-being. A constipated colon, for example, prevents the body from eliminating the waste products contained in feces. The retention of fecal matter in the lower intestine leads to a toxic environment in the entire gastrointestinal tract and, if the situation is not resolved, in the rest of the body. Chronic constipation can even make you feel unhappy, anxious, or depressed.

Crystal aggregations formed in the kidneys from dietary minerals can obstruct the flow of urine in the kidneys and urinary bladder, thereby causing kidney infection and kidney failure. The buildup of mineral deposits in the urinary system can also lead to fluid retention, weight gain, high blood pressure, and dozens of disease symptoms.

If acidic, toxic waste matter builds up in the chest and lungs, the body responds with mucus secretions to trap these noxious substances. As a result, the air passages of the lungs become congested, and the body runs out of breath/air. If the body is already very toxic and congested, a lung infection may result.

Lung infections occur to help destroy and remove any damaged, weak lung cells that otherwise would start rotting and form pus. Lung congestion prevents the natural removal of damaged or weak cells. If the congestion is not cleared up through natural means, such as coughing or draining, the pus may be trapped in the lung tissue. Naturally, infectious bacteria will increasingly populate the scene to assist the body in its desperate effort to clean out the congested area, filled with decomposing cells and waste

---

[4] For a complete understanding of what cancer actually is, and what causes it, see my book *Cancer is Not a Disease - It's Healing Mechanism*

products. Doctors call this healing mechanism *staph infection,* or pneumonia.

Poor hearing and ear infections may result if sticky mucus filled with toxins and/or dead or living bacteria enter the ducts that run from your throat to the ears (Eustachian tubes).

Likewise, thickening of the blood (platelets sticking together) caused by highly acid-forming foods or beverages may restrict its flow through the capillaries and arteries, and thereby lead to numerous conditions, ranging from simple skin irritation to arthritis or high blood pressure, even heart attack and stroke.

These or similar obstructions in the body are directly or indirectly linked to restricted liver performance - in particular, to an impasse caused by gallstones in the liver and gallbladder. The presence of chunks of hardened bile and other trapped organic or inorganic substances in these two organs greatly interferes with such vital processes as the digestion of food, elimination of waste, and detoxification of harmful substances in the blood.

By decongesting the liver bile ducts and the gallbladder, the body's 60 to 100 trillion cells will be able to *breathe* more oxygen, receive sufficient amounts of nutrients, efficiently eliminate their metabolic waste products, and maintain perfect communication links with the brain, nervous system, immune system, endocrine system, and all other parts of the body.

Almost every patient suffering a chronic illness has excessive amounts of gallstones in the liver. A doctor can easily confirm this by having a chronically ill patient do a liver flush. It is unfortunate that unless a specific liver disease is found, this vital organ is rarely considered a culprit for other diseases.

The majority of gallstones in the liver consist of the same harmless constituents as are found in liquid bile, with cholesterol being the main ingredient. A number of stones consist of fatty acids and other organic material that has ended up in the bile ducts. The fact that the majority of these stones are just congealed clumps of bile and other organic matter makes them practically invisible to x-rays, ultrasonic technologies, and computerized tomography (CT).

While populations in the Western Hemisphere rarely develop calcified stones in the liver, they are more frequently found in Asian populations, such as in Japan and China.

The situation is different with regard to the gallbladder, where up to about 20 percent of all stones can be made up entirely of minerals, predominantly calcium salts, cholesterol crystals and bile pigments. Whereas diagnostic tests can easily detect these hard, and possibly, large stones in the gallbladder, they tend to miss the softer, non-calcified stones in the liver.

Only when excessive amounts of cholesterol-based stones (85-95 percent cholesterol), or other clumps of fat, block the bile ducts of the liver may an ultrasound test reveal what is generally referred to as *fatty liver disease*. In such a case, the ultrasound pictures reveal a liver that is almost completely white (instead of black). A fatty liver can gather up to 70,000 stones before it succumbs to suffocation and ceases to function.

If you had a fatty liver and went to the doctor, you would be told that you had excessive fatty tissue in your liver. It is less likely, though, that you would be told that you had *intrahepatic gallstones* (stones obstructing the liver's bile ducts). As mentioned before, most of the smaller stones in the liver are not detectable through ultrasound or CT scans. Nevertheless, careful analysis of diagnostic images by specialists would show whether some of the smaller bile ducts in the liver were dilated because of obstruction.

A dilation of bile ducts caused by larger and denser stones or by clusters of stones may be detected more readily through magnetic resonance imaging (MRI). However, unless there is an indication of major liver trouble, doctors rarely check for intrahepatic stones. Unfortunately, although the liver is one of the most important organs in the body, its disorders are also underdiagnosed all too often.

Even if the early stages of a fatty liver or gallstone formation in the bile ducts were easily recognized and diagnosed, today's medical facilities offer no treatments to relieve this vital organ of the heavy burden it has to carry.

Most people in the developed world have accumulated hundreds and, in many cases, thousands of hardened bile and fat deposits in the liver. These stones continuously block the liver's bile ducts, which greatly stresses this vital organ and the rest of the body.

In view of the adverse effect these stones have on liver performance as a whole, their composition is quite irrelevant. Whether your doctor or you consider them conventional mineral-based gallstones, fat deposits, or clots of hardened bile, the net result is that they prevent the necessary amounts of bile from reaching the intestines.

The important question is how such a simple thing as obstructed bile flow can cause such complex diseases as congestive heart failure, diabetes, and cancer.

Liver bile is a bitter, alkaline fluid of a yellow, brown, or green color. It has multiple functions. Each one of these profoundly influences the health of every organ and system in the body. Apart from assisting with the digestion of fat, calcium, and protein foods, bile is needed to maintain normal fat levels in the blood, remove toxins from the liver, help maintain proper acid/alkaline balance in the intestinal tract, and keep the colon from breeding harmful microbes.

Bile prevents and possibly cures cancer and heart disease, the two leading causes of death! The importance of bile for maintaining good health has not been fully acknowledged yet, at least not by mainstream medicine. However, scientific evidence has been mounting that suggests the bile pigments bilirubin and biliverdin, which give color to bile, play an extremely important physiological role in humans.

According to a study published in 2008 in the prestigious medical journal *Mutation Research*, bile pigments possess strong anti-mutagenic properties[5]. The researchers stated that in the past, bile pigments and bilirubin, in particular, were thought of as useless by-products of heme[6] catabolism (breaking down) that can be toxic if they accumulate. "However, in the past 20 years, research probing the physiological relevance of bile pigments has been mounting, with evidence to suggest bile pigments possess significant antioxidant and anti-mutagenic properties," the study concludes.

Doctors tend to make you panic if your skin color or eyes turn yellow (jaundice). They won't tell you that your body is actually in the process of getting rid of dangerous peroxyl radicals and a number of classes of mutagens (polycyclic aromatic hydrocarbons, heterocyclic amines, oxidants), all chemicals known to cause cells to become cancerous. To say it differently, sometimes the body appears to make you ill so that it can make you truly healthy.

I consider this research finding to be one of most important discoveries in the field of medicine, something that the most ancient system of

---

[5]Mutat Res. 2008 Jan-Feb;658(1-2):28-41. Epub 2007 May 18
[6]Component of hemoglobin, the red pigment in blood

medicine (6,000-year-old Ayurveda) has known all along. Bile, unless trapped by stones in the bile ducts or by stones in the gallbladder, can prevent healthy cells from mutating into cancer cells. In fact, the research found that people with higher concentrations of bilirubin and biliverdin in their bodies have a lower incidence of cancer and cardiovascular disease.

According to Japanese research, the increased levels of bile pigments during jaundice can even resolve persistent, difficult to control asthma due to acute hepatitis B[7].

Naturally, these and similar findings, raise the question whether what medical science considers to be diseases may actually be complex survival and healing attempts by the body. When treated and suppressed with pharmaceutical drugs, the body's healing efforts may be completely compromised. Instead of waging a drug war against the body, we might just as well support it by removing unnecessary, accumulated obstructions. Given the immensely important role that bile and its components play in the body, it makes perfect sense to keep the bile flow unhindered at all times.

To maintain a strong and healthy digestive system, prevent cell mutation and oxidation damage, and feed body cells the right amount of nutrients, the liver has to produce 1–1.5 quarts of bile per day. Anything less than that is bound to cause problems with the digestion of food, elimination of waste, and the body's continual detoxification of the blood. Many people produce just about a cupful of bile or less per day. As will be shown in this book, nearly all health problems are a direct or indirect consequence of reduced bile availability.

People with chronic illnesses often have several thousand gallstones congesting the bile ducts of the liver. Some stones may have also formed in the gallbladder. By removing these stones from these organs through a series of liver flushes and maintaining a balanced diet and lifestyle, the liver and gallbladder can restore their original efficiency, and most symptoms of discomfort or disease in the body can start subsiding. You may find that any persistent allergies will lessen or disappear. Back pain will dissipate, while energy and well-being will improve.

Ridding the liver bile ducts of gallstones is one of the most important and powerful procedures you can apply to improve and regain your health.

In this book, you will learn how to remove painlessly up to several hundred gallstones at a time. The size of the stones ranges from that of a

---

[7]Tohoku J Exp Med. 2003 Mar;199(3):193-6

pinhead to a small walnut, and in some rare cases, a golf ball. The actual liver flush takes place within a period of less than 14 hours and can be done conveniently over a weekend at home.

Chapter 1 explains in detail why the presence of gallstones in the bile ducts, both inside and outside the liver, can be considered the greatest health risk and may cause almost every major or minor illness.

In Chapter 2, you will be able to identify the signs, marks, and symptoms that indicate the presence of stones in your liver or gallbladder.

Chapter 3 deals with the possible causes of gallstones.

In Chapter 4, you will learn the actual procedure to rid your liver and gallbladder of gallstones. It basically consists of a preparatory period of 6 days during which stones are being softened, and the actual flush procedure that involves the drinking of a mixture of olive and citrus juice.

Chapter 5 contains guidelines on what you can do to prevent new gallstones from forming.

Chapter 6, *What I Can Expect from the Liver and Gallbladder Flush*, covers some of the possible health benefits of this profound self-help tool.

Chapter 7 covers the many misconceptions laypersons and medical professionals still have about the liver flush, and the false information spread by those who have a financial and vested interest in keeping people away from cleansing their liver and proactively taking care of their own health.

Moreover, you can read what others have to say about their experiences with the liver flush on my website www.ener-chi.com, where you will also find a list of the most frequently asked questions pertaining to the flush

To reap the maximum benefit from this procedure, and to do it safely, I strongly encourage you to read this entire book before starting with the actual liver flush.

In addition to providing you with all the information you will need in order to have to safely and thoroughly cleanse your liver and gallbladder and restore your digestive health, this new edition is packed full with essential information about taking care of many other important aspects of your health and well-being.

"How does the liver and gallbladder flush work?" you may ask. The process is actually quite simple. Its cleansing effects are due to the ingested oil mixture prompting a powerful and quick discharge of bile from the liver and the gallbladder. The outpouring of bile takes along with it any toxins, cholesterol stones from the liver and calcified gallstones from the gallbladder, if present. Both, the liver and the gallbladder, release toxins and stones into the common bile duct.

The cleansing procedure also includes taking several doses of magnesium sulfate (Epsom salt) which relaxes the bile ducts and keeps them wide open during the release process while also ensuring easy passage of the stones through the intestinal tract[8]. The stones enter the duodenum (the first part of the small intestine) where the common bile duct joins the pancreatic duct. From there onwards, the stones and toxins travel into the large intestine for excretion.

The picture shown on the cover of the book is part of a series of energized oil paintings, known as Ener-Chi Art, which I created in order to help restore the life force energy (chi) in all the organs and systems of the body. The photographic print of this particular picture helps to restore chi flow in the liver and gallbladder.

Unfortunately, digital prints such as the one shown on the book cover do not have nearly this effect, although there are benefits. (To order photo prints, *see Other Books and Products by Andreas Moritz*) Viewing this picture for at least 30 seconds and preferably longer - before, sometimes during, and after the flush - energizes these two organs and may assist you in the process of cleansing and rejuvenating them. The picture, though, is not necessary to achieve excellent results.

I wish you great success on your journey to achieving the perpetual state of health, happiness, and vitality that you deserve!

---

[8]An Analysis of the Reaction of the Human Gall Bladder and Sphincter of Oddi to Magnesium Sulfate. *Surgery* 1943; 13:723-733. This effect has also been demonstrated by research published in the *American Journal of Digestive Diseases*; Volume 9, Number 5, 162-165, DOI: 10.1007/BF02997291

Chapter 1

*Successfully digesting your food protects you
against most illnesses; failing to digest it puts you
in an endless cycle of disease and suffering.*

Gallstones in the Liver: A Major Health Risk

Think of the liver as a large city with thousands of houses and streets. There are underground pipes for delivering water, oil, and gas. Sewage systems and garbage trucks remove the city's waste products. Power lines bring energy into the homes and businesses. Factories, transport systems, communication networks, and stores meet the daily living requirements of the residents.

The organization of city life is such that it can provide all that it needs for the continued existence of the population. But if a major strike, a power outage, a devastating earthquake, or a major act of terrorism, such as the one we witnessed in New York City on September 11, 2001, suddenly paralyzes city life, the population will begin to suffer serious shortcomings in all these vital sectors.

Like a city's infrastructure, the liver has hundreds of different functions and is connected with every part of the body. At every moment of the day, this vital organ is involved in manufacturing, processing, and supplying vast amounts of nutrients for the 60 to 100 trillion inhabitants (cells) of the body. Each cell is, in itself, a microscopic city of immense complexity that generates billions of biochemical reactions per second.

To sustain the incredibly diverse activities of all the cells of the body without disruption, the liver must supply them with a constant and uninterrupted stream of nutrients, enzymes, and hormones. With its intricate labyrinth of veins, ducts, and specialized cells, the liver needs to be completely unobstructed in order to maintain a problem-free production line and frictionless distribution system throughout the body.

The liver is not only the main organ responsible for distributing and regenerating the body's fuel supply, its activities also include the breaking down of complex chemicals and the synthesis of proteins.

The liver acts as a filtering or cleansing device for the blood; it even deactivates a limited amount of hormones, alcohol, and medicinal drugs. Its task is to modify these biologically active substances so that they lose their potentially harmful effects - a process known as detoxification. Specialized cells in the liver's blood vessels (Kupffer cells) mop up harmful elements and infectious organisms reaching the liver from the gut. The liver excretes the waste materials resulting from these actions via its bile duct network.

A healthy liver receives and filters 3 pints of blood per minute and produces 1 to 1.5 quarts of bile every day. This ensures that all the activities in the liver and in the rest of the body run smoothly and efficiently. As you will learn in this book, obstructive gallstones in its bile ducts greatly undermine the liver's ability to detoxify any externally supplied and internally generated harmful substances in the blood. These stones also prevent the liver from delivering the proper amounts of nutrients and energy to the right places in the body at the right time. This upsets the delicate balance in the body, known as *homeostasis*, thus leading to disruption of its systems and undue stress on its organs.

A clear example for such a disturbed balance is an increased concentration of the endocrine hormones estrogen and aldosterone in the blood. These hormones, produced in both men and women, are responsible for the correct amount of salt and water retention. When stones congest the gallbladder and the liver's bile ducts, these hormones may not be broken down and detoxified sufficiently. Hence, their concentration in the blood rises to abnormal levels, causing tissue swelling and water retention. Most oncologists consider elevated estrogen levels to be the leading cause of breast cancer among women. In men, high levels of this hormone can lead to excessive development of breast tissue and weight gain.

Over 85 percent of the American population is overweight or obese. Men, women, and children in this condition suffer mainly from fluid retention (with relatively minor fat accumulation). The retained fluids help trap and neutralize noxious substances that the liver can no longer effectively remove from the body. This unsightly side effect, however, helps the overweight or obese person to prevent or even survive a major toxicity crisis that could otherwise lead to a heart attack, cancer, or massive infection.

The problem with prolonged fluid retention in the tissues, though, is that it causes these toxins and other harmful waste matter (metabolic waste and dead cell material) to accumulate in various parts of the body and further congest the pathways of circulation and elimination. Wherever in the body the storage capacity for toxins and waste is exceeded, symptoms of illness begin to show up. These symptoms merely indicate that the body is desperately trying to correct these imbalances and heal itself.

My observations of hundreds of different diseases over the past 40 years have convinced me that disease is rather a highly sophisticated healing mechanism than an accidental mistake the body somehow makes. Oftentimes, though, this healing effort by the body constitutes an uphill battle, and we would be better off if we helped it along so we don't have to suffer needlessly.

Gallstones in the liver, which Johns Hopkins University and some medical schools refer to as *intrahepatic biliary gallstones* or *biliary stones*[9], tend to cluster together and form large obstructions that can lead to dilation of bile ducts (see **Figure 1a**). Intrahepatic gallstones are composed of mostly cholesterol and other bile constituents (see laboratory report - **Figure 1b**).

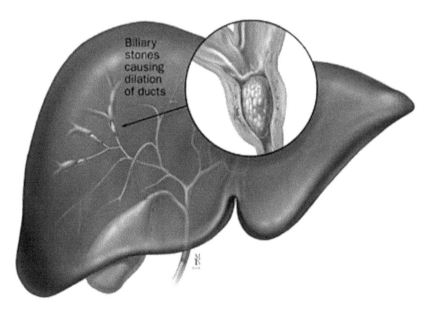

Figure 1a: Biliary stones (intrahepatic gallstones)
(By courtesy of Johns Hopkins University)

---

[9]Intrahepatic Biliary Gallstones, Johns Hopkins University, Gastroenterology & Hematology, Cholangiocarcinoma: Causes; http://www.hopkins-gi.org

Name: RYAN, SARAH JANE
Address: 17 DUNROBIN STREET
         SHEPPARTON. 3630
D.O.B.: 26/01/1977 Sex: F
Medicare No: 3242627517
Lab. Reference: 08097500
Date requested: 05/06/2008
Addressee: DR KRISTINA TAVCAR
Referred by: DR KRISTINA TAVCAR
Collected: 13/06/2008 17:16
Specimen:
Test name: CALCULUS

Requested: 05/06/2008
Performed: 13/06/2008
Test name: CALCULUS

```
SAMPLE 1

STONE ANALYSIS

ORIGIN                  :   Biliary
NUMBER OF STONES        :   Numerous gallstones and fragments
STONE SHAPE             :   Irregularly Shaped
STONE COLOUR            :   Light Green
STONE TEXTURE           :   Rough

WEIGHT TOTAL            :   0.2 g
CRUSHED APPEARANCE      :   Green, Soft
COMPOSITION             :   Predominantly Cholesterol
                            Not Detected Bilirubin

This specimen was collected on: 24/05/2008

SAMPLE 2
STONE ANALYSIS

ORIGIN                  :   Biliary
NUMBER OF STONES        :   Numerous gallstones and fragments
STONE SHAPE             :   Irregularly Shaped
STONE COLOUR            :   Light Green
STONE TEXTURE           :   Rough

WEIGHT TOTAL            :   <0.1 g
CRUSHED APPEARANCE      :   Green, Soft
COMPOSITION             :   Predominantly Cholesterol
                            Not Detected Bilirubin

This specimen was collected on: 13/06/2008

This test performed by Dorevitch Pathology
```

FILE
NORMAL
SPEAK TO PATIENT
SEE PATIENT
REQUIRE FILE

Figure 1b: Laboratory report (soft, green cholesterol stones)

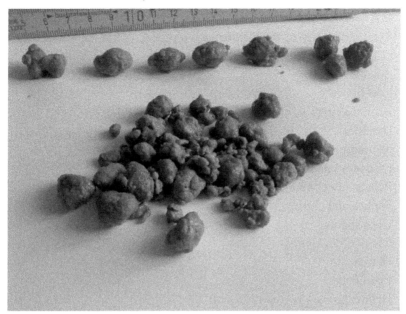

Figure 1c: Flushed out gallstones (soft cholesterol stones)

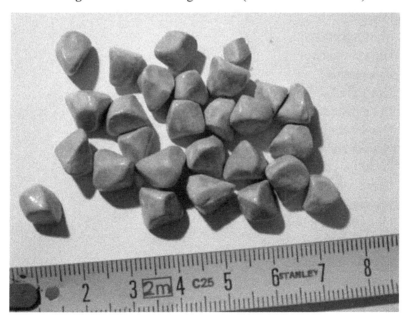

Figure 1d: Flushed out gallstones (hard, calcified gallstones)

If you suffer any of the following symptoms, or similar conditions, you most likely have numerous gallstones in your liver and gallbladder:

- Low appetite
- Food cravings
- Diarrhea
- Nausea
- Frequent vomiting
- Pain in upper abdomen
- Shakes and chills
- Constipation
- Clay-colored stool
- Hernia
- Flatulence
- Hemorrhoids
- Dull pain on the right side
- Difficulty breathing
- Liver cirrhosis
- Hepatitis
- Most infections
- High cholesterol
- Pancreatitis
- Heart disease
- Brain disorders
- Duodenal ulcers
- Nausea and vomiting
- A "bilious" or angry personality
- Depression
- Impotence
- Other sexual problems
- Prostate diseases
- Urinary problems
- Hormonal imbalances
- Menstrual and menopausal disorders
- Problems with vision
- Puffy eyes
- Any skin disorder

- Liver spots, especially those on the back of the hands and facial area
- Dizziness and fainting spells
- Loss of muscle tone
- Excessive weight or wasting
- Strong shoulder and back pain
- Pain at the top of a shoulder blade and/or between the shoulder blades
- Dark color under the eyes
- Morbid complexion
- Tongue that is glossy or coated in white or yellow
- Scoliosis
- Gout
- Frozen shoulder
- Stiff neck
- Asthma
- Allergies
- Headaches and migraines
- Tooth and gum problems
- Yellowness of the eyes and skin
- Sciatica
- Numbness and paralysis of the legs
- Joint diseases
- Knee problems
- Osteoporosis
- Obesity
- Chronic fatigue
- Kidney diseases
- Cancer
- Multiple Sclerosis and fibromyalgia
- Alzheimer's disease
- Cold extremities
- Excessive heat and perspiration in the upper part of the body
- Very greasy hair and hair loss
- Cuts or wounds that keep bleeding and do not heal
- Difficulty sleeping, insomnia
- Nightmares
- Stiffness of joints and muscles
- Hot and cold flashes
- Multiple chemical sensitivities

What Makes Bile so Important?

As already mentioned, one of the liver's most important functions is to produce bile, about 1 to 1.5 quarts (0.95 - 1.4 liters) per day. Liver bile is a viscous, yellow, brown, or green fluid that at a pH of 9.5 is highly alkaline and has a bitter taste. Without sufficient bile, hydrochloric acid entering the small intestine from the stomach can cause burns throughout the gastrointestinal tract. Also, ingested foods remain undigested or only partially digested. For example, to enable the small intestine to digest and absorb fat and calcium from the food you eat, the food must first combine with bile.

When bile secretion is insufficient, fat is not absorbed properly. The undigested fat remains in the intestinal tract. When undigested fat reaches the colon along with other waste products, intestinal bacteria break down some of the fat into fatty acids or excrete it with the stool. Since fat is lighter than water, having fat in the stool may cause it to float. When fat is not absorbed, calcium is not absorbed either, leaving the blood in a deficit. The blood subsequently takes its extra calcium from the bones.

Most bone density problems (osteoporosis) actually arise from insufficient bile secretion and poor digestion of fats, rather than from not consuming enough calcium. Few medical practitioners are aware of this fact and, hence, merely prescribe calcium supplements to their patients without addressing the underlying reason for calcium deficiency.

Likewise, the body also requires fats to help digest and make use of proteins and carbohydrates. To digest these fats, the liver and gallbladder must release sufficient amounts of bile. Poor bile secretion leaves these foods largely undigested, which subjects them to decomposition by bacteria. Persistent abdominal gas, discomfort, and bloating are among the first indications to show that this important liver function has been seriously compromised.

Besides breaking down the fats in our food, bile also removes toxins from the liver. The liver is the most important organ of detoxification, and the health of every cell depends on how effectively it rids itself of these toxins.

As already mentioned in the introduction, the important bile constituents, bilirubin and biliverdin, possess significant antioxidant and anti-mutagenic properties. Higher concentrations of bile pigments in the body have been linked with reduced prevalence of cancer and cardio-vascular disease.

One of the lesser-known but extremely important functions of bile is to deacidify and cleanse the intestines. Bile serves as the body's natural laxative. Constipation and sluggish bowel movements are the commonest consequences of impeded bile secretion.

When gallstones in the liver or gallbladder have critically obstructed bile flow, the color of the stool may be tan, orange-yellow, or pale as in clay, instead of the normal brown.

Gallstones are a direct product of an unhealthy diet and lifestyle. Even if someone has successfully dealt with all other causes of a chronic illness, if gallstones are still present in the liver or gallbladder, recovery may be short-lived or impossible.

Gallstones pose a considerable health risk and may lead to illness and premature aging. The following pages describe some of the main detrimental effects of gallstones on the different organs and systems in the body. When these stones are removed, the body as a whole can resume its normal, healthy activities.

Disorders of the Digestive System

The first part of the body affected by gallstones in the liver and gallbladder is the digestive system which can be compared to the root system of a plant or tree.

The alimentary tract of the digestive system maintains the following four main activities: ingestion, digestion, absorption, and elimination. The alimentary canal begins in the mouth; continues through the thorax, abdomen, and pelvic region; and ends at the anus (see **Figure2**).When you eat a meal, a series of digestive processes begin to take place. These can be divided into the mechanical breakdown of food through mastication (chewing) and the chemical breakdown of food through enzymes. These enzymes are present in the secretions produced by various glands of the digestive system.

Enzymes are minute chemical substances composed of proteins that cause or speed up chemical changes in other substances without themselves being changed. Digestive enzymes are contained in the saliva of the salivary glands of the mouth, the gastric juice in the stomach, the intestinal juice in the small intestine, the pancreatic juice in the pancreas, and the bile in the liver/gallbladder.

Absorption is the process by which tiny nutrient particles of digested food pass through the intestinal walls into the blood and lymph vessels, which help distribute them to the cells of the body.

The bowels eliminate as feces whatever food substances they cannot digest or absorb, such as the plant fiber cellulose. Fecal matter also contains bile, which carries toxins and the waste products resulting from the breakdown (catabolism) of red blood cells. Bile contains bilirubin that is derived from these dead red blood cells and gives stool its naturally brown color.

In a healthy digestive system, about one-third of the excreted fecal matter is made up of dead intestinal bacteria. The rest of the fecal matter is composed of indigestible fiber and sloughed off intestinal lining. The body can function smoothly and efficiently only if the bowel removes these daily-generated waste materials every day. Otherwise, the body can become a cesspool of waste, and gradually begin to suffocate in it.

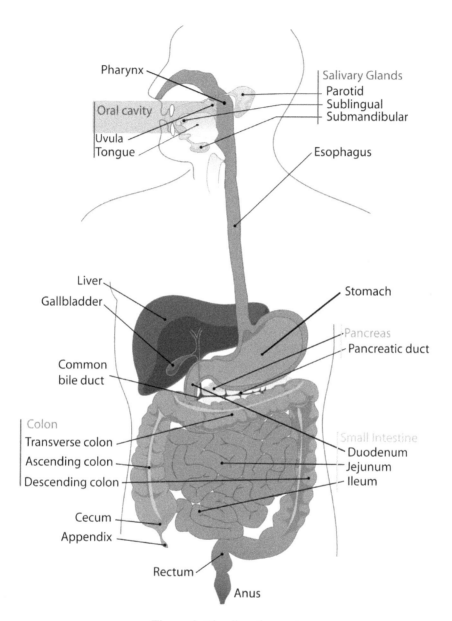

Figure 2: The digestive system
(Illustration by Mariana Ruiz Villarreal)

Good health results when each of these major activities in the digestive system is balanced and well coordinated with the rest of the body. By contrast, abnormalities begin to arise in the digestive system as well as in other parts of the body when one or more of these functions becomes impaired. The presence of gallstones in the liver and gallbladder has a disruptive influence on the digestion and absorption of food, as well as on the body's waste disposal system.

Diseases of the Mouth

Gallstones in the liver and gallbladder can be held responsible for most diseases of the mouth. The stones interfere with the digestion and absorption of food, which, in turn, forces waste products meant for elimination to remain in the intestinal tract. The storage of waste matter in the intestines creates a filthy, toxic environment that supports excessive breeding of destructive microorganisms and parasites and undermines preservation of healthy, resilient tissues.

Bacterial infection (thrush) and viral infection (herpes) in the mouth occur only when the intestines have accumulated considerable amounts of waste matter. Any amount of stagnant waste matter naturally attracts decomposing bacteria that start off the rotting process to break it down and reduce it. Particularly anaerobic organisms, originating in the gastrointestinal tract, begin to transform undigested carbohydrates, lipids, and proteins, to yield organic acids (propionic acid, lactic acid) and gases (methane, hydrogen sulphide, ammonia). This process of microbial proliferation, also referred to as putrefaction, leads to the highly uncomfortable condition known as bloating. You cannot help but notice when you are bloated because you will feel as though the joy of life is being sucked out of you.

Some of the powerful toxins and gases produced by decomposing bacteria in the intestines are absorbed into the blood and lymph fluids, which carry them to the liver and the brain, thereby causing energy loss and brain fog. The rest of the toxins remain in the intestines where they are a constant source of irritation to the intestinal lining (which begins in the mouth and ends in the anus). Eventually, parts of the intestinal wall become inflamed and develop ulcerous lesions. The damaged intestinal tissue begins to attract specific microbes to the scene of injury to help break down and dispose of any weak and damaged cells. We call this *infection*. Most doctors and laypersons will blame the germs for an infection; they do not even consider that there could be an underlying necessity for such a bacterial assistance.

Infection is a completely natural phenomenon seen everywhere in nature whenever there is something that needs to be decomposed. Bacteria never attack (infect) something that is as clean, vital, and healthy as a well-nourished fruit hanging on a tree. Only when the fruit becomes overripe, lacks nourishment, or falls to the ground can bacteria begin their clean-up job. While decomposing food or flesh, bacteria produce toxins. You can recognize these toxins by their unpleasant odor and acidic nature. A very similar process occurs when bacteria act on undigested food in the intestines. If this situation takes place day after day and month after month, the resulting toxins will lead to the appearance of symptoms of illness.

Thrush, which is a yeast infection that causes white patches in the mouth and on the tongue, indicates the presence of large quantities of yeast bacteria that have spread throughout the gastrointestinal tract (GI tract), including the mouth area. It shows up in the mouth because the mucus lining there is not as developed and resistant as in the lower parts of the GI tract.

The main source of thrush, though, is in the intestines. Since the largest part of the immune system in the body is located in the mucus lining of the GI tract, thrush indicates a major weakness in the body's general immunity to disease. The intestinal yeast can grow and spread unhindered.

Herpes, which doctors consider a viral disease, is similar to thrush, with the exception that, instead of bacteria attacking the cell exterior, viral materials attack the nucleus, or cell interior. In both cases, the *attackers* target only weak and unhealthy cells i.e. cells that are already damaged or dysfunctional and are potentially susceptible to mutate into cancerous cells.

Added to this survival drama, gallstones can harbor quantities of bacteria and viruses, which escape the liver via the secreted bile and affect those parts of the body that are the least protected or already weakened. The thing to keep in mind is that germs do not infect the body unless it requires their help. The intestinal tract needs bile to keep itself neat and clean. Lack of bile in the intestines prevents this from happening. The next best solution to removing harmful waste matter is to employ the assistance of germs for the purpose of decomposing it.

Gallstones in the liver bile ducts and gallbladder can also lead to other problems in the mouth. They inhibit proper bile secretion, which, in turn, subdues natural appetite and secretions of saliva from the salivary glands in the mouth. You need ample amounts of saliva to keep your mouth clean and its tissues soft and pliable. If your salivary glands produce too little of it, infectious germs begin to invade the mouth cavity. This can lead to tooth decay, gum destruction, and other tooth-related problems. However, to reiterate the previously made point, bacteria do not *cause* tooth decay or gingivitis. These germs are attracted only to those tissues in the mouth that are already affected by accumulated toxins or are otherwise undernourished and congested.

A bitter/sour taste in the mouth is caused by bile that has regurgitated into the stomach and, from there, into the mouth. This condition occurs because of major intestinal congestion, as seen, for example, during bouts of constipation. Instead of properly moving downward and out of the body, a portion of the intestinal content backs up. This backwashing of waste, in turn, may force bile, bile salts, bacteria, gas, toxins, and other irritating substances into the upper areas of the GI tract. Bile in the mouth, for example, drastically alters the pH value (acidity/alkalinity) of saliva, which inhibits its cleansing action and makes the mouth more susceptible to infectious germs.

A mouth ulcer in the lower lip indicates a similar inflammatory condition in the large intestine. A repeated occurrence of ulcers (in either one of the two corners of the mouth) points to the presence of duodenal ulcers (also see the following section, *Diseases of the Stomach*). Tongue ulcers, depending on their location on the tongue, indicate pockets of inflammation in corresponding areas of the alimentary canal, such as the stomach, small intestine, appendix, or large intestine.

Diseases of the Stomach

As already indicated, gallstones and subsequent digestive trouble can lead to regurgitation of bile and bile salts into the stomach. Such an occurrence adversely changes the composition of gastric juices and the amount of mucus generated in the stomach. The mucus is there to protect the surface stomach lining from the caustic effects of hydrochloric acid. The condition where this protective *shield* is broken or diminished is known as gastritis.

Gastritis can occur in acute or chronic form. When the surface cells (epithelium) of the stomach are exposed to acidic gastric juice, the cells absorb hydrogen ions. This increases their internal acidity, counterbalances their basic metabolic processes, and causes an inflammatory reaction. In more severe cases, there may be ulceration of the mucosa (peptic or gastric ulcer), bleeding, partial perforation of the stomach wall, and peritonitis, a condition that occurs when an ulcer erodes through the full thickness of the stomach and its contents enter the peritoneal cavity.

Duodenal ulcers develop when hydrochloric acid leaving the stomach erodes the duodenum's lining. In many cases, the acid production is unusually high. Eating too many foods that require strong acid secretions, as well as improper food combining (for more details, see my book *Timeless Secrets of Health and Rejuvenation*), often disturb balanced acid production. Esophageal reflux, commonly known as heartburn, is a condition in which stomach acid washes upward into the esophagus and causes irritation or injury to the delicate tissues lining the esophagus. Contrary to common belief, though, this condition is rarely due to the stomach's making too much hydrochloric acid, but instead due to backwashing of waste, toxins, and bile from the intestines into the stomach, and not having enough acid in the stomach.

The regurgitation of bile interferes particularly with gastric secretions, which, in turn, prevents the sphincter of the esophagus from properly closing. Hence, stomach acid may enter the esophagus, thereby causing the burning sensation so many people experience as heartburn. In most cases, acid reflux results when the stomach makes too little hydrochloric acid, thereby forcing food to remain there too long and to ferment. Taking antacids can further undermine the digestion of foods and cause serious corrosive damage to the stomach and the rest of the digestive system.

A number of other causes of gastritis and heartburn can be identified. They include overeating, consuming sugar, sweets, and fried foods, excessive alcohol consumption, heavy cigarette smoking, drinking too much coffee every day (more than 1-2 cups), drinking carbonated beverages, eating large quantities of animal protein and animal fats, and subjecting oneself to ionizing radiation (x-rays, CT scans, mammograms, etc.), immunosuppressive (cytotoxic) drugs, antibiotics, aspirin, and other anti-inflammatory drugs. At age 53, my father was treated for an entire year with antibiotics which perforated his stomach, causing him to bleed to death.

Food poisoning, very spicy foods, iced beverages, dehydration, and emotional stress also lead to gastric problems. Any of the above factors is capable of causing gallstones in the liver and gallbladder, thereby starting off a vicious cycle and creating major disruptions throughout the GI tract. In the final event, malignant stomach tumors may develop.

Most medical doctors now believe that the bacterium H. pylori is responsible for causing stomach ulcers. Combating H. pylori with antibiotic drugs usually brings relief and stops the ulcer. Although the drug does not prevent the ulcer from returning after discontinuation of the treatment, there is a high *recovery* rate. Still, these presumed recoveries may cause side effects that are often more serious than the original infection.

The infection by the H. pylori bug is only possible because factors other than a normally harmless germ have already weakened and damaged the stomach cells. In a healthy stomach, the same bug turns out to be completely innocuous. Most of us have lived with this bug without ever being troubled by it.

In fact, research now tells us we need this bug to regulate leptin. Leptin, a protein product of the obesity gene expressed primarily by adipocytes, is known to regulate food intake, energy expenditure, and body weight homeostasis. A 2001 study published in the medical journal *Gut* on the effect of H. pylori infection on gastric leptin expression[10] demonstrated that gastric leptin may play a role in weight gain after eradication of H. pylori infection.

Although these bugs can be found everywhere and in everyone, only a few people develop stomach ulcers. Why do H. pylori cause a gastric ulcer in 1 out of 20 people and not in the other 19, although the bacterium is found in all of them? Similarly, a trapped nerve can be seen as a cause of disease in the body, but not every trapped nerve results in disease. Instead of looking for an external culprit for such a problem, wouldn't it be far more important to find out *why* some trapped nerves produce pathological changes and others don't? Why does the same frightening situation cause a panic attack or an infarct in one person and not in another?

Conventional medicine erroneously assumes that removing a symptom of disease or infectious bacteria also removes the health condition. However, in reality, the *successful* removal of the symptoms usually creates a far more serious and often life-threatening situation.

As mentioned before, scientific research suggests that the disappearance of H. pylori, the bacterium present in peptic ulcers, may actually be contributing to the obesity epidemic. H. pylori regulates the

[10]Azuma *et al* (Gut 2001;49:324–9)

production of leptin and ghrelin. Leptin is a protein hormone with important effects in regulating appetite, body weight, metabolism and reproductive functions. Ghrelin, a circulating growth hormone-releasing peptide derived from the stomach, stimulates hunger and food intake.

Destroying H. pylori in the stomach can upset the balance of these hormones and lead to spiraling effects of weight gain and injury to all organs and systems in the body. Merely replacing one symptom of disease such as peptic ulcer with another one, such as obesity which can lead to cancer, diabetes or heart attack, is not only unwise but also very risky.

It is far better and easier to take care of the underlying causes of disease than merely shutting off its symptoms. Gallstones in the liver and gallbladder can cause intestinal congestion and thereby lead to frequent regurgitation of bile and toxins into the stomach, which may injure an ever-increasing number of stomach cells. In addition, antibiotics and other drugs destroy the natural stomach flora, including those bacteria that normally help to break down damaged cells or regulate important hormones such as leptin and ghrelin.

Although the antibiotic approach results in a quick relief of symptoms, it also lowers stomach performance permanently, which sets up the body for more severe challenges than just dealing with an ulcer[11].

According to a new research report published in *Nature*[12], titled "Stop the Killing of Beneficial Bacteria", antibiotics can permanently destroy gut flora balance, leading to lifelong illness. For one thing, use of antibiotics inevitably leads to Candida overgrowth and may cause obesity, type 1 diabetes, inflammatory bowel disease, allergies and asthma, disorders of the nervous system, and a permanently damaged immune system.

Author of the editorial, Professor Martin Blaser from New York University's (NYU) Langone Medical Center calls for a dramatic decrease in the use of antibiotics, especially in children and pregnant women. Blaser points out that antibiotics are routinely prescribed to children for ear infections and colds, although they have not been found to be of any significant benefit for either condition. On an average, children receive up to 20 courses of antibiotics before they reach adulthood.

In addition, up to one-half of women in developed countries receive antibiotics during pregnancy. Add to that the antibiotics that are added to

---

[11] For more details on the treatments of stomach ulcers and their consequences, see my book *Timeless Secrets of Health and Rejuvenation*

[12] Blaser MJ. Stop the killing of beneficial bacteria. Nature 476, 393–394 (25 August 2011). doi:10.1038/476393a

every vaccine and those that are found in all commercially-produced meat products, and you have a disease-generating disaster at hand. There is now even evidence of a close link between unbalanced intestinal flora and brain disorders, including autism and Alzheimer's disease.

Shortcuts to healing rarely pay off. A successful suppression of disease symptoms actually implies that the body's healing ability is being sabotaged. Symptoms of disease merely indicate that the body has responded to an existing imbalance and is actively engaged in healing itself. When doctors say, "Our treatment was a success," it actually translates as, "We were successfully able to stop the body's healing efforts." The main idea behind this symptom-oriented approach is that by ending or alleviating the symptoms of an illness, you also stop or control the illness. The only problem with shutting down disease symptoms like pain, infection, fever, inflammation, and thereby preventing the body from completing its healing efforts is that it leads to side effects that can ruin a person's health for life. In the United States, over 980,000 people die each year from the treatment of a disease, not the disease. For the vast majority of people, this makes medical treatment far more dangerous than doing nothing at all.

On the other hand, symptoms of stomach disorders, for example, tend to disappear spontaneously when all gallstones are removed and a healthy diet and balanced lifestyle are followed.

Diseases of the Pancreas

The pancreas is a small gland with its head lying in the curve of the duodenum. Its main duct joins the common bile duct to form what is known as the ampulla of the bile duct. The ampulla enters the duodenum at its midpoint. Apart from secreting the hormones insulin and glucagon, the pancreas produces pancreatic juice, which contains enzymes that digest carbohydrates, proteins, and fats. When the acidic contents from the stomach enter the duodenum, they combine with alkaline pancreatic juice and bile. This creates the proper acid/alkaline balance (pH value) at which the pancreatic enzymes are most effective.

Gallstones in the liver or gallbladder cut bile secretions from the normal amount of a quart or more per day, to as little as a cup or less per day. This severely disrupts the digestive process, particularly when fats or fat-containing foods are consumed. Subsequently, the duodenal pH remains too low, which inhibits the action of pancreatic enzymes, as well as those secreted by the small intestine. The net result is that food is only partially digested. Improperly digested food that is saturated with the stomach's hydrochloric acid can have a very irritating, caustic effect on the entire intestinal tract.

If a gallstone has moved from the gallbladder into the ampulla, where the common bile duct and the pancreatic ducts combine (see **Figure 3**), the release of pancreatic juice becomes obstructed and bile enters the pancreas. This causes a number of protein-splitting pancreatic enzymes, which are normally activated only in the duodenum, to be activated while still in the pancreas. This makes these enzymes highly destructive. They begin to digest parts of the pancreatic tissue, which can lead to infection, suppuration, and local thrombosis. This condition is known as pancreatitis.

Gallstones obstructing the ampulla release bacteria, viruses, and toxins into the pancreas, which can cause further damage to pancreatic cells, and eventually lead to malignant tumors. The tumors occur mostly in the head of the pancreas, where they inhibit the flow of bile and pancreatic juice. This condition is often accompanied by jaundice (for details, see the following section, *Diseases of the Liver*).

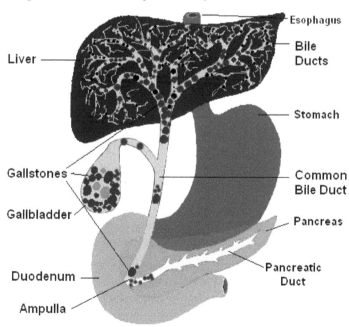

Figure 3: Gallstones in the liver and gallbladder

Gallstones in the liver, gallbladder, and ampulla may also be partly responsible for both types of diabetes: insulin-dependent and non-insulin-dependent. All the diabetic patients I have seen, including children, have had large quantities of stones in their liver. Each liver flush further improved their condition, provided that they followed a healthy daily regimen and ate a balanced diet void of refined sugar and animal products[13].

Diseases of the Liver

The liver is the largest gland/organ in the body. It weighs up to 3 pounds, is suspended behind the ribs on the upper right side of the abdomen, and spans almost the entire width of the body. Being responsible for hundreds of different functions, it is also the most complex and active organ in the body.

Since the liver is in charge of processing, converting, distributing, and maintaining the body's vital *fuel* supply (including nutrients, enzymes and energy), anything that interferes with these functions must have a detrimental effect on the health of the liver and the body as a whole. The strongest interference stems from the presence of gallstones.

Besides manufacturing cholesterol (an essential building material of organ cells, hormones, and bile), the liver also produces hormones and proteins that affect the way the body functions, grows, and heals. Furthermore, it makes new amino acids and converts existing ones into proteins. These proteins are the main building blocks of the cells, hormones, neurotransmitters, genes, and so forth. Other essential functions of the liver include breaking down old, worn-out cells, recycling proteins and iron, and storing vitamins and nutrients. Gallstones are tantamount to being a hazardous threat to all these vital tasks.

In addition to breaking down alcohol in the blood, the liver also detoxifies noxious substances, bacteria, parasites, and certain components of pharmaceutical drugs. It uses specific enzymes to convert waste and toxins into substances that can be safely removed from the body.

What's more, the liver filters more than a quart of blood each minute. Most of the filtered waste products leave the liver via the bile stream. Gallstones obstructing the bile ducts lead to high levels of toxicity in the liver and, ultimately, to liver diseases. This development is further

---

[13] See Overeating Protein in Chapter 3. Also, read more on diabetes in my books Timeless Secrets of Health and Rejuvenation, or Diabetes - No More!

exacerbated by regular intake of pharmaceutical drugs, initially broken down by the liver. The presence of gallstones prevents their detoxification, which can cause *overdosing* and serious side effects, even at low drug dosages. It also means that the liver is at risk for damage from the breakdown products of the drugs on which it acts. Alcohol that is not detoxified properly by the liver can critically injure or destroy liver cells.

All major liver diseases are preceded by extensive bile duct obstruction through gallstones. The gallstones distort the structural framework of the liver lobules (see **Figures 3** and **4a**), which are the main units constituting the liver; it contains more than 50,000 such units. Subsequently, the presence of stones makes blood circulation to and from these lobules increasingly difficult. In addition, they force liver cells to cut down bile production. An increasing amount of trapped bile becomes thick and turns into sludge and more stones (see **Figure 3b**). Nerve fibers also become damaged.

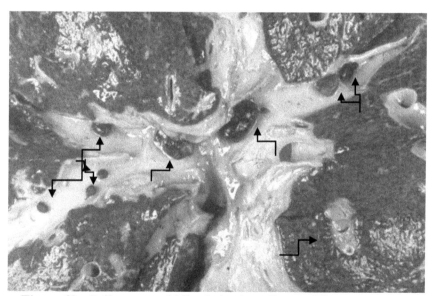

Figure 3b: Gallstones and bile sludge in a dissected liver

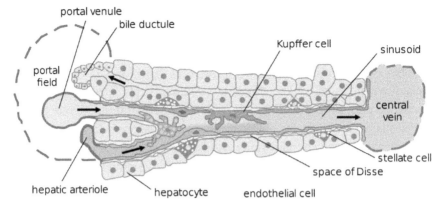

Figure 4a: A liver lobule

(Originally by Frevert U, Engelmann S, Zougbédé S, Stange J, Ng B, et al.)

Prolonged suffocation due to the presence of stones eventually damages or destroys liver cells. Fibrous scar tissue gradually replaces these cells, causing further obstruction and an increase in pressure on the liver's blood vessels. If the degree of regeneration of liver cells does not keep up with the degree of damage, liver cirrhosis (see **Figure 4b**) is imminent. Liver cirrhosis usually leads to death.

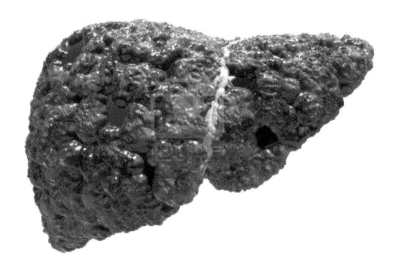

Figure 4b: Liver Cirrhosis
(Photograph by Sebastian Kaulitzki)

Liver failure occurs when cell suffocation destroys so many liver cells that the number of cells required to carry out the organ's most important and vital functions is insufficient. Consequences of liver failure include drowsiness, confusion, shaking of hands, tremors, drop in blood sugar, infection, kidney failure and fluid retention, uncontrolled bleeding, coma, and death. The capability of the liver to recover from major damage, though, is truly remarkable.

Once the liver flushes have removed all gallstones, and the afflicted person discontinues using alcohol and medicinal drugs, there usually are no significant long-term consequences, even though many of the liver cells may have been destroyed during the illness. When the cells grow again, they will do so in an ordered fashion that permits normal liver functions. This is possible because in liver failure (as opposed to liver cirrhosis) the basic structure of the liver has not been substantially compromised.

Fatty liver disease (see **Figure 4c**) is a common but reversible condition where large amounts of triglyceride fat accumulate in liver cells because of abnormal retention. In developed countries, fatty liver disease now affects 1 in every 10 people. Although, there are various primary reasons that can lead to this condition, they all share bile duct congestion as the immediate principal cause.

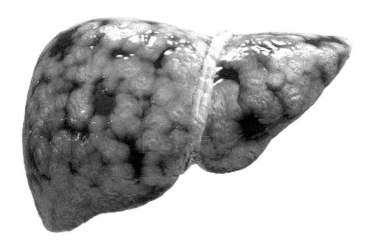

Figure 4c: Fatty Liver
(Photograph by Sebastian Kaulitzki)

The most well-known causes include excessive alcohol and fat consumption. Also drugs like amiodarone, methotrexate, diltiazem, expired tetracycline, highly active antiretroviral therapy, glucocorticoids, and tamoxifen can lead to fatty liver disease.

A healthy liver moves all excessive fat from the body via the bile ducts into the digestive tract. Gallstones in the liver's bile ducts, on the other hand, forces liver cells to accumulate fat, thereby making them *obese*. The fattier the liver gets, the less able it is to remove excessive fat from the rest of the body, regardless of dieting. This can make it increasingly difficult for a person to lose weight.

Fatty liver disease no longer just affects those who have abused alcohol for many years. Obesity levels among children are so high that many teenagers now develop cirrhosis and require liver transplants because of it. In fact, studies have shown that millions of children in the US are afflicted with *non-alcoholic liver disease* due to buildup of fat within liver cells[14]. On July 2, 2011, the *Telegraph* reported: "The condition increases the risks of heart disease, strokes and type 2 diabetes, and can lead to cirrhosis (scarring of the liver), which is often not detected until it is too late ... There is no medical treatment for the disease, but the extent of it can be reduced by weight loss and improvements in diet."

However, without first unclogging the bile ducts, weight loss may be difficult but if it occurs, it can actually cause further harm to the liver. Since all fats have to be processed by liver cells, releasing any accumulated fats from other parts of the body puts an extra burden on the liver, making it even more prone to congestion, even complete suffocation. Therefore, sudden weight loss should be avoided[15].

The popular gastric bypass operation can also increase the severity of fatty liver disease by causing a massive dumping of fats from around the body into the liver. Although the person may successfully lose weight, he puts the liver and the rest of the body at the risk of developing far more serious conditions than obesity, including heart disease, diabetes and cancer.

Acute hepatitis results when entire groups of liver cells begin to die off. Gallstones can harbor viral material, which can invade and infect liver cells, causing cell-degenerative changes. As gallstones increase in number and size, and as more cells become infected and die, entire lobules begin to

---

[14]Journal of Hepatology, July 2011; 55(1): 218–220; The Telegraph July 2, 2011
[15]For a balanced, natural weight loss program see my book *Feel Great, Lose Weight*

collapse, and blood vessels begin to develop kinks. This greatly affects blood circulation to the remaining liver cells.

The extent of the damage that these changes have on the liver and its overall performance largely depends on the degree of obstruction caused by the gallstones in the liver bile ducts. Cancer of the liver only occurs after many years of progressive occlusion of a large number of liver bile ducts. This applies also to tumors in the liver that emanate from primary tumors in the GI tract, lungs, or breast.

Most liver infections (type A, type B, type non-A, and type non-B) occur when the bile ducts in a certain number of liver lobules are congested with gallstones, which can even happen at a very early age for a number of reasons.

For example, clamping the umbilical cord too early, instead of the required 40-60 minutes after birth, can reduce the oxygenation of the blood in the baby by over 40 percent. This medical malpractice causes many toxins, normally filtered out by the placenta during the first hour after birth, to remain in the child's body, and it also leaves the child with fewer antibodies to protect it against disease.

It normally takes at least 40 to 60 minutes before the umbilical cord stops throbbing completely. Cutting the cord too early can affect the baby's liver right from the start and set it up for gallstone formation during childhood. This can subsequently lead to liver infections.

Furthermore, vaccine shots expose the baby's liver to the numerous carcinogenic toxins they contain[16]. Especially at an early age, the liver is unable to break down these toxic substances, thereby causing gallstones to form right after the first vaccine shot.

An inadequate diet that includes sugar, pasteurized cow's milk, animal proteins, fried foods, and other fast/junk foods, greatly affects the liver of children, too. And if the mother drinks alcohol, smokes, eats junk food, takes medication during pregnancy, or has been vaccinated herself, this also has detrimental effects on the child's liver.

One study by the Environmental Working Group (EWG) has shown that that blood samples from newborns contained an average of 287 toxins, including mercury, fire retardants, pesticides, food additives, chemicals from body care products, air pollutants, toxic plastic compounds, and Teflon chemicals. Many of these toxins are highly carcinogenic. It is

---

[16]For more details on the dangers of vaccines and their ingredients, see my book *Vaccine-nation: Poisoning the Population, One Shot at a Time*

impossible for a child's liver to detoxify blood filled with so many harmful chemicals. Forming gallstones to encapsulate some of these toxins is the only *remedy* the body has at its disposal.

According to the EWG report, in the month leading up to birth, the umbilical cord transfers the equivalent of at least 300 quarts of blood from the placenta to the developing child. This means, the new born child has the same chemical load as the mother. Furthermore, mothers who are not in good health and still breastfeed their babies, actually continue to contaminate them. All this overtaxes the small livers of these children.

Overall, the study detected a veritable chemical cocktail in 99-100 percent of pregnant women, sufficient to initiate the beginning stages of liver dysfunction, and even cancer growth, in unborn children.

In a series of new studies, the chemical toxin fluoride (its unnatural form), added to the municipal drinking water, toothpastes, and mouth rinses in the United States and other countries, has been clearly linked with causing brain damage, cancer of the bone (osteosarcoma), and other types of cancer. Of course, the liver is the only organ that can detoxify fluoride. However, fluoride cannot be broken down; to the contrary, this toxin accumulates in the body unchanged and can therefore damage the liver and other endocrine glands. As little as half a teaspoon can kill an adult. Regular fluoride ingestion can cause cancer, thyroidism, brain damage, and liver cirrhosis.

A healthy liver and immune system are perfectly able to destroy viral material, regardless of whether it has been picked up from the external environment or has entered the bloodstream in some other way, such as through vaccination or blood transfusion.

The majority of people exposed to hepatitis viruses never fall ill. In fact, we all have most viruses that exist outside the body in our body right now. However, when large amounts of gallstones are present, the liver becomes congested and toxic, which turns it into an environment conducive for increased viral activity.

Viruses are innate protein fragments that are believed to enter a host cell and cause it to produce copies of the same bits of protein (viruses). However, successive research by the scientists Antoine Béchamp (1816-1908), who originally discovered the so-called *germ*, Gunther Enderlein (1872-1968), and the biologist Royal Rife (1888-1971) led to the discovery that in a biological environment of increasing acidity, viruses can arise from fungi found within cells. Enderlein also showed that fungi developed from bacteria, depending on specific changes related to pH and the nutritive environment. In fact, depending on the internal environment, with the help of fungi, the body can develop and reproduce any kind of virus there is. Viruses don't possess reproductive capabilities and need host cells, bacteria, and fungi to reproduce them.

Contrary to popular assumption, viruses don't develop and attack the cell nucleus randomly. They tend to *hijack* the nuclei of only the weakest and most damaged cells to prevent them from mutating. Healthy cells also don't let viruses pass through to the cell nucleus. They produce interferons which are specific proteins that protect the cells against viruses, bacteria, parasites, and tumor cells by stimulating the defensive responses of the immune system. Not all viruses succeed, though, and liver cancer may result. I wish to point out that the presence of viruses in cancer cells does not mean viruses have cancer-producing effects. Besides, cancer cells have a purpose, too. They can mop up a lot toxins and thereby save organ tissues from sudden demise.

Gallstones can harbor plenty of viruses. Some of these viruses may break free and enter the blood. This is known as chronic hepatitis. Non-viral infections of the liver may be triggered (not caused) by bacteria that proliferate inside, and spread from, any of the bile ducts obstructed with gallstones.

The presence of gallstones in the bile ducts also impairs the liver cells' ability to deal with toxic substances such as chloroform, cytotoxic drugs, anabolic steroids, alcohol, aspirin, fungi, food additives, and the like. When this occurs, the body develops hypersensitivity to these predictable toxic substances and to other unpredictable ones contained in numerous pharmaceutical drugs. Many allergies stem from such conditions of hypersensitivity. For the same reason, there may also be a drastic increase in toxic side effects resulting from the intake of prescription medications and over-the-counter drugs, side effects that the Food and Drug Administration (FDA) or pharmaceutical companies may not even be aware of.

The most common form of jaundice results from gallstones being stuck in the bile duct leading to the duodenum, and/or from gallstones and fibrous tissue distorting the structural framework of the liver lobules. The movement of bile through the bile channels (canaliculi) is blocked, and the liver cells can no longer conjugate[17] and excrete bile pigment, known as bilirubin. Consequently, there is a buildup in the bloodstream of both bile and the substances from which it is made. As bilirubin begins to build up in the blood, it stains the skin.

Bilirubin concentration in the blood may be 3 times above normal before a yellow coloration of both the skin and the conjunctiva of the eyes becomes apparent. Unconjugated bilirubin has a toxic effect on brain cells. Jaundice may also result from a tumor in the head of the pancreas caused by bile duct congestion.

Many people have asked me if they can do liver flushes if they have liver cysts. Simple liver cysts are almost always asymptomatic and found incidentally during routine testing for something else. Sometimes, a test reveals one cyst, and another test a few days later shows five of them or none at all.

These cysts are not cancerous and not even dangerous. About 700 million people worldwide have them and only 250,000 of them will ever develop any complications like the cysts becoming too large and causing pressure.

Liver cysts are mostly filled with water. Medical science doesn't know how they originate. I believe that small lymph capillaries bulge out when temporarily congested, usually when the liver bile ducts are congested. If they remain bulged out for longer than a few weeks, they may remain that way and form into cysts.

Many people with liver cysts have done liver flushes without a problem, and in many, but not all cases, the cysts disappeared again. At least, that's what subsequent tests have revealed.

Diseases of the Gallbladder and Bile Ducts

Let me begin this section by explaining the two major roles of bile. Bile is produced by liver cells which secrete it into the liver's biliary network. It flows out of the liver within two major bile ducts and into the common hepatic duct, and finally into the common bile duct.

There are two possible directions that bile can take from there. The first direction is into the cystic duct, and from there, into the gallbladder. Most of the bile produced in the liver flows into the gallbladder. The gallbladder is a 4-inch pear-shaped pouch with a muscular wall that protrudes from the

---

[17] Conjugation is a biochemical process to bind a substance to an acid, thereby deactivating its biological activity, making it water-soluble, and facilitating its excretion

bile duct. It is attached to the posterior side of the liver (see **Figure5**). Bile that enters the gallbladder is altered there to make it suitable for being an effective digestive aid.

The second direction is down the common bile duct which leads into the duodenum, the first section of the small intestine. However, only a small amount of bile drains directly into the small intestine. Bile that takes this route is quite an inefficient digestive aid and is primarily used to carry away toxins and waste products.

A normal, healthy gallbladder generally holds about 2 fluid oz. (60 ml) of bile. Its walls are extremely flexible and allow the gallbladder to balloon out.

The bile stored in the gallbladder has a different consistency than the bile found in the liver. In the gallbladder, most of the salt and water contained in the bile is reabsorbed, thereby reducing it to a mere tenth of its original volume. Bile salts (as opposed to regular salt) are not absorbed, though, which means their concentration is increased about tenfold. The gallbladder also adds mucus to the bile, which turns it into a thick, mucus-like substance. Its high concentration makes bile the powerful digestive aid that it is.

The muscular wall of the gallbladder contracts and ejects bile when fat-containing foods and most protein foods enter the duodenum from the stomach. This function is regulated by the hormone cholecystokinin.

A more marked gallbladder activity is noted if food entering the duodenum contains a high proportion of fat. The body uses the bile salts contained in bile to emulsify the fat and facilitate its digestion.

Once the bile salts have done their job and left the emulsified fat for intestinal absorption, they travel on down the intestinal tract. Most of them are reabsorbed in the final section of the small intestine (ileum) and carried back to the liver. Once in the liver, the bile salts are collected again in the bile and secreted into the duodenum.

Inadequate bile secretion leads to improperly digested food which can clog up the intestines. Intestinal congestion leads to overgrowth of bacteria which de-conjugate bile salts. The reduced presence of bile salts further impedes fat digestion and absorption, thereby causing steatorrhea. Steatorrhea is a common condition among people eating fast foods or highly processed foods. It is recognized by the presence of excess fat in feces, causing them to float. Such stools typically have an oily appearance and are foul-smelling. Oily diarrhea is not uncommon. There may also be alternating diarrhea and constipation.

In addition to intestinal congestion and irritation, the breaking down of bile salts by intestinal bacteria leads to a shortage of bile salts in the liver. This, in turn, alters the balanced composition of bile ingredients. Diminished bile salt concentration in bile is the main cause for gallstones in the liver and the gallbladder.

People who have repeatedly taken medications such as antibiotics, often suffer from chronic proliferation of harmful intestinal bacteria, and therefore have a very high incidence of gallstones.

Liver, Gallbladder, Pancreas and Bile Passage

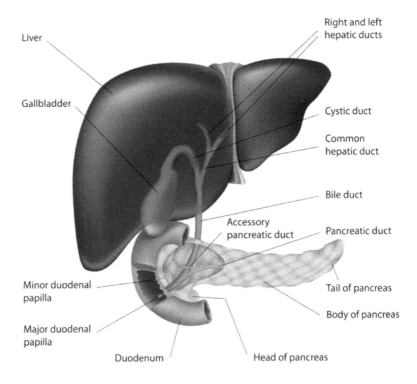

Figure 5: Liver, Gallbladder, Pancreas, and Bile Passage

What are gallstones?

Gallstones are soft or hard stones that only form in gall (bile).Gallstones in the gallbladder may be formed primarily of cholesterol crystals, calcium, long-chain fatty acids, and pigments such as bilirubin. Although cholesterol makes up only 5 percent of bile, it is the commonest component in at least 75 percent of all gallstones. Nevertheless, many of the stones are of mixed composition. Besides the above ingredients, gallstones may contain bile salts, water, mucus, as well as toxins, bacteria, and sometimes, dead parasites, as well as lecithin (a fat known as phospholipid).

In the liver, cholesterol is normally kept in soluble form, suspended in fluid. This is made possible through clusters of bile salts, called micelles. However, if the concentration of bile salts in bile diminishes, the bile fluid turns to thick sludge (see **Figure 3b**) Bile sludge consists of mostly cholesterol crystals, mucus and calcium bilirubinate (calcified bilirubin). Once cholesterol crystals reach a point of supersaturation, cholesterol stones start being formed.

Cholesterol stones are more readily formed when liver bile ducts have already accumulated some stones. Bile duct congestion causes the liver to accumulate bilirubin, which in turn may increase the incidence of cholesterol stones.

Some other types of stones consist of 50-100 percent amorphous materials, according to research published in the *World Journal of Gastroenterology*[18]. They are resistant like solids but, like liquids, lack a crystalline structure (see some gel-like stones in **Figure13a**). Ultrasound and other diagnostic methods do not detect them.

Gallstones can range in size from a pinhead to a golf ball.

Calcified gallstones in the gallbladder can be of varied consistency and are usually made of calcified bilirubin, called bilirubinate. They can be light-brown (see **Figure 1d**) or black, or any color in between, depending on bilirubin concentration. People with hemolytic anemia (a relatively rare type of anemia in which red blood cells are being destroyed), or cirrhosis (scarred liver), tend to have black stones of the calcified variety. Brown stones contain more cholesterol and calcium than black stones.

Gallstones can be formed in both the liver's intrahepatic bile ducts and the gallbladder. Stones in the liver are rarely recognized. Likewise, most

---

[18]World J Gastronternol 2004;10(2)303-305

people with gallstones in the gallbladder are unaware that they have them. However, in some cases a stone may irritate or inflame the gallbladder wall, resulting in painful spasms, infection, and other complications. Occasionally, gallstones can also form in the extra-hepatic bile ducts, such as the common bile duct. This condition is called choledocholithiasis. It occurs only in about 10 percent of patients with gallstones. Most hard stones originate in the gallbladder.

Not all gallbladder diseases are directly caused by hard gallstones. In a condition called acalculous gallbladder disease, a person has symptoms of gallbladder stones, yet there is no evidence of hard stones in the gallbladder or biliary tract. However, bile sludge or soft bile stones impacting the gallbladder or common bile duct may cause this *phantom* symptom of a gallstone attack. Ultrasound scans tend to miss the obstruction since it consists of merely congealed bile, and the sound waves go right through it. The symptoms can be acute or persistent, depending on the severity of the obstruction. They can also occur when the blood supply to the gallbladder is inadequate or the gallbladder is unable to properly eject bile.

In the German medical textbook, *Pathologie der Leber und Gallenwege* (Pathology of the Liver and Bile Ducts)[19], on page 1067, the authors explain that gallstones can occur in the bile ducts of the liver for many months or years without any symptoms or apparent abnormal liver performance tests. They state that it can be very difficult to detect these stones with ultrasound, routine x-rays, or computer tomography (CT scans). This is a very important finding which explains why intrahepatic gallstones are so rarely diagnosed and why most medical doctors are not even aware of their existence.

The bottom line is that the occurrence of intrahepatic gallstones can be extremely common, unbeknownst to the vast majority of medical professionals.

Usually, stones in the gallbladder keep growing in size for about 8 years before noticeable symptoms begin to appear. Larger stones are generally calcified or semi-calcified (like the stones shown in **Figures 6a**

---

[19]Published by Springer Verlag, ISBN, By Helmut Denk, J. Düllmann, H -P Fischer, O Klinge, W Lierse, K -H Meyer Zum Bueschelfelde, U Pfeifer, K H Preisegger, G Ramadori, A Tannapfel, C Wittekind, U Wulfhekel, H Zhou, Springer Verlag, ISBN 3-540-65511-5

and 6d) and can be detected easily through radiological means or by using ultrasound. Some 85 percent of the gallstones found in the gallbladder measure about ¾ inches across (see **Figures 6b and 6c**), although some can become as large as 2 to 3 inches across. (See **Figure 6d** of a large calcified gallstone that I personally examined and photographed, moments after my wife released it without any pain during her 9th liver flush. This stone emitted an extremely noxious odor unlike any I had ever come across. Also see **Figure 6e** of more large calcified stones.) The stone material matched what I have seen in a dissected gallbladder. Such stones form when, for reasons explained in Chapter 3, bile in the gallbladder becomes too saturated and its unabsorbed constituents begin to harden.

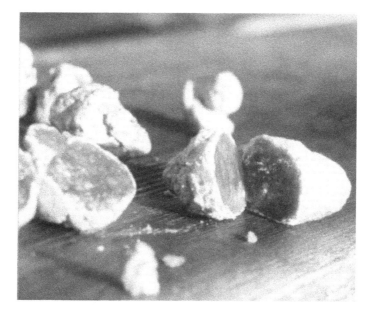

Figure 6a: Semi-calcified gallstones

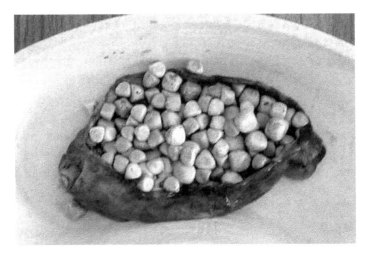

Figure 6b: Fully calcified gallstones in a dissected gallbladder
(Photograph by Alex Khimich)

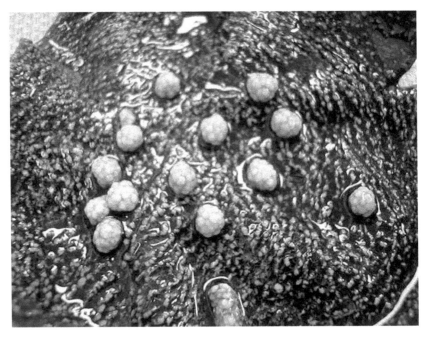

Figure 6c: Hundreds of gallstones and sludge in a dissected gallbladder

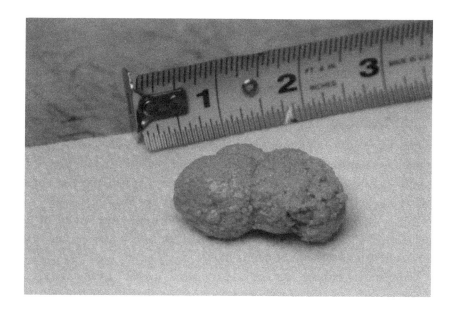

Figure 6d: One large, semi-calcified gallstone

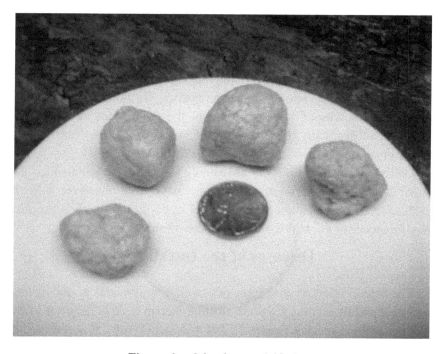

Figure 6e: Other large calcified stones

If a gallstone slips out of the gallbladder and becomes impacted in the cystic bile duct, it is called biliary colic. Cholecystitis results from obstruction of the cystic duct with inflammation of surrounding tissue. There may also be superimposed microbial infection. It is quite common to encounter ulceration of the tissues between the gallbladder and the duodenum or colon, with fistula formation and fibrous adhesions.

If a stone gets trapped in the common bile duct, choledocholithiasis results (see **Figure 3**). All biliary tree obstructions that include stones are usually associated with **colicky** pain. The strong spasmodic and painful contraction helps to move the trapped stones onward.

Biliary colic is accompanied by considerable distension of the gallbladder. If the gallbladder is packed with gallstones, it can suffer extremely painful spasmodic contractions.

Gallbladder disease generally originates in the liver. When the occurrence of gallstones in the bile ducts of the liver and, eventually, the development of fibrous tissue, distort the structure of liver lobules, venous blood pressure starts to rise in the portal vein. This, in turn, increases the blood pressure in the cystic vein, which drains venous blood from the gallbladder into the portal vein. The incomplete elimination of waste products through the cystic duct causes a backup of acidic waste in the tissues composing the gallbladder. This gradually reduces the stamina and performance of the gallbladder and also decreases the ability of the gallbladder to expel bile (gallbladder ejection fraction). This results in increasing amounts of bile remaining in the gallbladder and becoming stagnant. Subsequently, the formation of mineralized gallstones is just a matter of time.

Gallstones in the gallbladder are usually formed in the gallbladder. It is possible, though, that some stones may pass from the liver into the gallbladder if the common bile duct is clogged up and there is no other way for stones to go. In this situation, there would also be jaundice.

Diseases of the Intestines

The small intestine is continuous with the stomach at the *pyloric sphincter* and its average length in an adult human male is 22 feet 6 inches (6.9 m), and in the adult female 23 feet 4 inches (7.1 m). It is followed by the large intestine, which is about 3.5 to 5 feet (1-1.5 m) (see **Figure 2**). It is divided into 3 structural parts: duodenum, jejunum, and ileum.

The small intestine is where most of the digestion and absorption of food takes place. It secretes intestinal juice to complete the digestion of carbohydrates, proteins, and fats. It also absorbs nutrient materials necessary for nourishing and maintaining the body, and protects it against infection by microbes that have survived the antimicrobial action of hydrochloric acid in the stomach.

When acid food from the stomach enters the duodenum, it combines first with bile and pancreatic juice, and then with intestinal juice. One of bile's most important roles is to activate pancreatic enzymes. Gallstones in the liver and gallbladder drastically reduce the secretion of bile, which impairs the ability of pancreatic enzymes to digest carbohydrates, proteins, and fats. This, in turn, prevents the small intestine from properly absorbing the nutrient components of these foods (such as monosaccharides from carbohydrates, amino acids from protein, and fatty acids and glycerol from fats). The resulting poor absorption of nutrients can lead to malnourishment and subsequent food cravings.

Since the presence of bile in the intestines is essential for the absorption of life-essential fats, calcium, and the fat-soluble vitamins A, D, E, and K, gallstones can lead to life-threatening diseases, such as heart disease, osteoporosis, and cancer. For example, the liver uses the vitamin K to produce the compounds responsible for the clotting of blood. In case of poor vitamin K absorption, hemorrhagic disease may result.

Likewise, poor absorption of vitamin D, which is actually a steroid hormone, can cause havoc throughout the body. Vitamin D regulates thousands of genes and the immune system. A deficiency of this vital hormone increases the risk of death from cardiovascular disease and serious infections, causes cognitive impairment in older adults, leads to severe asthma in children, and is responsible for many types of cancer.

On the other hand, in a study published in the September, 2011 issue of the *European Journal of Clinical Nutrition*, W. B. Grant of the Sunlight, Nutrition and Health Research Center in San Francisco demonstrated that increased vitamin D in blood can not only add years to life but also prevent many common diseases.

According to the researchers, conditions and diseases responsive to vitamin D account for over half of the world's mortality include cancer, cardiovascular disease, diabetes, tuberculosis and respiratory diseases and infections. By restoring normal vitamin D levels, these conditions and diseases can be prevented or eliminated.

A recent study published in the medical journal *PLoS ONE*[20] shows how a lack of vitamin D promotes DNA damage and colon cancer risk. Colon cancer is the third most commonly diagnosed cancer in the world. It therefore stands to reason that we not only ensure to produce enough of the sunshine vitamin in our body but also absorb it properly.

Vitamin D is also essential for healthy calcification of bones and teeth[21]. Calcium is essential for the hardening of bone and teeth, the coagulation of blood, and the mechanism of muscle contraction. Poor bile secretion can, therefore, undermine the uptake of calcium, a mineral the body requires for some of its most vital activities. (**Note:** Tooth problems can interfere with the important mastication process and lead to numerous gastrointestinal disturbances)

Insufficient bile secretion can also prevent the small intestine from absorbing vitamin A and carotene at the required amounts. If vitamin A absorption is inadequate, the epithelial cells become damaged. These cells play an essential role in all the organs, blood vessels, lymph vessels, and other important parts in the body. Vitamin A is also necessary to maintain healthy eyes and protect against microbial infection. It is of great importance to realize that supplementing these vitamins alone does not resolve the problem of deficiency. Quite to the contrary, vitamin supplementation often causes the very deficiency it is supposed to end, especially if it involves synthetic vitamins[22].

In short, the body is unable to fully absorb these vitamins when fats can no longer be digested properly. The main cause of inadequate absorption of the 4 essential, fat-soluble vitamins is an insufficient supply of bile, pancreatic lipase, and pancreatic fat. Bile secretion occurs in response to ingesting dietary fats or oils. It stands to reason that following a low-fat or no-fat diet can actually endanger your life. The misinformation that even unrefined, natural fats are bad for us has greatly contributed to the massive increase in cardiovascular disease in the world.

To sum up, without normal bile secretions and fat intake, the body cannot digest and absorb enough of these vitamins, which, in turn, can

---

[20] PLoS ONE 6(8): e23524. doi:10.1371/journal.pone.0023524
[21] The only truly safe way to get enough vitamin D is from exposure to sunlight and certain foods. See more details in my book *Heal Yourself with Sunlight*
[22] Most commercial vitamin products contain synthetic vitamins which are useless and potentially very harmful to the body. See more details on the vitamin controversy in my book *Timeless Secrets of Health and Rejuvenation*

cause considerable damage to the circulatory, lymphatic, immune, digestive, respiratory, and skeletal systems.

Inadequately digested foods tend to ferment and putrefy in the small and large intestines. They attract a vast number of bacteria to help speed up the process of decomposition. The by-products of putrefaction are often extremely toxic, and so are the excretions produced by the bacteria.

All of this strongly irritates the mucus lining, which constitutes the body's foremost line of defense against disease-causing agents (pathogens).

Regular exposure to these toxins impairs the body's immune system, 60 percent of which is located in the intestines. Overburdened by a constant invasion of toxins, the small and large intestines may be afflicted with a number of disorders, including diarrhea, constipation, abdominal gas, Crohn's disease, irritable bowel syndrome (IBS), ulcerative colitis, diverticular disease, hernias, hemorrhoids, polyps, dysentery, appendicitis, volvulus, and intussusceptions, as well as benign and malignant tumors.

A number of these conditions lead to artificial stomas, such as colostomy and ileostomy (see **Figure** 7). These surgically-created openings in the intestines allow the removal of fecal wastes from the body, to drain into a pouch.

There were an estimated 800,000 ostomy patients in the US in 2000. Over 120,000 new surgeries were performed since then each year. At this rate increase, by the end of 2011 an estimated 2 million patients should have received a stoma.

The noxious toxins that cause intestinal inflammation and damage usually result from the putrefaction and fermentation of improperly digested foods by bacteria. There can be dozens of highly toxic substances, such as sepsin, skarol, indican, putrescine, cadaverine, and octopamine; the latter has been shown to affect important brain functions, and in children, they can contribute to developmental problems and even autism[23].

---

[23]Link between bowel disease and autism:
http://www.dailymail.co.uk/news/article-388051/Scientists-fear-MMR-link-autism.html#ixzz1Bajg4Fra

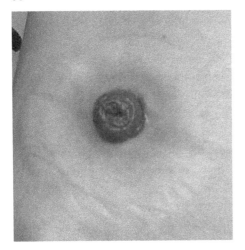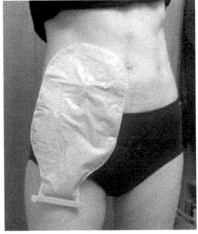

Figure 7: Ileostomy and ileostomy bag

Typical indications for toxins afflicting the intestines include the following conditions: foul-smelling breath and/or body odor, coated tongue, mouth and tongue ulcers, sinus congestion, acid reflux, nausea, weak immune system, kidney and bladder problems, headaches, gas, bloating, abdominal distention, abdominal cramping, weight grain, pain in joints, muscle stiffness, constantly feeling drained or tired, mental disorders, depression, anxiety, nervousness, poor memory and concentration, schizophrenia, autism-like symptoms, brain fog, insomnia, signs of premature aging such as loss of skin elasticity and wrinkles, neurodermatitis, eczema, psoriasis, eye disorders, menstrual cramps, tilted uterus, hormonal imbalances, and prostate enlargement.

Ample bile flow maintains good digestion and absorption of food and has a strong cleansing action throughout the intestinal tract. Every part of the body depends on the basic nutrients made available through the digestive system, as well as the efficient removal of waste products from that system. Gallstones in the liver and gallbladder considerably disrupt both these vital processes. Therefore, they can be held accountable for most, if not all, of the different kinds of ailments that can afflict the body. Removal of gallstones helps to normalize the digestive and eliminative functions, improve cell metabolism, and maintain balance in body and mind.

Important Note on Squatty Toilet Stools: Sitting on a Western style toilet seat forces one to strain, making waste elimination difficult and incomplete. Human beings were designed to perform their bodily functions in the squatting position, as seen in all native populations. In order to be squeezed empty, the colon needs to be compressed by the thighs. Furthermore, for complete elimination of the fecal mass, the puborectalis muscle must be relaxed and the ileocecal valve from the small intestine needs to be closed. By ignoring these requirements, the sitting toilet makes it nearly impossible to empty the colon completely. In the sitting position, the puborectalis muscle forces the rectum out of its natural position and *chokes* it. Thus, air and fecal movements become blocked. This leads to fecal stagnation and the development of hemorrhoids, appendicitis, polyps, ulcerative colitis, irritable bowel syndrome, diverticular disease and colon cancer. On the other hand, squatting relaxes the puborectalis muscle and straightens the rectum. Infants of every culture instinctively adopt this posture to relieve themselves. As research has shown, if they don't get *trained* to sit on Western style toilet bowls, they rarely develop these intestinal disorders, unless their dietary and lifestyle habits are unbalanced. (To find a good toilet squatting stool, see *Product Information*)

Disorders of the Circulatory System

For descriptive reasons, I have divided the circulatory system into two main parts: the blood circulatory system and the lymphatic system.

The blood circulatory system consists of the heart, which acts as a pump, and the blood vessels, through which the blood circulates.

The lymphatic system consists of lymph nodes and lymph vessels, through which colorless lymph flows. Lymph has multiple interrelated functions. It is responsible for the removal of fluid surrounding the cells from tissues and takes fatty acids from the intestinal tract and transports them to the liver. It also takes white blood cells to and from the lymph nodes into the bones.

The body contains 3 times more lymph fluid than blood. Lymph takes up waste products from the cells, as well as cellular debris, and removes these from the body.

The lymphatic system is the primary circulatory system used by all immunological cells: macrophages, T cells, B cells, lymphocytes, and so forth. An obstruction-free lymphatic system is necessary to maintain strong immunity and homeostasis.

Coronary Heart Disease

Heart attacks take more American lives than any other cause. Although it occurs suddenly, a heart attack is actually the final stage of an insidious disorder that has been years in the making. This disorder is known as coronary heart disease. Since the disease plunders mostly prosperous nations and rarely killed anyone before 1900, we have to hold our modern lifestyle, unnatural foods, and unbalanced eating habits responsible for today's literally heartsick society. However, long before the heart begins to malfunction, the liver loses much of its vitality and efficiency.

The liver influences the entire circulatory system, including the heart. In fact, the liver is the greatest protector of the heart. Under normal conditions, the liver thoroughly detoxifies and purifies venous blood that arrives via the portal vein from the abdominal part of the digestive system, the spleen, and the pancreas.

In addition to breaking down alcohol, the liver detoxifies noxious substances, such as toxins produced by microbes. It also kills harmful bacteria and parasites and neutralizes certain drug compounds with the help of specific enzymes. One of the liver's most ingenious feats is to remove the nitrogenous portion of amino acids, since nitrogen is not required for the formation of new protein. The liver forms urea from this waste product. The urea ends up in the bloodstream and is excreted in the urine. The liver also breaks down the nucleoprotein (nucleus) of worn-out cells of the body. The by-product of this process is uric acid, which is excreted with the urine as well.

The liver filters more than a quart of blood per minute, leaving only the acidic carbon dioxide for elimination through the lungs (see **Figure 8**).

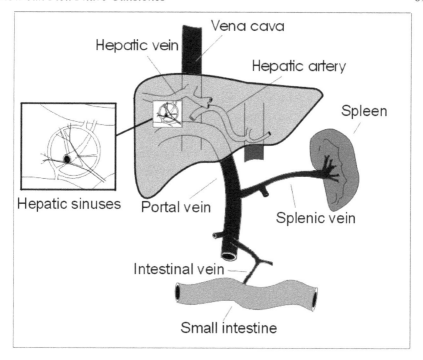

Figure 8: The way the liver circulates and filters blood

After it is purified in the liver, the blood passes through the hepatic vein into the inferior vena cava, which takes it straight into the right side of the heart. From there the venous blood is carried to the lungs, where the interchange of gases takes place: carbon dioxide is excreted and oxygen absorbed. After leaving the lungs, the oxygenated blood passes into the left side of the heart. From there it is pumped into the aorta, which supplies all body tissues with oxygenated blood.

The presence of gallstones in the bile ducts of the liver distorts the basic framework of the liver cell units (lobules). Consequently, the blood vessels supplying these cell units develop kinks, which greatly reduce internal blood supply. Liver cells become weakened or damaged, and harmful cellular debris begins to enter the bloodstream. This further affects the liver's ability to detoxify the blood. As a result, more and more harmful substances are retained both in the liver and in the blood.

A congested liver can obstruct the venous blood flow to the heart, leading to heart palpitation or even heart attack. It is obvious that toxins that are not neutralized by the liver end up damaging the heart and blood vessel network.

Another consequence of liver congestion is that proteins from dead cells (which the body has to remove at a rate of about 30 billion cells per day) and unused food proteins are not sufficiently broken down, which, in turn, raises protein concentrations in the blood. This can thicken the blood and cause platelet aggravation. As a result, the body tries to store these proteins in the basal membranes of the blood vessel walls (a detailed explanation of this scenario is provided below).

Once the body's storage capacity for protein is exhausted, any new proteins taken up by the blood remain trapped in the bloodstream. This can cause the number of red blood cells to increase, which raises the packed cell volume of the blood, called hemocrit, to abnormal levels. At the same time, the concentration of hemoglobin in the blood begins to increase, which may give rise to a red complexion of the skin, particularly in the face and upper chest. (**Note**: Hemoglobin is a complex protein that combines with oxygen in the lungs and transports it to all body cells) As a result, the red blood cells become enlarged and are, therefore, too big to pass through the tiny vessels of the capillary network. Evidently, this causes the blood to become too thick and slow moving, thereby increasing its tendency toward clotting (platelets sticking together).

The formation of blood clots is considered to be the main risk factor for heart attack or stroke. Since fat has no clotting ability, this risk stems mainly from the high concentration of protein in the blood and blood vessel walls.

Researchers have discovered that the sulfur-containing amino acid homocysteine (HC) promotes the tiny clots that initiate arterial damage and the catastrophic ones that precipitate most heart attacks and strokes[24]. Be aware that HC is up to 40 times more predictive than cholesterol in assessing cardiovascular disease risk. HC results from the normal metabolism of the amino acid methionine, which is abundant in red meat, milk, and dairy products. High concentrations of protein in the blood hinder the continuously required distribution of important nutrients, especially water, glucose, and oxygen to the cells.

Excessive amounts of proteins in the blood are also responsible for blood dehydration, i.e. blood thickening - one of the leading causes of high blood pressure and heart disease. Furthermore, these proteins undermine complete elimination of basic metabolic waste products (see the following section, *Poor Circulation*).

---

[24] Ann Clin & Lab Sci 1991; Lancet 1981

If the liver, due to bile duct congestion, is unable to remove excessive uric acid from the blood, the extra amount of uric acid can also lead to blood vessel damage. At normal blood levels, uric acid serves as an antioxidant and prevents injury to our blood vessel linings. Too much of it, though, causes the damage leading to cardiovascular disease, heart attack, stroke and arthritis-like conditions (gout).

Diet often plays a major role causing excessive uric acid levels. Besides, foods high in purines such as sea food and red meat, as well as beer and sugary soft drinks (containing high fructose corn syrup) are major culprits for increasing blood uric acid levels.

Any one of these or all these factors combined coerce the body to raise its blood pressure. This condition, which is commonly known as hypertension, reduces the life-endangering effect of blood thickening, to some extent. It also permits enough nutrient-rich blood to circulate through the congested body. However, this life-saving response to a life-threatening situation unduly stresses and damages the blood vessels.

On the other hand, the body's raising of the blood pressure may still be a better development than the one that occurs when the blood pressure is lowered through medication. Leading health experts now recognize hypertensive drugs to be a major cause of congestive heart failure and other debilitating illnesses. Congestive heart failure is a progressive condition of *slow death*, whereby every small movement, every breath taken, or every word uttered requires huge effort, and the body becomes unable to perform even the simplest of tasks.

One of the body's first and most efficient approaches for avoiding the danger of an imminent heart attack is to take excessive proteins out of the bloodstream and store them elsewhere, for the time being (see **Figure 9**).

Thickening of Blood Capillary Wall

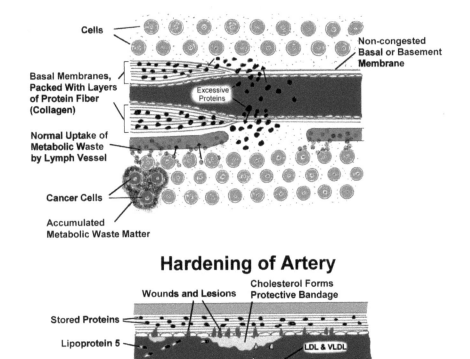

Hardening of Artery

Figure 9: The early stages of heart disease

The only place where protein can be accommodated in large quantities is in the blood vessel network. The capillary walls are able to absorb most of the excessive, unused, or unusable protein. The body converts the soluble protein into collagen fiber, which is 100 percent protein, and stores it in the basal membrane of the blood vessel walls. The basal membrane has the capacity to increase its thickness by 8 to 10 times before its storage capacity for protein is exhausted.

This emergency response by the body, though, comes with a hefty price tag. Storing proteins in the blood vessel walls means that the body can no longer pass adequate amounts of oxygen, glucose, and other essential nutrients to the cells. The cells affected by such a *famine* may include those that make up the heart muscle. The result is heart muscle weakness and reduced performance of the heart. This, in turn, contributes to degenerative illnesses, including diabetes, fibromyalgia, arthritis, and cancer. In other words, whenever the heart is affected, the entire body suffers.

Once the capillary walls have no space left to accommodate excessive protein, the basal membranes of the arteries themselves start taking up protein. The beneficial effect of this action is that the blood remains thin enough to avert the threat of a heart attack, at least for some time. Eventually, though, the very same tactic that prevents the threat of sudden death also damages the blood vessel walls. (**Note**: Only the more primary survival mechanisms of the body, such as the fight-or-flight response, the common cold, and diarrhea are without significant, long-term side effects) The inner lining of the arterial walls becomes rough and thick, like rust in a water pipe. Cracks, wounds, and lesions begin to appear at various locations.

Smaller blood vessel injuries are dealt with by blood platelets. These tiny blood components release the hormone serotonin, which helps to constrict the blood vessels and reduce bleeding. However, larger wounds, as are typically found in diseased coronary arteries, cannot be sealed by platelets alone; they require the body's more complex process of blood clotting. If a blood clot breaks loose, it can enter the heart and result in myocardial infarction, commonly called a heart attack. A clot that reaches the brain results in a stroke. A blood clot entering the opening of a pulmonary artery that delivers used blood to the lungs can be fatal.

To prevent this danger before it arises, the body uses an entire arsenal of first aid measures, including the release of the blood chemical lipoprotein 5(LP5) and cholesterol. Owing to its sticky nature, LP5 works as a Band-Aid to create a firmer seal around the wounds and lesions within the arteries.

As a secondary but equally important rescue operation, the body attaches specific types of cholesterol to the injured areas of an artery (more on this in the section *High Cholesterol*). This acts as a more reliable bandage than LP5 can provide. Since cholesterol deposits still are not protection or fortification enough, extra connective tissue and smooth muscle cells begin to grow inside the blood vessel.

In addition, the body deposits calcium in these softer bandages to provides them with the necessary rigidity and stability. Called atherosclerotic plaques, these calcium-rich deposits can eventually block an artery completely, thereby severely obstructing the flow of blood to the heart. In response to this grave situation - unless interfered with through a bypass operation, angioplasty, or the insertion of a stent - the body makes its own bypasses by turning existing or new capillaries into small, blood-supplying arteries. Although this option is better than surgery, it still does not significantly reduce the danger of a heart attack.

Contrary to common assumption, a heart attack does not occur as a result of blood vessel obstruction, but rather because of blood clots and/or soft fragments of atherosclerotic deposits making their way into the heart. The blood clots and soft pieces of cholesterol implicated in triggering heart attacks are almost never released from the rock-hard structures of the more occluded sections of an artery, but tend to be released from newly created lesions and their protective cholesterol patches. For this reason, stent or bypass operations, which do not address the numerous smaller, soft patches of arterial deposits, have neither reduced the incidence of heart attacks nor lowered the mortality rate from these attacks.

Don't take my word for it, but listen to Dr. Dwight Lundell, one of the world's greatest heart surgeons, who has been a heart specialist M.D. and surgeon for 25 years, having performed 5,000 open heart surgeries. Dr. Lundell was Chief Surgeon at the Banner Heart Hospital in Mesa, AZ.

Dr. Lundell writes in a letter published online in *Prevent Disease*[25] in March 2012: "Simply stated, without inflammation being present in the body, there is no way that cholesterol would accumulate in the wall of the blood vessel and cause heart disease and strokes. Without inflammation, cholesterol would move freely throughout the body as nature intended. It is inflammation that causes cholesterol to become trapped."

He goes on to say, "I have peered inside thousands upon thousands of arteries. A diseased artery looks as if someone took a brush and scrubbed repeatedly against its wall. Several times a day, every day, the foods we eat create small injuries compounding into more injuries, causing the body to respond continuously and appropriately with inflammation."

Although the gradual destruction of blood vessels, known as atherosclerosis, initially protects a person's life against a heart attack caused by a blood clot, it is in due course also responsible for weakening the heart and the rest of the body. Most forms of coronary heart disease

---

[25] World Renown Heart Surgeon Speaks Out On What Really Causes Heart Disease, News, March 1, 2012, http://preventdisease.com

can be reversed by cleansing the liver and by clearing out any existing protein deposits in the capillaries and arteries. Other dietary and lifestyle changes may be necessary as well (see Chapter 3).

Cholesterol-lowering drugs have now been shown to cause cancer, diabetes, liver damage, and even dementia, and they do nothing to protect the heart against heart attack, but instead increase the risk of heart failure. Dr. Lundell put it this way: "Despite the fact that 25% of the population takes expensive statin medications and despite the fact we have reduced the fat content of our diets, more Americans will die this year of heart disease than ever before." He asks this important question: "How much lower must we go before admitting there is no correlation between lowering cholesterol and heart attack risk?"

According to the American Heart Association, more than 75 million Americans currently suffer from heart disease, 20 million have diabetes and 57 million have pre-diabetes. As you are about to find out, cholesterol-lowering drugs have a lot to do with it.

Unraveling the Lies about Cholesterol

According to a Norwegian study published in *the Journal of Evaluation in Clinical Practice* on 25 Sept, 2011[26], if you have cholesterol levels above 5.0 mmol/l (193 mg/dl), you will live longer.

Women especially benefit from higher cholesterol levels. For example, compared with women whose cholesterol was under 5.0 mmol/l (193 mg/dl), those with a level over 7.0 mmol/l (270 mg/dl) enjoyed a 28 percent reduction of death and 26 percent reduction of cardiovascular diseases. While men appear to have less striking benefits from higher cholesterol levels than women, they clearly benefit from them. Compared with men whose cholesterol was under 5.0 mmol/l (193 mg/dl), those with a level up to 5.0 mmol/l (228 mg/dl) enjoyed an 11 percent reduction of death and 20 percent reduction of cardiovascular diseases.

The findings of this study titled, "Is the Use of Cholesterol in Mortality Risk Algorithms in Clinical Guidelines Valid?" contradict the medical theory that lowering total cholesterol levels reduces mortality rates from cardiovascular disease and other causes.

The team of researchers from the Norwegian University of Science and Technology followed 52,087 individuals (24,235 men and 27,852 women)

[26] Journal of Evaluation in Clinical Practice, 25 SEP 2011; DOI: 10.1111/j.1365-2753.2011.01767.x;

aged 20-74 years and free from known cardiovascular disease at the start of the study for a total period of 10 years.

The researchers discovered major flaws in previous cholesterol studies that linked high cholesterol levels with increased risk of cardiovascular disease. These previous studies included thousands of individuals aged 75 years or more with established cardiovascular diseases and a history of heart attack, stroke and angina pectoris. Furthermore, such important data on serum cholesterol, systolic blood pressure and smoking status was not provided for thousands more. All of these factors play a leading role in the cause of death from heart disease. Including this manipulative strategy in such important clinical studies tips the balance of the cholesterol-heart disease link toward cholesterol being a risk factor of cardiovascular disease and death.

"Our study provides an updated epidemiological indication of possible errors in the CVD risk algorithms of many clinical guidelines," the researchers stated. They suggest that "...clinical and public health recommendations regarding the 'dangers' of cholesterol should be revised. This is especially true for women, for whom moderately elevated cholesterol (by current standards) may prove to be not only harmless but even beneficial."

This piece of research bares a lifesaving truth and confirms what I have believed in and written about in my book *Timeless Secrets of Health and Rejuvenation* almost 15 years ago when the anti-cholesterol campaigns gained their greatest momentum. In the book, I argue that people with higher total cholesterol must have lower levels of cancer, heart attack, stroke, and mental disorders. I showed that it is perfectly healthy for a person aged 60 to have a cholesterol level of 260. The older a person gets, the higher his cholesterol needs to be in order for him to remain healthy. A 90-year-old could have a cholesterol level of 290 and be in perfect health, cancer-free.

Thankfully, all the cholesterol lies are about to be laid bare.

What Cholesterol Does for You

Cholesterol is an important building block of every cell in the body and is essential for all metabolic processes. It is particularly important in the production of nerve tissue, bile, and hormones. Without it, you cannot even think a single thought, digest a single milligram of fat, or make a single hormone.

On the average, our body produces about half a gram to one gram of cholesterol per day, depending on how much of it the body needs at the time. The adult human body is able to produce 400 times more cholesterol per day than what it would obtain from eating 3.5 oz. of butter. The main cholesterol producers are the liver and the small intestine, in that order. Normally, they are able to release cholesterol directly into the bloodstream, where it is instantly tied to blood proteins. These proteins, which are called lipoproteins, are in charge of transporting the cholesterol to its numerous destinations. Three main types of lipoproteins are in charge of this function: low density lipoprotein (LDL), very low density lipoprotein (VLDL), and high density lipoprotein (HDL).

In comparison to HDL (upon which researchers bestowed the name *good* cholesterol), LDL and VLDL are both relatively large cholesterol molecules; in fact, they are the richest in cholesterol and so there is good reason for their large size. Unlike their smaller cousin, which easily passes through blood vessel walls, the LDL and VLDL versions of cholesterol are meant to take a different pathway; they leave the bloodstream in the liver.

The blood vessels supplying to the liver have a quite different structure than the ones supplying to other parts of the body. They are known as sinusoids. Their unique, grid-like structure permits the liver cells to receive the entire blood content, including the larger cholesterol molecules. The liver cells rebuild the cholesterol and excrete it, along with bile, into the intestines. Once the cholesterol enters the intestines, it first combines with fats, then it is absorbed by the lymph, and finally it enters the blood, in that order.

Gallstones in the bile ducts of the liver inhibit bile secretion and partially, or even completely, block the cholesterol's escape route. Owing to backup pressure on the liver cells, bile production drops.

Typically, a healthy liver produces over a quart of bile per day. When the major bile ducts are blocked, barely a cup of bile, or even less, will find its way to the intestines. This prevents much of the VLDL and LDL cholesterol from being excreted with the bile. As you will see, this can have catastrophic consequences for the entire body.

Gallstones in the liver bile ducts distort the structural framework of the liver lobules, which damages and congests the sinusoids. A sinusoid is a small blood vessel similar to a capillary but with a fenestrated endothelium. Fenestrations are pores or small holes in the blood vessel wall that greatly increase their permeability. The liver, spleen, and bone marrow contain sinusoids instead of regular capillaries to allow for larger molecules and wastes to be exchanged through the thin walls of the sinusoids. Deposits of excessive protein can close the grid holes of these blood vessels (see more detailed explanations in the previous section, or in my book *Timeless Secrets of Health and Rejuvenation*).

Whereas the *good* cholesterol HDL has small enough molecules to leave the bloodstream through ordinary capillaries, as a result of the sinusoid congestion, the larger LDL and VLDL molecules cannot, and are more or less trapped in the blood. Consequently, LDL and VLDL concentrations begin to rise in the blood to levels that seem potentially harmful to the body. Yet even this situation is merely part of the body's survival tactics.

The body needs the extra cholesterol to patch up the increasing number of cracks and wounds that are formed because of the accumulation of excessive protein in the blood vessel walls or other adverse dietary/lifestyle reasons. Eventually, though, even the life-saving *bad* cholesterol, which rushes to every wound or injured site in the body, cannot completely prevent blood clot formation in a coronary artery, in which event one of the escaping blood clots may enter the heart and cut off its oxygen supply.

In addition to this complication, reduced bile secretion impairs the digestion of food, particularly fats. Fats are necessary to maintain proper metabolism. Therefore, if not enough cholesterol is available, metabolic disorders may result, including diabetes. (see also the following section, *The Statin Deception*) They can lead to serious cell damage in the organs and systems of the body.

When the liver cells no longer receive sufficient amounts of LDL and VLDL molecules, they assume that the blood is deficient in these types of cholesterol. This stimulates the liver cells to increase the production of cholesterol, further raising the levels of LDL and VLDL cholesterol in the blood. However, the *bad* cholesterol is trapped in the circulatory system because its escape routes - the bile ducts and the liver sinusoids - are blocked or damaged.

In the meanwhile, the arteries attach as much of the *bad* cholesterol to their walls as they possibly can to patch up the wounds and lesions caused by advanced cell damage. Calcium is integrated into the cholesterol patches which make the arterial walls increasingly rigid and hard. This protective measure is still better, though, than having all their wounds and lesions exposed to the gushing blood stream.

Coronary heart disease, regardless of whether it is caused by smoking, drinking excessive amounts of alcohol, sugar, overeating protein foods, stress, medication, or any other reason, usually does not occur unless gallstones have impacted the bile ducts of the liver.

Removing gallstones from the liver and gallbladder cannot only prevent a heart attack or stroke, but can also help reverse coronary heart disease and heart muscle damage. Cholesterol levels begin to normalize as the distorted and damaged liver lobules regenerate themselves and the wounds and lesions in the blood vessels heal up.

The Statin Deception

Cholesterol-lowering drugs (statins) don't bring the body back to a healthful condition in which the liver can naturally normalize blood cholesterol. Instead, statins artificially lower the level of cholesterol in the blood by blocking the enzyme in the liver that is responsible for making cholesterol. However, by creating such an artificial *cholesterol famine* in the liver, bile is not formed properly, which increases the risk of gallstones and hinders the proper digestion of food.

As I will demonstrate below, there is no proof that taking statins reduces your risk of heart attack or death, especially if you are either a healthy young woman with high cholesterol, or a man or a woman over 69 years of age with high cholesterol. In fact, older patients with lower cholesterol have a higher risk of dying than those with higher cholesterol. This applies to entire countries. Populations with higher average cholesterol than Americans, such as Spain and Switzerland, also have less heart disease.

You should also know that 75 percent of people who have heart attacks have normal cholesterol. Although there is no scientific evidence to show that high cholesterol has anything to do with causing a heart attack (it is now well understand that blood vessel inflammation is the main culprit) many doctors continue pushing statin drugs on their patients.

If your doctor has prescribed you two medications (Zocor and Zetia) to achieve a more *successful* cholesterol reduction, you need to know that this only leads to more plaque buildup in the arteries and no fewer heart attacks. There is a hefty price to be paid for letting toxic drugs manipulate such an important substance as cholesterol. Cholesterol is the precursor to all steroid hormones in the body; to forcefully cause any of these to fluctuate up or down without involving the body's own regularity mechanisms can have disastrous consequences.

Accordingly, the side effects of statins are numerous; they include diabetes, kidney failure, liver disease, and ironically, even heart disease.

A 2011 meta-analysis report published in the *Journal of the American Medical Association*[27] has demonstrated that taking statin drugs increases the risk of developing new-onset diabetes. The data involving 32,000 people showed that the risk of diabetes increased in direct proportion with higher dosage used. The huge number of statin prescriptions handed out to large portions of the population during the past 15-20 years may therefore be a major contributing factor to the current epidemic of adult-onset diabetes.

According to a new Harvard Medical School report[28], women over the age of 45 are 50 percent more likely to develop diabetes if they are taking a statin drug.

Diabetes is no longer considered a disease that affects the elderly. It is now more commonly found among the working age group or younger. According to the International Diabetes Federation, type 2 diabetes in children is becoming a global public health issue[29]. Now, statins are even prescribed for kids as young as 8 years old.

Diabetes takes about 3.8 million lives per year worldwide, which is in the range of the magnitude of deaths due to HIV/AIDS. Globally, it is estimated that more than 250 million people are afflicted with diabetes and an additional 380 million suffer from pre-diabetes.

Statins cannot be considered *preventive* medicine when they actually cause, or contribute to, some of the most serious illnesses prevalent among modern societies.

There are now over 900 clinical studies that have shown numerous disastrous adverse effects (AEs) caused by statins, according to a large study by the *American Journal of Cardiovascular Drugs*[30]. Common adverse effects include cognitive loss, neuropathy, muscle destruction,

---

[27]JAMA, June 22, 2011; 305(24): 2556-2564
[28]Study - statin drugs linked to higher diabetes risk (naturalnews.com)
[29]International Diabetes Federation, "Backgrounder," *Diabetes Atlas, Third Edition (2006)*, p. 2, [online, cited August 18, 2008]
[30]Statin adverse effects: a review of the literature and evidence for a mitochondrial mechanism. Am J Cardiovasc Drugs. 2008;8(6):373-418. doi:

pancreatic and hepatic dysfunction, and sexual dysfunction; yet these are rarely acknowledged by physicians.

The authors of the study from the Department of Medicine at the University of California, San Diego, said, "Physician awareness of statin AEs is reportedly low even for the AEs most widely reported by patients."

Case in point, patients may experience severe muscle problems or develop cancer[31] as a result of taking a statin drug, but most doctors won't blame this drug for it. And they may falsely assume that the patient just contracted another illness, when it is the statin that is responsible for it.

It is particularly disturbing to give statins to young people, especially women who intend to become pregnant and want to give birth to healthy children. Statins are actually classified as a *pregnancy Category X medication,* meaning, statins cause serious birth defects! However, there is hardly an obstetrician who is unwilling to prescribe a statin to a pregnant woman or a woman planning a pregnancy who also has elevated cholesterol levels.

Statins are not even effective for the reasons they are intended for. It has been shown that 155 people prone to having a cardiovascular event, such as a heart attack, need to take intensive-dose statins for one year for just one person to prevent a cardiovascular event. Of course, all of them increase their risk of developing diabetes or other similar devastating AEs.

One major serious side effect of statins is that they deplete the body of vitamin D, an essential steroid hormone that the body uses to regulate thousands of genes, the immune system, and some of the most important processes. The body also uses vitamin D to prevent or reduce insulin resistance - the main cause of diabetes. In order to make vitamin D, the body needs cholesterol. Artificially lowering cholesterol equates to draining the sap out of a plant, without which the plant cannot grow.

Statins Cause Heart Disease and Liver Damage

Ironically, statins also increase a person's risk for chronic heart failure, high blood pressure, and heart attack. They do this by blocking the pathway involved in cholesterol and CoQ10 production. CoQ10 is a powerful antioxidant that protects cells and mitochondrial DNA. By reducing blood cholesterol, statins hinder CoQ10 and other fat-soluble antioxidants from reaching muscle cells, including those that make up the

---

[31]*Mail Online,* **Sep 29, 2011**

heart. The result is increased free radical activity and mitochondrial damage. In short, a heart starved of cholesterol and CoQ10 cannot perform, and it dies.

A 2009-study conducted at Michigan State University and published in *Clinical Cardiology*[32], found that heart muscle function was *significantly better* in the placebo group than in those taking statin drugs. In the conclusion, the researchers noted: "Statin therapy is associated with decreased myocardial [heart muscle] function." In other words, if you take statins, you can expect to weaken your heart and cause it to fail.

Of course, drug companies cannot make any legitimate claims that the use of statins reduces the risk of heart disease and stroke, but they have somehow succeeded in generating this mindset among the general population. If your doctor has told you that lowering your cholesterol with statins will protect you against heart attacks, you have been grossly misled.

The #1 prescribed cholesterol-lowering medicine is Lipitor. I suggest that you read the following warning statement, issued on the official Lipitor website:

"LIPITOR® (atorvastatin calcium) is a prescription drug used with diet to lower cholesterol. LIPITOR is not for everyone, including those with liver disease or possible liver problems, and women who are nursing, pregnant, or may become pregnant. LIPITOR has not been shown to prevent heart disease or heart attacks."

Also take note that the LIPITOR website, like all other statin sites, makes the following or a similar statement: "Along with diet and exercise, LIPITOR is proven to lower *bad* cholesterol by 39 to 60 percent (average effect depending on dose)." The drug makers know that there is no real proof that statins alone can lower *bad* cholesterol. In fact, it is diet and exercise that has a proven track record of significantly reducing cholesterol, with or without taking a statin drug. And if a patient who takes the drug without also exercising and changing his diet, the doctor and the drug maker are off the hook and cannot be blamed for the possible absence of expected benefits.

Have you ever wondered why these drug makers are so actively promoting a healthy diet and exercise program along with the advice to take their drug when they are really only interested in selling their drugs,

---

[32]Statin therapy decreases myocardial function as evaluated via strain imaging. Rubinstein J, Aloka F Cardiology Division, Department of Medicine, Michigan State University, Abela GS. *Clin Cardiol*.2009 Dec;32(12):684-9

not diet books or exercise machines? Well, without the two, the statins are quite useless.

Also, there is no real clinical evidence that statins lower cholesterol. All statin studies so far were done using an undisclosed placebo. Typically, drug companies use a placebo that makes the subjects in the placebo have worse results than the subjects in the group that receives the actual drug. So when the drug fares *better* than the placebo, it is automatically considered efficacious. The trick is to choose a placebo that consists of a highly-concentrated cholesterol-elevating fatty substance.

With authentic studies (unlike those sponsored by pharmaceutical companies), you may get completely different results. As shown in the Michigan University study, heart health is significantly better among subjects who do not receive statins than among those taking them.

The desperate propaganda effort by the medical industry to prevent a decline in statin sales, and to actually increase it, is reflected in a December 2011 study that attempts to link statin use with other benefits than just lowering of blood cholesterol. In the conclusion of the study[33], published in the *Journal of Infectious Diseases* in January 2012, the researchers claim that "statin use may be associated with 50% reduced mortality in patients hospitalized with influenza." Accordingly, the mass media promptly announced: "Statins reduce flu death risk by half, study shows."

The abstract of the study omitted to mention that while 33 percent of the patients were given statins, the rest were given antiviral medications. In other words, this wasn't a clinical study at all. All scientific studies now must include a placebo group to determine the efficacy and efficiency of a particular drug treatment. In this study, statin drugs were compared to toxic antiviral drugs, not a placebo.

In other words, what the study really found is that antiviral drugs kill people infected with the flu virus twice as quickly as the statins. This could hardly be a surprise, for *side effects* of antivirals like Tamiflu and Relenza can be very serious, especially in individuals already hospitalized for a different illness or otherwise immune-compromised. There is nothing mentioned in this study that could explain why statins would be able to prevent flu deaths.

The researchers grossly neglected to make the obvious assumption that more sick patients taking antivirals die than sick patients taking statins.

---

[33] J Infect Dis. 2012 Jan;205(1):13-9. Epub 2011 Dec 13

But obviously misleading claims made by these researchers didn't discourage them from crediting statins with another *unexpected* benefit: "If you are lucky enough to be on a statin drug, you will have the advantage of being twice as protected against dying from a bout of influenza than those who choose not to take it." Who wants to die from the flu?!

All of this fraud is topped by the more recent discovery that 2 employees of a communications company admitted that they had been paid to ghostwrite some of the studies done on Tamiflu, with explicit instructions to come to the *correct* conclusion regarding Tamiflu's effectiveness[34]. You may remember George W. Bush had spent more than $1 billion of taxpayers' money to stockpile the drug, to help ward off the H1N1 pandemic that never happened.

According to a 2012 *Los Angeles Times* article by David Finkelstein titled, "No Magic Bullet on the Flu[35]," "After reanalyzing the raw data finally made available (they still don't have it all) ... there was no proof that Tamiflu reduced serious flu complications like pneumonia or death. In short, it appears the pharmaceutical companies had been ... conning the public on matters of health..."

Science fraud is widespread. New discoveries made by researchers at the University of California, published in the *Annals of Medicine* in October 2010, have shown that 92 percent of about 145 clinical trials conducted between 2008 and 2009, for example, are invalid because they didn't disclose the type of placebo they used. By choosing a placebo that actually raises cholesterol levels in the member of the control group, researchers can easily *prove* that a statin drug is more effective than the placebo. The Federal Drug Administration (FDA) has sanctioned this obviously completely unscientific practice of *objective* scientific investigation. It's not difficult to see why. The FDA receives its funding mainly from drug companies.

Many doctors and scientists refer to the infamous JUPITER study[36] to justify statin treatment. This study, which was published in the *New England Journal of Medicine* in 2008, boasted that statins could lower the risk of heart attack by 54 percent, and the risk of stroke by 46 percent. The research was funded by Astra-Zeneca, the maker of the statin drug Crestor.

---

[34]Doctors outraged after recommending a drug (that you may be taking), Dr. Joseph Mercola, February 07, 2012 http://www.mercola.com/
[35]No magic bullet on the flu, Los Angeles Times, January 15, 2012
[36]JUPITER study, N Engl J Med 2008; 359:2195-2207November 20, 2008

Of course, the *positive* outcome of the study boosted statin sales throughout the world, and everyone was happy. However, two years later, trouble showed up in the house of the drug-maker. The claims that statins could prevent heart attacks and strokes were refuted in three articles published in the *Archives of Internal Medicine*.

Particularly, one of the three studies that reviewed the methods and results of the JUPITER trial found that the study was flawed. According to its abstract, "The possibility that bias entered the trial is particularly concerning because of the strong commercial interest in the study." The statin trial was discontinued after less than 2 years of follow-up, with no differences between the two groups (drug subjects and placebo subjects) on the most objective criteria.

The researchers concluded: "The results of the trial do not support the use of statin treatment for primary prevention of cardiovascular diseases and raise troubling questions concerning the role of commercial sponsors[37]." In the meanwhile, the drug maker made billions of dollars from selling a snake oil purported as a preventive for heart attack and stroke. While patients get no such benefits, they may still receive serious adverse effects. Nicknamed the *gorilla statin*, or the *super-statin*, Crestor has done extremely well at Wall Street and the lucrative cholesterol marketplace. Who cares if the drug is useless or even harmful as long as it is selling well?

The patient population and medical professionals are not only being deceived by fraudulent research, but even the scientific theories supporting standardized research methods are flawed and unproven. Prominent researchers from the University of Oxford, University Medical Center Hamburg-Eppendorf, Cambridge University, and Technical University, Munich, found that the ultimate and most influential determining factor of whether a drug treatment is, or isn't, effective is nothing less than the patient's own mind. Their research, published on February 16, 2011 in the medical journal, *Science Translational Medicine*[38], removes any doubt that it is the placebo effect that is responsible for healing, and not a drug treatment or even a surgical procedure.

The researchers state in the study's abstract: "Evidence from behavioral and self-reported data suggests that the patients' beliefs and expectations

---

[37]Cholesterol lowering, cardiovascular diseases, and the rosuvastatin-JUPITER controversy: a critical reappraisal. Arch Intern Med. 2010 Jun 28;170(12):1032-6.
[38][Sci Transl Med 16 February 2011: Vol. 3, Issue 70, p. 70ra14, DOI: 10.1126/scitranslmed.3001244]

can shape both therapeutic and adverse effects of any given drug." They discovered how divergent expectancies in patients alter the analgesic efficacy of a potent opioid (painkilling drug) in healthy volunteers by using brain imaging.

In this study, when test subjects were told that they were not receiving painkiller medications (even though they were), the medication proved to be completely ineffective. In fact, the research showed that the benefits of painkillers could be boosted or completely wiped out by manipulating the subjects' expectations, which basically means it is entirely up to the patient whether he gets relief, or not.

The most common adverse statin reactions received by the *Swedish Adverse Drug Reactions Advisory Committee* from 1988-2010 is severe liver injury. Even though doctors are taught to ask their patients about any preexisting liver conditions, they rarely tell them that taking a statin can lead to jaundice, liver transplantation, and death from acute liver failure. Such reactions, which can occur very suddenly and without any warning signs, account for 57 percent of all statin-related side effects.

All kinds of other ill-effects can occur when your cholesterol levels get too low, including depression, anxiety, episodes of violent behavior, hormonal imbalances, sexual dysfunction, anemia, immune-suppression, cataracts, dysfunction of the pancreas, Parkinson's disease, nerve damage in hands and feet, increased cancer risk (the lower the cholesterol, the higher the risk), and stroke.

According to a large study published in the *Journal of the American Medical Association*[39,] men with cholesterol of 330 mg/dl had less hemorrhagic stroke than men with cholesterol less than 180 mg/dl. It is obvious that higher serum cholesterol levels provide protection from hemorrhagic stroke.

When statin use pushes LDL cholesterol too low, patients develop memory problems or pre-Alzheimer's, or even complete amnesia. Is it a coincidence that the incidence of Alzheimer's disease increased so dramatically ever since statins became the most popular drugs of all time?

It is important to realize that cholesterol is essential for the normal functioning of the immune system, particularly for the body's response to the millions of cancer cells that every person's body makes each day (for more detailed information about what causes cancer and how to heal it, see my book *Cancer Is Not A Disease - It's A Survival Mechanism*).

---

[39]JAMA, Nov 28, 1986 - Vol. 296, No 20

Despite all the health problems seemingly associated with high cholesterol levels, this important substance is *not* something we should try to eliminate from our bodies. Just because cholesterol is found at the crime scene doesn't mean it is a culprit. Cholesterol does far more good than harm. The harm is generally symptomatic of other problems. I wish to emphasize, once again, that *bad* cholesterol only attaches itself to the walls of arteries to avert immediate heart trouble, and not cause it. The body has no intention to commit suicide, even if doctors like to imply this by the use of suppressive, intervening treatments.

The fact that cholesterol never attaches itself to the walls of veins should be part of the cholesterol discussion. When a doctor tests your cholesterol levels, the blood sample is taken from a vein, not from an artery. Because blood flow is much slower in veins than in arteries, cholesterol should obstruct veins much more readily than arteries, but it never does. There simply is no need for that. Why? Because there are no abrasions and tears in the lining of the vein that require patching up. Cholesterol only affixes itself to arteries in order to coat and cover the abrasions and protect the underlying tissue like a waterproof bandage. Veins do not absorb proteins in their basal membranes like capillaries and arteries do and, therefore, are not prone to this type of injury.

Bad cholesterol saves lives; it does not *take* lives. LDL allows the blood to flow through injured blood vessels without causing a life-endangering situation. The theory that high LDL is a major cause of coronary heart disease is unproved and unscientific. It has misled the population to believe that cholesterol is an enemy that has to be fought against and destroyed at all costs. Human studies have not shown a cause-and-effect relationship between cholesterol and heart disease.

There are hundreds of studies that were intended to prove that such a relationship exists, but all they revealed was a statistical correlation between cholesterol and heart disease - quite fortunately, I might add. If there were no *bad* cholesterol molecules attaching themselves to injured arteries, we would have millions more deaths from heart attack than we already have. By contrast, dozens of conclusive studies have shown that the risk of heart disease increases significantly in people whose HDL levels decrease. It would be much wiser to find out what keeps HDL levels normal than to inhibit cholesterol production in the liver and thereby destroy this precious organ. Elevated LDL cholesterol is not a cause of heart disease; rather, it is a consequence of an unbalanced liver, of a congested, dehydrated circulatory system, and of an inadequate diet and lifestyle.

According to a study published in the Journal *of the American Medical Association*, titled "Cholesterol and Mortality", after age 50, there is no increased overall death rate associated with high cholesterol. The same study showed that for every 1 mg/dl drop in cholesterol in your body, your risk of death soared by a whopping 14 percent. In other words, taking statins can kill you.

My question is this: Why risk a patient's health or life by giving him a drug that has no effect whatsoever in preventing the problem for which it is being prescribed? The reason why the lowering of cholesterol levels cannot prevent heart disease is that cholesterol does not cause heart disease.

On the contrary, high cholesterol is a life saver, according to the recently published Norwegian HUNT 2 study[40]. Researchers at the Norwegian University of Science and Technology found that women with elevated cholesterol (more than 270 mg/dl) had a 28 percent lower risk of dying than women with low cholesterol (under 193 mg/dl). Risk for heart disease, cardiac arrest and stroke, which are leading causes of death, also declined as cholesterol levels rose. In other words, telling women to lower their cholesterol is extremely dangerous medical advice - but try telling that to statin-prescribing doctors!

The most important issue with regard to cholesterol is how efficiently a person's body uses cholesterol and other fats. The body's ability to digest, process, and utilize fats depends on how clear and unobstructed the bile ducts of the liver are. When bile flow becomes unrestricted through a series of liver flushes, both the LDL and the HDL levels are naturally balanced, provided diet and lifestyle are balanced as well. In addition, regular full body sun exposure has been shown to keep cholesterol levels where they need to be[41]. Taking these basic precautions are some of the best things you can do to prevent coronary heart disease.

---

[40]High Cholesterol Actually Saves Lives, J Eval Clin Pract. 2012 Feb;18(1):159-68. doi:
[41] See details about how sun exposure normalizes blood cholesterol in my book *Heal Yourself With Sunlight*

Poor Circulation, Enlargement of the Heart andSpleen, Varicose Veins, Lymph Congestion, Hormonal Imbalances

Gallstones in the liver may lead to poor circulation, enlargement of the heart and spleen, varicose veins, congested lymph vessels, and hormonal imbalances. When gallstones have grown large enough to seriously distort the structural framework of the lobules (units) of the liver, blood flow through the liver becomes increasingly difficult. This not only raises the venous blood pressure in the liver, but also raises it in all the organs and areas of the body that drain used blood through their respective veins into the liver's portal vein (see **Figure 8**). Restricted blood flow in the portal vein causes congestion, particularly in the spleen, stomach, esophagus, pancreas, gallbladder, and small and large intestines. This can lead to an enlargement of these organs, due to a reduction of their ability to remove cellular waste products, and to a clogging of their respective veins.

A varicose vein is one that is so dilated that the valves do not sufficiently close to prevent blood from flowing backward. Sustained pressure on the veins at the junction of the rectum and anus in the large intestine leads to the development of hemorrhoids, a type of varicose vein. Other common sites of varicose veins are the legs, the esophagus, and the scrotum. Dilation of veins and venules (small veins) can occur anywhere in the body. It always indicates an obstruction of blood flow[42].

Poor blood flow through the liver also affects the heart. When the organs of the digestive system become weakened by an increase in venous pressure, they become congested and begin to accumulate harmful waste materials, including metabolic waste and debris from cells that have been broken down. The spleen becomes enlarged while it is dealing with the extra workload associated with removing damaged or worn-out blood cells. This further slows blood circulation to and from the organs of the digestive system, which stresses the heart, raises blood pressure, and injures blood vessels.

---

[42] Prescribed by doctors in Germany as a highly successful alternative to surgery for varicose veins, the herbal remedy *horse chestnut seed*, or *conkers*, has shown success in the treatment of "heavy legs", hemorrhoids, and cramps. In combination with cleansing of the liver, colon, and kidneys, conkers can lead to complete recovery. Taking ¼ to ½ teaspoon of cayenne pepper in water or in the form of capsules each day can also help clear up hemorrhoids and varicose veins.

The right half of the heart, which receives venous blood via the inferior vena cava from the liver and all other parts of the body located below the lungs, becomes overloaded with toxic, sometimes infectious, material. This eventually causes enlargement, and possibly infection, of the right side of the heart.

Almost all types of heart disease have one thing in common: blood flow is being obstructed. But blood circulation does not become disrupted easily. It must be preceded by a major congestion of the bile ducts in the liver. Gallstones obstructing the bile ducts dramatically reduce or cut off the blood supply to many liver cells. Reduced blood flow through the liver affects the blood flow in the entire body, which, in turn, has a suppressive effect on the lymphatic system.

The lymphatic system, which is closely linked with the immune system, helps to clear the body of harmful metabolic waste products, foreign material, and cell debris. All cells release metabolic waste products into, and take up nutrients from, a surrounding solution, called extracellular fluid or connective tissue. The degree of nourishment and efficiency of the cells depends on how swiftly and completely waste material is removed from the extracellular fluid. Since most waste products cannot pass directly into the blood for excretion, they accumulate in the extracellular fluid until they are removed and detoxified by the lymphatic system. The potentially harmful material is filtered and neutralized by lymph nodes that are strategically located throughout the body. One of the key functions of the lymphatic system is to keep the extracellular fluid clear of toxic substances, which makes this a system of utmost importance.

Poor circulation of blood in the body causes an overload of foreign, harmful waste matter in the extracellular tissues and, consequently, in the lymph vessels and lymph nodes as well. When lymph drainage slows down or becomes obstructed, the thymus gland, tonsils, and spleen start to deteriorate quite rapidly. These organs form an important part of the body's system of purification and immunity. In addition, microbes harbored in gallstones can be a constant source of recurring infection in the body, which may render the lymphatic and immune systems ineffective against more serious infections, such as infectious mononucleosis (also known as EBV infectious mononucleosis or glandular fever), measles, typhoid fever, tuberculosis, syphilis, and the like.

Owing to restricted bile flow in the liver and gallbladder, the small intestine is limited in its capacity to digest food properly. This permits substantial amounts of waste matter and poisonous substances, such as cadaverines and putrescines (foul-smelling compounds produced during putrefaction of animal protein), to seep into the lymphatic ducts.

These toxins, along with fats and proteins, enter the body's largest lymph vessel, the thoracic duct, at the cysterna chyli. The cysterna chyli (or cisterna chyli, also called receptaculum chyli) is a dilated sac at the lower end of the thoracic duct into which lymph from the intestinal trunk and two lumbar lymphatic trunks flows. It is situated in front of the first two lumbar vertebrae at the level of the belly button (see **Figure 10**) and it forms the primary lymph vessel transporting lymph and fatty chyle from the abdomen via the aortic opening to the junction of left subclavian vein and internal jugular veins.

Although the cysterna chyli/thoracic duct complex is the most common drainage trunk of most of the body's lymphatic activities, most medical doctors rarely even recognize its congested state to be a major cause of disease. You will, however, see here that it plays one of the most important roles in the body.

Toxins, antigens, and undigested proteins from animal sources, including fish, meat, poultry, eggs, and dairy foods, as well as leaked plasma proteins, cause these lymph sacs to swell and become inflamed. As soon as an animal is slaughtered, its cells die and their protein bonds are broken down by cellular enzymes. Most of these so-called *degenerate* proteins are difficult for the body to utilize, and they become outright harmful unless they are promptly removed by the lymphatic system.

Dead flesh also invites enhanced microbial activity. According to a study by the US Department of Agriculture, nearly 80 percent of ground beef is contaminated with disease-causing microbes. The contamination continues or worsens once the flesh food arrives in the intestines where bacteria, fungi, worms, and parasites feed on the pooled wastes.

Since the human body can only digest between 15 and 20 percent of an average size hamburger (2.5 oz. or about 70 grams) at a time, most of it turns into waste that becomes subject to putrefaction. For more information about the risks of eating flesh foods, see this article titled "Eating Meat Kills More People Than Previously Thought[43]."

---

[43] http://www.naturalnews.com/025957_meat_eating_cancer.html#ixzz1ZvgwuBNQ

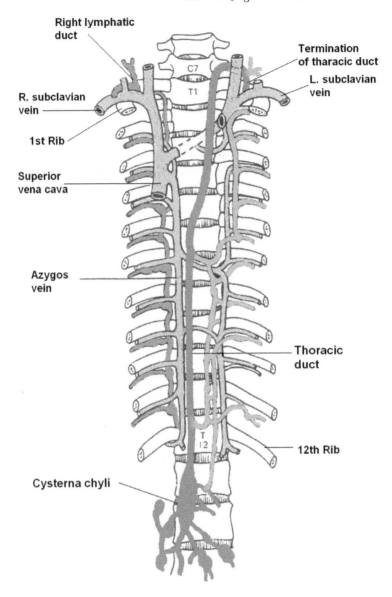

Figure 10: Cysterna chyli and the thoracic duct

The decomposing flesh food becomes source of degenerate proteins and highly toxic substances which are absorbed and end up congesting the cysterna chyli vessel. In some cases, allergic reactions occur.

When the cysterna chyli vessel is overtaxed and congested, the lymphatic system is no longer able to sufficiently remove even the body's own degenerate proteins (from worn-out cells). This results in lymph edema.

While lying on the back, existing lymph edema can be felt as hard knots, sometimes as large as a fist, in the area of the belly button. These *rocks* are a major cause of middle and low back pain and abdominal swelling, and, in fact, of most symptoms of ill health. Many people who have *grown a tummy* consider this abdominal extension to be just a harmless nuisance or a natural part of aging. They don't realize that they are breeding a living time bomb that may go off some day and injure vital parts of the body. In reality, every person with a bloated abdomen suffers from major lymph congestion.

The body's immune system and lymphatic system are intrinsically connected. Some 80 percent of the lymphatic system is associated with the intestines, making this area of the body the largest center of immune activity. This is no coincidence. The part of the body where most disease-causing agents are neutralized is, in fact, the intestinal tract. However, the same part of the body can become a cesspool of toxins and pathogens if it doesn't function properly. Any lymph edema, or other kind of obstruction in this important part of the lymphatic system, can lead to potentially serious complications elsewhere in the body.

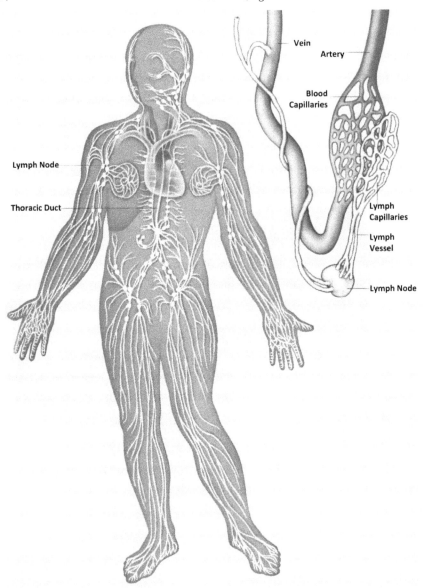

Figure 10: Lymphatic system and lymph nodes

Given that the thoracic duct has to remove nearly 85 percent of the body's daily-generated cellular waste and other potentially hazardous material, a blockage there causes backing up of toxic waste into other, more distant parts of the body.

When the daily-generated metabolic waste and cellular debris are not removed from an area in the body for a certain length of time, symptoms of disease start to manifest. The following are but a few typical examples of illness indicators that result directly from chronic, localized lymph congestion: obesity, cysts in the uterus or ovaries, enlargement of the prostate gland, rheumatism in the joints, enlargement of the heart, congestive heart failure, congested bronchi and lungs, swelling or enlargement of the neck area, stiffness in the neck and shoulders, backaches, headaches, migraines, dizziness, vertigo, ringing in the ears, earaches, deafness, dandruff, frequent colds, sinusitis, hay fever, certain types of asthma, thyroid enlargement, eye diseases, poor vision, swelling in the breasts, certain breast cancers, kidney problems, lower back pains, swelling of the legs and ankles, scoliosis, brain disorders, memory loss, stomach trouble, enlarged spleen, irritable bowel syndrome, hernia, polyps in the colon, and others.

The thoracic duct normally empties its detoxified waste contents into the left subclavian vein at the root of the neck. This vein enters the superior vena cava, which leads straight into the heart. In addition to blocking proper lymph drainage from the various organs or parts of the body, congestion in the cysterna chyli and thoracic duct permits toxic materials to be passed into the heart and heart arteries. This unduly stresses the heart. It also allows these toxins and disease-causing agents to enter the general circulation and spread to other parts of the body.

Hardly a disease can be named that is *not* caused by lymphatic obstruction. Lymph blockage, in most cases, has its origin in a congested liver that, in turn, may result in digestive problems, such as constipation, diarrhea, malabsorption of nutrients, leaky gut, irritable bowel syndrome, a disturbed gut flora, food allergies, Candida overgrowth, parasitic infections, etc. In the extreme eventuality, lymphoma or cancer of the lymph may result, of which Hodgkin's disease is the most common type.

When the circulatory system begins to malfunction because of gallstones in the liver, the endocrine system starts to be affected as well. The endocrine glands produce hormones that pass directly from the glandular cells into the bloodstream, where they influence bodily activity, growth, and nutrition. The glands most often affected by lymphatic congestion are the pancreas, adrenal cortex, ovaries, testes, and, foremost of all, the thyroid and parathyroid.

An underactive thyroid is particularly concerning in that it can lead to a large number of disease conditions that may not even be recognized as being caused by gallstones and the resulting lymphatic congestion.

In a German study, researchers found there is an association between thyroid and gallstone disease with a gender-specific relation between hypothyroidism and cholelithiasis[44]. My experience with individuals who had suffered from an underactive thyroid, and who, after doing a series of liver and gallbladder flushes subsequently restored normal thyroid functions, gives me reason to believe that this *association* is actually a cause-effect association.

That said, I agree with the authors of the study that once the thyroid is deficient in thyroid hormone, a delayed emptying of the biliary tract may occur, but my findings clearly show that poor liver and gallbladder performance leads to the thyroid dysfunction and the many related symptoms, such as the following: fatigue, dry skin and hair, hair thinning/hair loss, depression, morning headaches that get better through the day, brain fog, loss of memory, hoarse voice, difficulty concentrating, intolerance to cold, low body temperature, poor circulation/numbness in hands and feet, muscle cramps with no exertion, weight gain and difficulty losing it, decreased appetite, constipation, gallbladder diseases such as gallstones, chronic digestive problems such as low stomach acid.

A more severely disrupted circulatory function leads to imbalanced hormone secretions by the islets of Langerhans in the pancreas, and the pineal and pituitary glands.

Blood congestion, which is characterized by the thickening of the blood, prevents hormones from reaching their target places in the body in sufficient amounts and on time. Consequently, the glands go into hypersecretion (overproduction) of hormones.

When lymph drainage from the glands is inefficient, the glands themselves become congested. This brings about hyposecretion (lack) of hormones. Diseases related to imbalances of the thyroid gland include toxic goiter, Graves' disease, cretinism, myxoedema, tumors of the thyroid, and hypoparathyroidism. Thyroid disorders can also reduce

---

[44]*World J Gastroenterol* 2005;11(35):5530-5534

calcium absorption and cause cataracts, as well as hair loss, behavioral disorders, and dementia. Poor calcium absorption, alone, is responsible for numerous diseases, including osteoporosis (loss of bone density). If circulatory problems disrupt the secretion of balanced amounts of insulin in the pancreatic islets of Langerhans, diabetes may result.

Gallstones in the liver can cause liver cells to cut down protein synthesis. Reduced protein synthesis, in turn, prompts the adrenal glands to overproduce cortisol, a hormone that stimulates protein synthesis. Too much cortisol in the blood, however, gives rise to atrophy of lymphoid tissue and a depressed immune response, which is considered the leading cause of cancer and many other major illnesses.

(**Note**: Please let me mention at this point that my interpretation of *disease* differs from the one upheld by mainstream medicine. I have reasons to believe that the symptoms of disease, such as a cancerous tumor, is an adequate and useful healing attempt initiated by the body to try balance and rectify an otherwise very difficult and potentially life-endangering underlying condition. Conventional medicine is mostly dedicated to treating away the symptoms of disease, not the disease itself.)

An imbalance in the secretion of adrenal hormones can cause a wide variety of disorders, as it leads to weakened febrile response (fever) and diminished protein synthesis. Proteins are the major building blocks for tissue cells, hormones, and so forth. The liver is capable of producing many different hormones. Hormones determine how well the body grows and heals.

The liver also inhibits certain hormones, including insulin, glucagon, cortisol, aldosterone, thyroid, and sex hormones. Gallstones in the liver impair this vital function, which may increase hormone concentrations in the blood. Hormone imbalance is an extremely serious condition and can easily occur when gallstones in the liver have disrupted major circulatory pathways that are also hormonal pathways.

For example, by failing to keep blood cortisol levels balanced, a person may accumulate excessive amounts of fat in the body. If estrogens are not broken down properly, the risk of breast cancer increases. If blood insulin is not broken down properly, the risk of cancer rises, and the cells in the body may become resistant to insulin, which is a major precursor of diabetes.

Disease is naturally absent when blood flow and lymph flow are both unhindered and normal. Both types of problems - circulatory and lymphatic - can be improved or eliminated through a series of liver flushes and prevented by following a balanced diet and lifestyle.

Disorders of the Respiratory System

Both mental and physical health depend on the effectiveness and vitality of the cells in the body. The cells of the body derive most of their energy from biochemical reactions that take place in the presence of oxygen. One of the resultant waste products is carbon dioxide. The respiratory system provides the routes by which oxygen is taken into the body and carbon dioxide is excreted. Blood serves as the transport system for the exchange of these gases between the lungs and the cells.

Gallstones in the liver can impair respiratory functions and cause allergies, disorders of the nose and nasal cavities, and diseases of the bronchi and lungs. When gallstones distort or injure the lobules (units) of the liver, the blood-cleansing ability of the liver, small intestine, lymphatic system, and immune system diminishes. Toxic waste material, normally rendered harmless by these organs and systems, now begins to seep into the heart, lungs, bronchi, and other respiratory passages. Constant exposure to these irritating substances lowers the resistance of the respiratory system to them. Lymph congestion in the abdominal region, particularly in the cysterna chyli and thoracic duct, interferes with proper lymphatic drainage from the respiratory organs. Most respiratory ailments occur because of such lymph blockages.

Pneumonia results when the body's natural protective measures fail to prevent inhaled or blood-borne microbes from reaching and colonizing the lungs. Gallstones in the bile ducts of the liver harbor harmful microbes, as well as highly toxic, irritating material that can enter the blood via areas in the liver that are damaged by the presence of these stones. They also hamper the liver's ability to filter out and neutralize toxins. Gallstones are a constant source of immune suppression, which leaves the body, and particularly the upper respiratory tract, susceptible to both internal and external disease-triggering factors. These include blood-borne and airborne microbes (believed to cause pneumonia), cigarette smoke, alcohol, x-rays, corticosteroids, allergens, antigens, common air pollutants, chemicals found in foods and drinking water, toxic waste matter from the GI tract, and the like.

Further respiratory complications arise when handfuls of gallstones that have accumulated in the liver bile ducts lead to liver enlargement. The liver, situated in the upper abdominal cavity, spans almost the entire width of the body. Its upper and anterior surfaces are smooth and shaped to fit under the surface of the diaphragm. When enlarged, the liver obstructs the movement of the diaphragm and prevents the lungs from extending to their normal capacity during inhalation.

By contrast, a smooth, healthy liver permits the lungs to easily extend into the abdominal region, which puts pressure on the abdomen and squeezes the lymph and blood vessels to force lymph and blood toward the heart. This breathing mechanism is often called *belly breathing*, and it can be easily observed in healthy babies, especially.

An enlarged liver prevents the full extension of the diaphragm and lungs, which causes reduced exchange of gases in the lungs, lymphatic congestion, and the retention of excessive amounts of carbon dioxide in the lungs. The restricted uptake of oxygen negatively affects cellular functions throughout the body.

Most people in the industrialized world now have an enlarged liver, especially those who are overweight or obese. What doctors generally consider a *normal-sized* liver is actually oversized. Once all gallstones are removed through a series of liver flushes, the liver can gradually return to its original size.

Almost all diseases of the lungs, bronchi, and upper respiratory passages are either caused or worsened by gallstones in the liver and can be improved or eliminated by removing these stones through liver cleansing.

Disorders of the Urinary System

The urinary system is an extremely important excretory and regulatory system of the body. It consists of the following: two kidneys, which form and excrete urine; two ureters, which convey the urine from the kidneys to the urinary bladder; a urinary bladder, where urine collects and is temporarily stored; and a urethra, through which urine passes from the urinary bladder to the exterior of the body (see **Figure 12**).

Smooth functioning of the urinary system is essential for maintaining an appropriate fluid volume by regulating the amount of water that is excreted in the urine. It is particularly involved in regulating the concentrations of various electrolytes[45] in the body fluids and maintaining normal pH (acid/alkaline balance) of the blood. This system is also involved in the disposal of waste products resulting from the breakdown (catabolism) of cell protein in the liver, for example.

Most diseases of the kidneys and other parts of the urinary system are related to an imbalance of the simple filtration system in the kidneys. About 26 to 40 gallons of dilute filtrate are formed each day by the two kidneys. Of these, only 34 to 52 oz. are excreted as urine (the rest is absorbed and recirculates). With the exception of blood cells, platelets, and blood proteins, all other blood constituents must pass through the kidneys. The process of filtration is disrupted and weakened when the digestive system - and in particular, the liver - perform poorly.

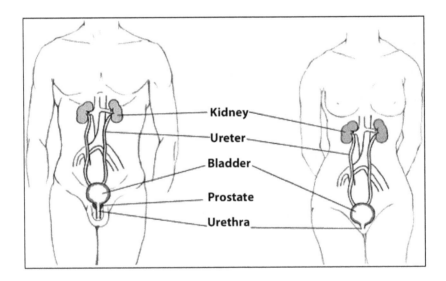

Figure 12: The urinary system

Gallstones in the liver and gallbladder reduce the amount of bile that the liver is able to produce. Thus, it becomes difficult to digest food properly. Much of the undigested food begins to ferment and putrefy, leaving toxic waste matter in the blood and lymph. The body's normal excretions, such as urine, sweat, gases, and feces, do not usually contain

---

[45]Electrolytes are substances that become ions in solution and are able to conduct electricity. In the human body, the balance of the electrolytes is essential for normal function of cells and organs. The most common electrolytes include sodium, potassium, chloride, and bicarbonate.

disease-generating waste products; that is, of course, for as long as the passages of elimination remain clear and unobstructed and these waste products can easily leave the body.

Disease-causing agents consist of tiny molecules that appear in the blood and lymph. They are visible only through powerful electron microscopes. These molecules have a strong acidifying effect on the blood. To avoid a life-threatening disease or coma, the blood must rid itself of these minute toxins. Accordingly, it dumps these unwanted intruders into the connective tissue of the organs. The connective tissue consists of a gel-like fluid (lymph) that surrounds all cells. The cells are *bathed* in this connective tissue.

Under normal circumstances, the body knows how to deal with acidic waste material that has been dumped into the connective tissue. It releases an alkaline product, sodium bicarbonate ($NaHCO_3$), into the blood that is able to retrieve the acidic toxins, neutralize them, and then eliminate them through the excretory organs. This ingenious cleaning system, though, begins to fail when toxins are deposited faster than they can be retrieved and eliminated. In due course, the connective tissue may become as thick as jelly. Nutrients, water, and oxygen can no longer pass freely, and the cells of the organs begin to suffer malnutrition, dehydration, and oxygen deficiency.

Some of the most acidifying compounds for the human body are proteins from flesh foods. Gallstones inhibit the digestive system's ability to properly digest these proteins and break them down into usable amino acids. Amino acids must be whole and undamaged to be rapidly transported across the digestive membrane in order for the body to derive benefits from them.

Heating animal proteins foods such as meat, poultry, fish, eggs, and cheese during cooking, baking, or frying destroys their three-dimensional structures and causes them to coagulate. For example, a normally liquid egg becomes hard when boiled; the heat tears apart the bonds of protein molecules. This change is known as protein denaturation.

The denaturation of proteins also means loss of solubility in water and dilute salt solutions. However, solubility is essential for proper utilization and transportation of the amino acids across the digestive membrane and the cell membranes. Denatured proteins constitute a serious health risk in that they trigger inflammatory responses in blood vessels, lymph vessels, joints, nerves, and other parts for the body. They can be held responsible for numerous disease processes, including cancer, coronary heart disease, arthritis, disorders of the nervous system, and others.

Heat is not the main cause of protein coagulation and denaturation. However, certain toxic salts, alcohol, physical injury, ionizing radiation (x-rays, CT scans), and ultrasonic vibrations (ultrasounds) can also denature the protein and render it insoluble in the body.

We must remember that proteins are the basic building blocks of cells. Frequent medical radiation and exposure to ultrasounds can cause serious, irreversible damage to the clusters of proteins making up our cells.

Regardless, the body has a rescue program in place that helps it keep as many of these damaged proteins out of the bloodstream as possible. Denatured and excessive proteins are temporarily stored in the connective tissues and then converted into collagen fiber. The collagen fiber is then built into the basal membranes of the capillary walls (see **Figure 9**).

The basal membranes may become up to 10 times thicker than normal. A similar situation occurs in the basal membranes of arteries. As the blood vessel walls become increasingly congested, fewer proteins are able to escape the blood stream. This leads to blood thickening, making the blood more and more difficult for the kidneys to filter. (**Note**: The kidneys filter only the plasma part of the blood, which contains all the nutrients, antibodies, waste products, hormones, minerals, vitamins, etc., but no blood cells)

At the same time, the basal membranes of the blood vessels supplying the kidneys also become congested, making them harder and more rigid. As the process of hardening of the blood vessels progresses further, blood pressure begins to rise and overall kidney performance drops. More and more of the metabolic waste products excreted by the kidney cells, which would normally be eliminated via venous blood vessels and lymphatic ducts, are now retained and adversely affect the performance of the kidneys even further.

Through all this, the kidneys become heavily overburdened and can no longer maintain normal fluid and electrolyte balances in the body.

In addition, urinary components, such as salts and minerals, may precipitate and form into crystals and pebbles of various types and sizes (see **Figure 13a**) from as small as a grain of sand to the size of a golf ball. These kidney stones can trigger severe pain in the abdomen, flank, or groin and be the cause of blood in the urine. Crystal-shaped stones (see **Figure**

13b) are especially damaging since they easily rupture blood vessels and inflame the delicate kidney tissue.

One in every 20 people develops a kidney stone at some point in their life, usually due to dietary reasons.

The most common type of stone is formed when uric acid concentration in the urine exceeds 2 to 4 mg percent. This amount was considered within the range of tolerance until the mid-1960s, when it was adjusted upward. Uric acid is a by-product of the breakdown of protein in the liver. Since meat consumption rose sharply in that decade, the *within the norm* level was adjusted to 7.5 mg percent. Increased sugar consumption (high fructose corn syrup) in soft drinks also greatly contributed to an overall rise of uric acid levels in the general population[46].

The upward adjustment, however, does not make the lower levels of uric acid between 4 mg and 7.5 mg percent any less harmful to the body. All stones formed from excessive uric acid concentrations of 4 mg percent and higher (see *Bladder stones* in **Figure 13c**) can lead to urinary obstruction, kidney infection, and, eventually, kidney failure.

As kidney cells become increasingly deprived of vital nutrients, especially oxygen, malignant tumors may develop. In addition, tiny uric acid crystals that are not eliminated by the kidneys can settle in the joints and cause rheumatism, gout, and water retention.

Symptoms of impending kidney trouble are often deceptively mild in comparison to the potential severity of kidney disease. The most observable and common symptoms of kidney problems are abnormal changes in the volume, frequency, and coloration of the urine. These are usually accompanied by swelling of the eyes, face, and ankles, as well as pain in the upper and lower back. If the disease has progressed further, there may be blurred vision, tiredness, declined performance, and nausea.

The following symptoms may also indicate malfunctioning of the kidneys: high blood pressure, low blood pressure, pain moving from the upper to lower abdomen, dark-brown urine, pain in the back just above the waist, excessive thirst, increase in urination (especially during the night), less than 500 ml of urine per day, a feeling of fullness in the bladder, pain while passing urine, drier and browner skin pigment, ankles being puffy at night, eyes being puffy in morning, bruising, and hemorrhaging.

---

[46]Fructose is found to increase cardiovascular and diabetes risk in adolescents, www.naturalnews.com

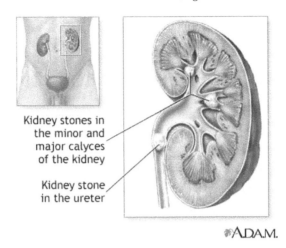

Kidney stones in
the minor and
major calyces
of the kidney

Kidney stone
in the ureter

⚛A.D.A.M.

Figure 13a: Kidney stones embedded in the kidney

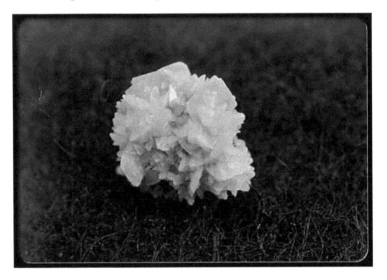

Figure 13b: Crystal-shaped kidney stone
Image Source: Flickr / Ken Gantz

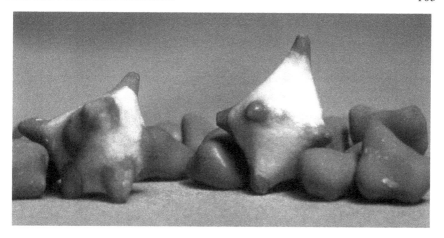

Figure 13c: Bladder stones

All major diseases of the urinary system are caused by toxic blood; in other words, by blood filled with tiny molecules of waste material and excessive or denatured proteins. Gallstones in the liver and gallbladder can impair digestion, cause blood and lymph congestion, and disrupt the entire circulatory system, including that of the urinary system.

When the gallstones are removed, the urinary system has a chance to recuperate, rid itself of accumulated toxins and stones, and maintain fluid balance and normal blood pressure. This is necessary for all the processes in the body to run smoothly and efficiently.

Recommendations: Make sure to be well hydrated by drinking 6-8 glasses of water each day and to avoid becoming overweight. Dehydration and weight gain are major risk factors for developing kidney stones, and so are a high intake of animal protein, a diet high in refined salt and other processed foods, excessive sugar consumption, and excessive vitamin D supplementation. If you have kidney stones, you may need to cleanse the kidneys, in addition to the liver and gallbladder (see *Keep Your Kidneys Clean*, Chapter 5).

Disorders of the Nervous System

Our persona, the way we carry ourselves, our interactions with other people, our moods, desires, patience and tolerance levels, and our reactions to life's occurrences - are all strongly influenced by the state of the health of our nervous system. In today's fast-paced world, we are exposed to a variety of stressful conditions that can wreak havoc on our bodies. The brain is the control center of the body, and unless it receives proper nourishment and undergoes regular cycles of restfulness and revitalization, we can easily be overwhelmed and thrown off balance. Constant nervousness, anxiety, impatience, anger, irritability, aggressiveness, depression etc., are all indications that the nervous system is weak and overtaxed.

Brain cells are normally easily capable of manufacturing the huge number of neuropeptides (powerful brain hormones) they need for the complex tasks they must perform, day after day, year after year. However, their life support depends on the continuous supply of nutrients necessary to produce those hormones. Modern intensive agriculture has nearly depleted farm soil of all its basic nutrients (see *Eat Ionic, Essential Minerals*, Chapter 5).

Stripping the soil of its nutrients and loading it up with chemical poisons (pesticides), and doing the same to foods through modern food processing methods has certainly added to the nutritional deficiencies so prevalent among the populations in industrialized nations. However, most nutrient deficiencies still result from poor performance of the digestive system and, particularly, of the liver. Lack of such nutrients can hinder the ability of our brains to manufacture the hormones they need in order to function efficiently.

The brain can operate for quite some time with substandard amounts of nutrients, but the price one pays includes fatigue, lack of energy, mood swings, depression, sickness, aches and pains, and general discomfort. Some extreme deficiencies may manifest in mental disorders, such as schizophrenia, autism, and Alzheimer's.

The health of the nervous system, which includes the brain, the spinal cord, pairs of spinal and cranial nerves, and autonomic functions, largely depends on the quality of the blood. Blood is composed of plasma (a straw-colored transparent fluid) and cells. The constituents of plasma are water, plasma proteins, mineral salts, hormones, vitamins, nutrient materials, organic waste products, antibodies, and gases. There are 3 varieties of blood cells: white cells (leukocytes), red cells (erythrocytes), and platelets (thrombocytes). Any abnormal changes in the blood affect the nervous system as well as the rest of the body.

All 3 types of blood cells are formed in the red bone marrow, which is nourished and maintained by the nutrients supplied by the digestive system. Gallstones in the liver interfere with the digestion and assimilation of food, which fills the plasma of the blood with excessive waste material and reduces nutrient supplies to the red bone marrow. This, in turn, upsets the balance of blood cell constituents, disrupts hormonal pathways, and causes abnormal responses in the nervous system.

Most diseases afflicting the nervous system are rooted in improperly formed blood, brought about by a dysfunctional liver and resulting imbalance in the gut's bacteria population.

Each of the numerous functions of the liver has a direct influence on the nervous system, particularly the brain. Liver cells convert glycogen (complex sugar) into glucose, which, besides oxygen and water, serves as the most important nutrient for the nervous system. Glucose covers most of that system's energy requirements.

The brain, although it constitutes only one-fiftieth of the body's weight, contains about one-fifth of the total blood volume in the body. It uses up vast amounts of glucose. Gallstones in the liver drastically reduce glucose supplies to the brain and the rest of the nervous system. This, in turn, can affect the performance of the organs, senses, and mind. Have you ever felt completely drained of energy for no apparent reason? The reason is a temporary shortage of glucose to the cells. At the early stages of imbalance, you may develop food cravings, particularly for sweet or starchy foods, and experience frequent mood swings or emotional stress.

There are other, even more serious problems resulting from occurrence of gallstones in the liver. The liver forms the plasma proteins and most of the blood-clotting factors from the body's amino acid pool. Presence of gallstones in the bile ducts of the liver increasingly inhibits this important function. When the production of clotting factors drops, platelet count drops, too, and there may be spontaneous capillary bleeding or hemorrhagic disease.

If a hemorrhage occurs in the brain, it may lead to destruction of brain tissue, paralysis, or death. The severity of the bleeding may be determined by such variable triggers as hypertension and alcohol abuse. Platelet counts also drop when the production of new cells does not keep pace with the destruction of damaged or worn-out cells; this occurs when gallstones cut off the blood supply to the liver cells.

Vitamin K is another element essential for the synthesis of major clotting factors. It is a fat-soluble vitamin stored in the liver. To absorb fats in the intestines, the body requires bile salts that are made available through bile secretions. Gallstones in the liver and gallbladder obstruct bile flow, which leads to inadequate fat absorption and subsequent vitamin K deficiency.

As discussed earlier, gallstones in the liver can lead to disorders of the vascular system. When the blood undergoes changes and becomes too thick, blood vessels begin to harden and become damaged. If a blood clot forms in an inflamed/injured artery, a piece of that blood clot (embolus) may lodge in a small artery distant from the injury and obstruct the blood flow, causing ischemia and infarction. If the infarction occurs in a brain artery, it is called a stroke.

All circulatory disturbances affect the brain and the rest of the nervous system. The disruption of liver functions particularly affects astrocytes, the cells that make up the main supporting tissue of the central nervous system. This condition is characterized by apathy, disorientation, brain fog, delirium, muscular rigidity, and coma.

Nitrogenous bacterial waste absorbed from the colon, unless detoxified by the liver, may reach the brain cells via the blood. Other metabolic waste products, such as ammonia, may reach toxic concentrations and change the permeability of the blood vessels in the brain, thus reducing the effectiveness of the blood-brain barrier. This may permit various noxious substances to enter the brain and cause further damage.

Atrophy of neural tissue, which is the main cause of dementia or Alzheimer's disease, results when a large number of neurons of the brain no longer receive enough nourishment. When a certain class of neurons that are responsible for producing the brain hormone and neurotransmitter dopamine suffer malnourishment, Parkinson's disease results. Repeated exposure to certain environmental or internally produced toxins can also be responsible.

Multiple sclerosis (MS) occurs when the cells that produce myelin (a sheath of fatty material that surrounds most axons of nerve cells) suffer malnutrition and insufficient lymph drainage. The myelin sheath diminishes, and axons become injured. MS patients usually suffer from progressive intestinal congestion, which prevents proper nutrient absorption. Cleansing the eliminative organs and improving nutrition are among the most powerful approaches to halt and possibly reverse MS.

The liver controls the digestion, absorption, and metabolism of fatty substances throughout the body. Gallstones interfere with fat metabolism and affect cholesterol levels in the blood. Cholesterol is an essential building block of all our body cells and plays an essential role in cell metabolism. Our brains consist of more than 10 percent pure cholesterol (all water removed). Cholesterol is important for brain development and brain function. It protects the nerves against damage or injury.

An imbalance of blood fats and cholesterol levels can profoundly affect the brain and nervous system and, thereby, cause almost any type of illness in the body. Removing gallstones from the liver and gallbladder increases nutrient supplies to all the cells, rejuvenates the nervous system and improves all functions in the body.

Disorders of the Bone

Although bone is the hardest and densest tissue in the body, it is, nevertheless, very much alive. Human bone consists of 20 percent water, 30-40 percent organic material such as living cells; and 40-50 percent inorganic material, such as calcium. Bone tissue contains many blood and lymph vessels and nerves. The cells responsible for balanced bone growth are osteoblasts and osteoclasts. Osteoblasts are the bone-forming cells, whereas osteoclasts are responsible for reabsorption of bone materials to maintain optimum shape. A third group of cells, known as chondrocytes, are in charge of forming cartilage. The less dense parts of the bone, called cancellous bone, contain red bone marrow, which produces red and white blood cells.

Most bone diseases occur when bone cells no longer receive enough nourishment. Balanced bile secretion plays a key role, for example, in the digestion and absorption of essential minerals such as calcium, magnesium and zinc - important building materials for healthy bone.

Good bone health results from the sustained balance between the functions of osteoblast and osteoclast cells. This delicate balance becomes upset when nutrient supply is deficient and thereby slows the production of new bone tissue by osteoblasts. Osteoporosis results when the amount of bone tissue is reduced because the growth of new bone does not keep pace with the destruction of old bone. Cancellous bone is usually affected before compact bone is. Compact bone makes up the outer layer of the bone. This makes it harder for an individual to notice when osteoporosis actually occurs.

In generalized osteoporosis, excessive calcium is reabsorbed from bone, thereby raising the calcium levels of blood and urine. This may predispose a person to form stones in the kidneys and, possibly, suffer renal failure. Excess blood calcium can also lead to calcified gallstones in the gallbladder. Gallstones substantially reduce bile production. Since bile is essential for the absorption of calcium from the small intestines, a vicious cycle begins to unfold that leads to more calcifications and less bone building.

Even if the body received more than enough calcium from foods or mineral supplements, a shortage of bile would render much of the ingested minerals useless for bone building and other important metabolic processes.

Furthermore, the presence of gallstones in the liver prevents it from removing acidic metabolic wastes and toxins, thereby leaving excessive amounts of harmful acids in the blood. To avoid a dangerous alteration of blood pH (acid/alkaline balance) the blood leaches minerals from the bones and teeth. A similar principle is at work when a person drinks cow's milk. To neutralize the highly acidic phosphorus that abounds in the milk, the body uses not only the milk's calcium but also calcium from the bones and teeth.

Eventually, the body's calcium reserves become depleted, diminishing bone density or bone mass. This may lead to bone and hip fractures, and even death. With more than half of all women over age 50 already affected by osteoporosis (albeit only in industrialized nations), it is obvious that the current medical advice of taking hormones or calcium supplements and drinking milk is a shot in the dark; it in no way addresses the imbalance in the liver and gallbladder caused by reduced bile output due to gallstones.

Prescription drugs to slow the body's breakdown of bone have miserably failed to reduce the incidence of osteoporosis. In fact, they often produce horrendous side effects that include severely brittle bones that can shatter to pieces at the slightest impact.

Rickets and osteomalacia are diseases that affect the calcification process of bones. In either case, the bones become soft, especially those of the lower limbs, which are bowed by the weight of the body. The fat-soluble vitamin D, calciferol, is essential for balanced calcium and phosphorus metabolism and, therefore, healthy bone structures.

Insufficient bile secretion and disturbance of the cholesterol metabolism, both of which are caused by gallstones in the liver, lead to vitamin D deficiency. Lack of regular exposure to sunlight or the use of sunscreens can, in fact, cause or further aggravate these conditions.

Infection of bones, or osteomyelitis, may result when there has been a prolonged lymphatic obstruction in the body, especially in or around bone tissues. Consequently, blood-borne microbes gain unhindered access to bones. As mentioned before, infectious microbes only attack cell tissues that are acidified, weak, unstable, or damaged. The microbes may originate from gallstones, a tooth abscess, or a boil.

Malignant tumors of the bone can occur when lymphatic congestion in the body and the bones, especially, has reached extreme proportions. The immune system is suppressed and malignant tumor particles from the breasts, lungs, or prostate gland can spread to or develop in those parts of the bones that have the softest tissue and are more prone to congestion and acidification, i.e. the cancellous bone.

Bone cancer and all other diseases of the bone indicate lack of nourishment of bone tissue. Such diseases usually defy treatment unless all gallstones in the liver are removed and all other organs and systems of elimination are cleared of any existing congestion as well.

Disorders of the Joints

Our body contains three types of joints: fibrous or fib joints, cartilaginous or slightly movable joints, and synovial or freely movable joints. The most susceptible to disease are the joints of the hands, feet, knees, shoulders, elbows, and hips. Rheumatoid arthritis, osteoarthritis, and gout are among the most commonly found joint disorders.

Most people stricken with rheumatoid arthritis have a long history of intestinal complaints: bloating, flatulence, heartburn, belching, constipation, diarrhea, coldness and swelling of hands and feet, increased perspiration, general fatigue, loss of appetite, weight reduction, and more. It is reasonable, therefore, to conclude that rheumatoid arthritis is linked with any of these, or similar, symptoms of major intestinal and metabolic disturbances.

I have personally experienced all the symptoms mentioned above when I suffered painful bouts of juvenile rheumatoid arthritis during my childhood years. I was also afflicted with numerous digestive disorders, including acid reflux, constipation with alternating diarrhea, and malabsorption. My arthritis symptoms completely vanished soon after I was able to restore healthy digestive functions.

Since I consider arthritis to be the combined result of many different health conditions and specific root causes, I shall elaborate on this important topic in the following section on autoimmune disease.

Autoimmune Disease Myths Unraveled

The GI tract is constantly exposed to a large number of viruses, bacteria, and parasites. In addition to these and many other natural *antigens* (foreign materials) contained in plant and flesh foods, the digestive system may also have to deal with chemical insecticides, pesticides, hormones, antibiotic residues, preservatives, and colorings contained in so many processed foodstuffs today. In addition, there is the organic plastic compound bisphenol A (BPA) - an antioxidant in plastic bottles and food packaging - leaching BPA into our food and beverages. This harmful ingredient is also found in the liners of metal food and beverage cans.

Many people are still exposed to the highly toxic chemical fluoride added to municipal water in the United States and other countries.

Some large-molecule medical drugs such as penicillin also act as toxins.

Possible naturally occurring antigens include pollen from flowers, plants, plant antibodies and enzyme inhibitors, fungi, mold, and the like.

It is the task of the immune system (most of it is located in the intestinal lining) to protect us against all these potentially harmful invaders and substances. To be able to accomplish this task every day, both the digestive and lymphatic systems must remain unobstructed and efficient. Gallstones in the liver seriously disrupt the digestive process, which leads to an overload of toxic substances in the gut, blood and lymph.

Most doctors consider arthritis an autoimmune disease affecting the synovial membrane. Autoimmunity is thought to be a condition in which the immune system develops immunity to its own cells. It results when antigen/antibody complexes (*rheumatoid factors*) are formed in the blood.

Naturally, the B-lymphocytes (immune cells) in the intestinal wall become stimulated and produce antibodies (immunoglobulins) when coming into contact with these antigens. However, a normal immune system requires the activation of these B cells by T cells (special lymphocytes that play a central role in cell-mediated immunity) before the former can produce antibodies in large quantities.

It is important to know that T cells must be triggered first before the immune system can mount an inflammatory response in the intestines or elsewhere in the body. In spite of this well-established medical fact, modern medicine still hypothesizes that this kind of inflammatory response means the body is mistakenly attacking its own cells. However, there are major flaws in this theory, which proposes that the body is capable of making grievous mistakes. However, we cannot draw the conclusion that the body is erroneous in its activities just because we don't know why the body behaves in this way. Our lack of insight and understanding of the true mechanisms of disease and healing should not be misconstrued as incompetency on behalf of the body.

Taking Lessons from the Body

The actions the body takes during an autoimmune response are far from being miscalculated, accidental occurrences; in fact, they are based on the body's innate wisdom, and they are intentional.

The T cell activated immune cells circulate in the blood, and some settle in the lymph nodes, spleen, mucus membranes of the salivary glands, lymphatic system of the bronchial tubes, vagina or uterus, milk-producing mammary glands of the breasts, and capsular tissues of the joints.

If there is repeated exposure to the same types of toxic antigens in the gut lining, antibody production will increase dramatically, particularly in areas of the body where immune cells have settled because of a previous encounter with foreign, potentially harmful, invaders. Accordingly, the body goes into its inflammatory mode.

There are now 101 different diseases considered autoimmune diseases, including autistic disorder, Alzheimer's disease, multiple sclerosis, ulcerative colitis, Crohn's disease, lupus, encephalomyelitis, alopecia, type 1 diabetes, epilepsy, Chronic Fatigue Syndrome, Graves' disease, Guillain-Barré Syndrome, Parkinson's disease, psoriasis, thyroiditis, myocarditis, and arthritis - a general term for more than 100 different diseases that affect the joints.

Since all these autoimmune diseases exhibit the same fundamental mechanism, allopathic medicine treats them basically in the same way, using IVIG, steroids, plasmapheresis or other cytotoxic and immunosuppressive treatments. These treatments often result in severe side effects that include kidney failure, fluid retention, liver tumors, heart attack, stroke, and death.

The standard medical approaches ignore the fact that autoimmune diseases are actually triggered by a protein on the surface of a virus, bacteria, food or other substance. T cells only activate B cells into action *after* an infection has occurred or they made contact with harmful chemicals or proteins in your food. By avoiding the food or substance that provokes the antibody/antigen complex, the autoimmune response abates. The trick is finding out which proteins could serve as a trigger for an autoimmune response.

Eating cooked meat creates excess uric acid and ammonia in the body, both of which are toxic to the system. As a result of the applied heat, this protein food becomes coagulated (hardened) and denatured. Another example is the boiling of an egg; the heat causes its liquids to become hard. As a result, the polypeptide bonds cannot be broken down into amino acids. The immune system treats these damaged polypeptides as harmful invaders, and reacts by first engaging its T cells, and then producing antibody complexes leading to inflammation.

Pasteurization of dairy products, such as milk, cheese and yoghurt also causes damage to the food's polypeptides, and therefore may lead to autoimmune responses in the body. I have repeatedly witnessed a spontaneous recovery from the debilitating and often deadly autoimmune Crohn's disease in patients after I recommended that they stop eating dairy products (or peanuts - a legume responsible for millions of serious allergic reactions each year). No other treatment was necessary.

The person who is most likely to develop an autoimmune disease tends to have low vitamin D levels due to insufficient, regular sun exposure or use of sunscreens. Another reason is high toxicity evoking a bacterial, viral or fungal infection that causes the immune system to overreact to environmental toxins or foods. A third reason is significant immune deficiency. Immune deficiency is not an exclusive condition found only among older people, but it is becoming increasingly common among young adults and now even children.

The Vaccination Dilemma

Besides low levels of vitamin D, the commonest cause of immune deficiency and immune-suppression is vaccination. Vaccines are filled with dozens of carcinogenic chemicals, toxic metals, and protein fragments from animal parts, foreign DNA, formaldehyde, antibiotics like neomycin and streptomycin, and adjuvants known to cause an abnormal hyperactivation of the immune system, which always leads to weakening and suppression of natural immunity in the body.

The most commonly given adjuvants contain aluminum salt (aluminum phosphate), which is well-known for being a powerful neurotoxin, linked to Alzheimer's disease and other neurological disorders[47].

The body is designed to create natural immunity by using a different system from the one activated when a vaccine is injected into the body. This primary immune system, also known as IgA immune system, is strategically located in the body's mucus membranes where pathogens and antigens normally make contact with the body.

The mucus membranes constitute the body's first line of defense. It is here that invading organisms (pathogens) and toxins are analyzed and dealt with in the most appropriate ways, usually without requiring an activation of the immune system. In other words, with relatively few exceptions like a few immunity-boosting infections (auto-immunization) during childhood, you would not even notice when your body encounters pathogens.

The situation, however, is very different when a virus is injected into your body in a vaccine, especially when combined with an adjuvant like aluminum phosphate or squalene. Your IgA immune system is not only bypassed but actually becomes suppressed, and your body's immune system is forced into high gear in response to harmful vaccine ingredients. When injected, the body considers adjuvants to be foreign bodies and, thus, it quickly elicits an intense, abnormal, and long-lasting immune response.

Adjuvants help vaccine-manufacturers to drastically cut production costs. They allow them to produce more of the multiple-dose vials versus single-dose vials and to facilitate shipping large amounts of vaccines to

---

[47]Aprile, M.A. and Wardlaw, A.C., 1966. Aluminium compounds as adjuvants for vaccines and toxoids in man: A review Can. J. Public Health 57:343

doctors' offices and clinics. Adjuvants in vaccines also reduce the amount of vaccine serum needed to evoke the same response. However, adjuvants in vaccines carry serious health risks, including autoimmune diseases, coma, and death.

Adjuvants are so dangerous that it may just take one vaccine shot to permanently damage the immune system. According to a 2000 study published in the *American Journal of Pathology*, a single injection of the adjuvant squalene into rats triggered "chronic, immune-mediated joint-specific inflammation", also known as rheumatoid arthritis.

It has been known since the 1930s that adjuvants can cause autoimmune disease. If scientists want to induce an autoimmune disease in a lab animal, they simple inject it with the adjuvant *Freund's Complete Adjuvant*. If injected into humans via a vaccine, an adjuvant can trigger such a strong overreaction of the immune system that it loses its ability to distinguish what is *foreign* from what is *self*. This is the breaking point of tolerance where the overwhelmed immune system begins its indiscriminate assault on friend and foe alike - friend being the body's own cells[48]. It is like a bull that is being speared by a Spanish bullfighter. In its utter state of desperation, the bull will attack anything that moves.

Even foreign, harmless substances which the immune system would not normally react against are now being attacked, too. That's why allergies are so much higher among vaccinated than non-vaccinated individuals. In 1992, a study by the New Zealand Immunization Awareness Society (IAS) found that vaccinated children suffered 5 times more asthma and nearly 3 times more allergies than non-vaccinated ones.

An allergy is a hypersensitivity disorder of the immune system which causes the body to react to normally harmless substances in the environment. Adjuvants in vaccines are among the main culprits behind a hyperactive and overly sensitive immune system.

Of course, adding the mercury-containing preservative thimerosal to vaccines and other medical drugs only further sensitizes the immune system. Thimerosal is now the fifth most common allergen, according to the North American Contact Dermatitis Group (NACDG)[49]. Most of the flu vaccines given to millions of children and adults each year contain this

---

[48]Adverse effects of adjuvants in vaccines, by Viera Scheibner, Ph.D. 2000,
http://www.whale.to/vaccine/adjuvants.html
[49] Marks JG, Belsito DV, DeLeo VA, et al. North American Contact Dermatitis Group Patch-Test Results, 1998-2000. Am J Contact Dermat 2003;14:59-62

neurotoxin and are much responsible for the massive allergy epidemics afflicting the immunized population.

Flu vaccines can do more than just cause autoimmune diseases. The flu vaccine may even pose an immediate risk to your cardiovascular system. One 2007 study published in the *Annals of Medicine*, concluded: "Abnormalities in arterial function and LDL oxidation may persist for at least two weeks after a slight inflammatory reaction induced by influenza vaccination. These could explain in part the earlier reported increase in cardiovascular risk during the first weeks after an acute inflammatory disorder."

How many people die from a heart attack after receiving a flu shot? I don't think we'll ever find out. However, we now know for certain that the true risks of vaccination have been deliberately kept from us by those very agencies that are responsible for public health.

CDC Caught Deliberately Falsifying Vaccine Research Data

The Centers for Disease Control and Prevention (CDC) have for many years denied a possible link between mercury in vaccines and autism spectrum disorder (ASD). However, in October 2011, the CDC has been caught deliberately fudging data to try to cover up evidence linking mercury in vaccines with ASD[50].

To conceal any incriminating vaccine data, the CDC had handed its massive database of vaccine records over to a private company, effectively pronouncing it off-limits to researchers and preventing dissemination of the data through the Freedom of Information Act (FOIA).

However, this didn't stop the Coalition for Mercury-Free Drugs (CoMeD). During an enquiry through FOIA it was discovered, as suspected, that the same original Danish study which the CDC referred to as "definitive evidence" that thimerosal does not increase a child's chances of developing ASD, actually revealed its exact opposite to be true. The Danish research is irrefutably clear about the findings: Thimerosal in vaccines increases a person's chances of developing autism and other neurological diseases (see *Vaccines - A Death Trap*, Chapter 3, for more detailed information about this fraud which is misleading millions of

---

[50]http://www.naturalnews.com/034038_vaccines_autism.html

unsuspecting parents into believing that mercury in vaccines is safe for their children).

In the US, at least 1 in every 100 fully vaccinated children is afflicted with ASD, while only 1 in every 2,000 non-vaccinated children has the disease. In European countries like Iceland, where children receive one-third the number of vaccine shots, only 1 in 30,000 children has ASD. In the US, now 1 in every 88 children has ASD, according to a statement made by the CDC in March 2012, citing statistics from the year 2008. In those US states where children receive the most vaccines, or where relatively more children become vaccinated, as for example in Utah and New Jersey, as many as 1 in 47 children develop ASD. By comparison, in the mostly rural state of Iowa where fewer children become vaccinated, 1 in 718 children has autism[51].

If the overall trend increase has been consistent since 2008, which appears to be the case, then 1 in every 63 children in the US now has ASD (year 2012). One doesn't need to be a scientist to make sense of this man-made tragedy.

The FDA is not an innocent bystander in this conspiracy against the health of the American people. Both the CDC and FDA have tried to conceal from concerned parents that vaccines still contain mercury. In a recent court hearing the FDA unintentionally admitted that flu vaccines now routinely given to babies as young as 6 months of age contain it, according to *Courthouse News Service* on Friday, March 23, 2012[52].

"The Food and Drug Administration is not liable for approving a mercury-based vaccine preservative because more expensive, mercury-free vaccines are available upon request," a federal judge ruled. "Thimerosal-preserved flu vaccines are necessary to ensure sufficient supply at a reasonable price," according to the judgment.

The problem with this questionable *solution* to allegedly avoid mercury poisoning of American babies is that most doctors neither inform parents about what flu vaccines really contain, nor recommend the other, less toxic options. Most parents still trust their child's pediatrician and do what they are told. And why pay for an expensive vaccine, when there is a cheaper one available, especially when the doctor insists that the vaccine (containing mercury) is completely safe? The FDA has no intention of

---

[51] Autism Rates in US States, http://www.stellamarie.com/
[52] FDA admits mercury is contained in common flu vaccines given to children. *Courthouse News Service* Friday, March 23, 2012

hanging a poster on the wall of a pediatrician's office that could say something like this: "Attention parents: Beware, the flu shot your child may be receiving today contains brain-damaging mercury!"

"While the use of mercury-containing preservatives has declined in recent years with the development of new products formulated with alternative or no preservatives, thimerosal has been used in some immunoglobulin preparations, anti-venins, skin test antigens, and ophthalmic and nasal products, in addition to certain vaccines", writes the FDA on its *Thimerosal in Vaccines* web page (www.fda.gov).

Thimerosal is a mercury-based compound that is FDA-approved as a vaccine preservative, which makes it perfectly legal for doctors to inject this powerful neurotoxin into babies. Besides, doctors and pharmaceutical companies are no longer liable for causing vaccine injuries, including death.

One average flu vaccine contains 25 micrograms of mercury and the Environmental Protection Agency (EPA) stipulates a safety limit of 5 micrograms. Case in point, children who are vaccinated against the flu receive over 500 percent more mercury in one day than is considered safe by the very governmental agency responsible for keeping us safe from environmental toxins.

What is most remarkable about all this is that FDA seems to be far more concerned about mercury in skin products that come from overseas than the mercury injected into the body. These products are a threat to the profits of large US companies which obviously want the FDA to take action. Accordingly, the FDA recently announced that mercury poisoning has been linked to skin products[53]. The products in question are primarily skin lighteners and anti-aging creams.

"Exposure to mercury can have serious health consequences," says Charles Lee, M.D., a senior medical advisor at FDA. "It can damage the kidneys and the nervous system, and interfere with the development of the brain in unborn children and very young children."

The following statement by FDA toxicologist Mike Bolger, Ph.D. is even more disturbing: "You don't have to use the product yourself to be affected."

"People - particularly children - can get mercury in their bodies from breathing in mercury vapors if a member of the household uses a skin cream containing mercury. Infants and small children can ingest mercury

---

[53]Mercury Poisoning Linked to Skin Products, FDA Consumer Update, March 6, 2012

if they touch their parents who have used these products, get cream on their hands and then put their hands and fingers into their mouth, which they are prone to do," adds Bolger.

These are truly remarkable admissions coming from a health agency that has repeatedly refused to acknowledge the dangers inherent with dental amalgams, and that claims mercury in tooth fillings is perfectly safe for the human body. Experimental research has clearly demonstrated that mercury vapor escaping from dental amalgams[54] can easily enter the lungs and the brain. Shouldn't the FDA tell parents to stop kissing their babies or being too close to them? Exhaling mercury vapor from their teeth may just as likely enter their children's mouth and settle on their skin, and thus endanger their health, no?

If mercury vapor from skin creams is so dangerous for children, any kind of mercury vapor from any other source must be equally harmful. And if mercury vapor is, in fact, as dangerous as the FDA claims it to be, injecting even miniscule amounts of this deadly toxin into the blood of a young child must obviously be even far more dangerous to its brain, nervous system, and kidneys than the tiny amounts that it may inhale when a mother with some hand cream on her hands touches her child. It doesn't require rocket science to figure this out.

The FDA also avoids informing the public that the aluminum phosphate added to these vaccines greatly increases the toxicity of mercury, thereby turning the minimum mercury tolerance level into a complete joke - a joke that can cause severe brain damage to an unsuspecting child, and untold suffering and financial hardship to the parents. After millions of parents found that their children became autistic after receiving vaccine shots, there was a massive increase in class action lawsuits against the vaccine-producing pharmaceutical companies Wyeth, GlaxoSmithKline Plc, Merck & Co. and Sanofi-Aventis S.A. As a result, the vaccine makers threatened the Obama administration that they would stop producing vaccines altogether unless they received complete immunity from prosecution for vaccine injuries.

In 2010, the US Supreme Court has guaranteed vaccine manufacturers a free pass in the civil court system if the vaccine they make and sell in the US ends up crippling or killing a child or adult. Pediatricians and other medical workers giving vaccines don't need to be concerned either; they are also protected from civil liability if vaccines hurt someone they

---

[54]Smoking Teeth = Poison Gas - YouTube

vaccinate. In other words, the US Supreme Court's ruling granted these drug giants the perfect immunity from the consequences of wrongdoing; they have free rein in packing any kind of toxic compounds into their vaccine products, and nobody can stop them.

By adding toxic, carcinogenic ingredients to their vaccines, they generate an ever-increasing number of new patients that require medical treatments which mostly consist of medical drugs that they also produce.

The cover-ups by the CDC and FDA have let off the hook those responsible for the huge autism epidemic, which began when mercury and adjuvants were first added to vaccines. Without this elaborate conspiracy against the people, lawsuits resulting from permanent vaccine injuries in children would bankrupt numerous governments, including the US and the UK, and almost the entire pharmaceutical industry. The cost for life-long care and treatment of an autistic person is incredibly high and often astronomical for any family, but it would simply be unaffordable for any government and pharmaceutical company.

Donald Trump Speaks Out

Thankfully, some very influential spokespeople and celebrities are now coming to the aid of the ostracized vaccine safety awareness movement, including business mogul Donald Trump. During an interview with Fox News on April 2, 2012, the anniversary of the fifth annual World Autism Awareness Day, Trump unexpectedly raised serious concern about vaccinations. He told viewers: "I *strongly* believe that Autism Spectrum Disorders are linked to exposure to vaccines[55]."

Trump has been actively engaged in helping children with autism for many years. During the interview, the tycoon explained that a series of casual observations had led him to the conclusion that *monster* vaccinations cause autism.

Trump's remarks must have been a bombshell for the most aggressive vaccine-pushers, including doctors, pharmaceutical companies, government health agencies, and of course, the most powerful vaccine advocate, Bill Gates. They all deny the existence of a vaccine-autism link by referring to the fraudulently altered research data the CDC had released in 2008. They have applied monumental efforts in trying to suppress and delegitimize the work that has been done on vaccine-caused autism by

---

[55] Trump warns Fox News viewers: Autism caused by vaccines, April 2, 2012, see interview at www.rawstory.com

researchers at several universities and, most notably, by Dr. Andrew Wakefield. Fortunately, through a ruling by Britain's High Court, Dr. Wakefield's key research colleague, Professor John Walker-Smith, has recently been vindicated of having falsified research proving the vaccine-autism link[56]. In other words, the work by these two scientists is now considered genuine and valid.

While Trump acknowledged that speaking out against vaccines and the vaccine schedule is controversial, he said, "...I couldn't care less. I've seen people where they have a perfectly healthy child, and they go for the vaccinations and a month later the child is no longer healthy."

"I've gotten to be pretty familiar with the subject," Trump went on to say. "You know, I have a theory - and it's a theory that some people believe in - and that's the vaccinations. We never had anything like this. This is now an epidemic. It's way, way up over the past 10 years. It's way up over the past two years. And, you know, when you take a little baby that weighs like 12 pounds into a doctor's office and they pump them with many, many simultaneous vaccinations - I'm all for vaccinations, but I think when you add all of these vaccinations together and then two months later the baby is so different, then lots of different things have happened. I really...I've known cases."

Usually, the media which are sponsored, in large part, through advertisements paid for by pharmaceutical companies, have a financial interest in keeping their sponsors happy. I personally would like to thank Donald Trump for bringing this important issue, which concerns so many millions of individuals and their families, back into the minds of the people. He has clearly shown that he is not afraid of surprising one of the world's leading news channels by issuing such as stern warning.

All vaccines significantly alter the immune system and, therefore, play a major role in triggering autoimmune diseases and numerous other health conditions. In a 2005 epidemiological study covering over 151 previously conducted studies, researchers from the Department of Healthcare and Epidemiology, University of British Columbia, found an inverse association between acute infections and cancer development[57]. The study found that suppressing childhood infections with vaccines significantly increases one's risk of developing cancer later in life.

56Doctor from MMR controversy wins High Court appeal - next up, Dr. Andrew Wakefield himself, www.naturalnews.com
[57]Cancer Detect Prev 2006; 30(1):83-93. Epub 2006 Feb 21.

Chronic diseases were extremely rare over 100 years ago when few vaccines were given to the population. The more vaccines are administered, the more compromised the immune system becomes[58]. Most diseases back then used to be acute infections resulting from poor hygiene and nutrition, contaminated drinking water, and overcrowded cities.

Even the CDC admits on their website that clean water is more effective in preventing infectious diseases than vaccines. The only problem with using clean water as the preferred medicine is that, unlike with mass vaccination, one cannot make the same billions of dollars of profit year after year by installing some simple water purification devices in affected communities, or by educating people that drinking clean, non-fluoridated water is what keeps the body healthy and the immune system strong (for additional information on the subject of vaccination, see Chapter 3). To remove thimerosal and other toxic vaccine ingredients from the body, I strongly recommend taking organic sulfur crystals (see Chapter 5 for details). A colleague of mine has seen the complete reversal of autism in 16 people, simply through the long-term use of organic sulfur crystals.

Smart Gut Reactions

Science is beginning to recognize that damaging the intestinal lining through harsh, erosive chemicals, dehydration and poor nutrition is causing far more diseases than previously thought. Recently, researchers at UT Southwestern Medical Center in Dallas, Texas, discovered that a once mysterious cell population lurking in the intestinal lining is essential for preventing normally beneficial bacteria from invading into deeper tissue where they can cause debilitating conditions like inflammatory bowel disease (IBD)[59].

According to the research findings, people suffering from the disease frequently have more bacteria that adhere to, or invade, their gut lining. When their immune system mounts an attack on these microbial invaders, they can develop painful ulcers and bloody diarrhea.

The researchers also found that a specialized T cell normally present on body surfaces such as the skin and the gastrointestinal tract patrols intestinal borders, sensing when microorganisms have invaded the epithelial cells lining the intestine. "When this happens, these T cells

---

[58]For details see my book Vaccine-nation: Poisoning the Population, One Shot at a Time
[59] UT South western scientists unmask mysterious cells as key 'border patrol agents' in the intestine, May 9, 2011 in Health & Medicine

swing into action, making antibiotic proteins that kill the rogue bacteria and prevent their entry into deeper tissue," said Dr. Hooper, who is also an investigator for the Howard Hughes Medical Institute at UT Southwestern. This action lasts for several hours until other immune cells can be recruited as backup. However, there are consequences when the intestinal tract becomes a constant battleground.

A battleground is recognized by its devastated environment. Overexposure to toxins, food additives, trans fatty acids (as found in fast foods, such as hamburgers and French fries), medical drugs, alcohol, undigested putrefied foods, denatured proteins, and more, can easily cause what is known as *leaky gut*, a condition where bacteria and toxins enter the intestinal tissues, blood, and lymph. An initially limited and localized immune reaction may then escalate and spread to other areas in the body. T cells are only supposed to deal with foreign invaders, but they will need to be activated against the body's own tissues when toxins (antigens) begin to accumulate there.

The encounter with the antigens raises the level of antigen/antibody complexes in the blood and upsets the fine balance that exists between the immune reaction and its suppression. Autoimmune diseases, which indicate an extremely high level of toxicity in the body, directly result from a disturbance of this balance. If antibody production is continually high in synovial joints, inflammation becomes chronic, leading to gradually increasing deformity, pain, and loss of function.

The overuse of the immune system leads to self-destruction in the body. If this form of self-destruction occurs, for example, in the fatty myelin sheath of nerve tissue, it is called Multiple Sclerosis. However, we know that fat tissue is capable of absorbing a large amount of toxins and harmful heavy metals, thereby keeping them from doing direct harm.

Naturally, toxins migrate toward fatty tissue. A fatty liver is a merely a survival attempt by the body to deal with the load of toxins the liver can no longer break down and remove because of chronic congestion of its bile ducts. Yet, seen from a deeper perspective, what appears to be the body's act of self-destruction is but a final attempt at self-preservation. The body only *attacks* itself if the toxicity has increased to such a degree that it could cause more damage than an autoimmune response would.

The body certainly has no intention of committing suicide, although the term autoimmune disease implies just that. When the body's cell membranes are clogged with foreign, harmful chemicals, foreign protein fragments and toxic particles like trans fatty acids, it is an absolutely normal response by the immune system to attack these contaminants. The resulting inflammation provides it with the opportunity to wash out and remove at least some of the toxins. To call this survival response a *disease* makes no sense, is unscientific, and reflects a lack of knowledge of the true nature of the body.

Gallstones inhibit the body's ability to keep it well nourished and clean, which makes them a leading cause of toxicity. They prevent the liver from adequately taking noxious substances out of the bloodstream. If the liver cannot filter out toxins from the blood, they end up being dumped into the extracellular fluid. The more toxins accumulate in the extracellular fluid, the more severely the cell membranes become clogged with injurious materials. An autoimmune response may be necessary to destroy the most contaminated cells and thereby save the rest of the body, at least for a while. When all gallstones are removed from the liver and gallbladder, the immune system does not have to take recourse to such extreme measures of defending the body on the cellular level.

A healthy, balanced diet can, of course, greatly support the body in maintaining a balanced immune system. For example, research conducted at the University of Cambridge and published in the journal *Cell* in October 2011 revealed that compounds found in cruciferous vegetables, such as broccoli, kale, bok choy, and many varieties of leafy greens act as chemical signals necessary for a fully functioning immune system[60].

Osteoarthritis is a degenerative, non-inflammatory illness. It occurs when the renewal of articular cartilage (a smooth, strong surface, covering bones that are in contact with other bones) does not keep pace with its removal. The articular cartilage gradually becomes thinner until, eventually, the bony articular surfaces come into contact, and the bones begin to degenerate. Abnormal bone repair and chronic inflammation may follow this form of damage.

Like most diseases, this symptom results from a long-standing digestive disorder. As fewer nutrients are absorbed and distributed for tissue building, it becomes increasingly difficult to maintain healthy sustenance of bone and articular cartilage. Gallstones in the liver impair

---

[60]Ying Li, Silvia Innocentin, David R. Withers, Natalie A. Roberts, Alec R. Gallagher, Elena F. Grigorieva, Christoph Wilhelm, Marc Veldhoen. **Exogenous Stimuli Maintain Intraepithelial Lymphocytes via Aryl Hydrocarbon Receptor Activation**. *Cell*, 13 October 2011 DOI: 10.1016/j.cell.2011.09.025 - For dietary recommendations, see my book *Timeless Secrets of Health and Rejuvenation*

the basic digestive processes and, therefore, play perhaps the most important role in the development of osteoarthritis.

Gout, which is another joint disease connected to poor liver performance, is caused by sodium urate crystals in joints and tendons. Gout occurs in some people whose blood uric acid is abnormally high. When gallstones in the liver begin to affect blood circulation in the kidneys (see Chapter 1, *Disorders of the Urinary System*), uric acid excretion becomes inefficient. This also causes increased cell damage and cell destruction in the liver and kidneys, as well as in other parts of the body.

Uric acid is a natural waste product resulting from the breakdown of purines in cell nuclei; it is produced in excess with increased cell destruction. Purines are part of all human tissue and found in many foods. Excess amounts can be caused by either an over-production of uric acid by the body or the under-elimination of uric acid by the kidneys. Smoking cigarettes, overconsumption of alcohol, using stimulants, and so forth, can all cause marked cell destruction, which releases large quantities of purines and degenerate cell proteins into the bloodstream. When alcohol is present in the blood or remains there too long because the liver cannot break it down efficiently enough, or a person drinks too much of it, not all uric acid becomes dissolved, and the excess crystallizes and settles in joints.

In addition, uric acid production rises sharply with higher levels of meat, seafood and egg yolk consumption[61]. While higher levels of meat and seafood consumption are associated with an increased risk of gout, moderate intake of purine-rich vegetables is not associated with an increased risk of gout. Fructose, a sugar found in commercial sugar products and fruits, and added to thousands of processed foods and beverages in the form of high fructose corn syrup (HFCS), is also a major cause of uric acid buildup in the body. (**Note**: While fruits eaten in moderation don't seem to pose a problem for the body, fruit juices contain concentrated amounts of fructose which can easily elevate uric acid levels in the blood to abnormal levels)

Incidentally, all the aforementioned foods and substances can lead to gallstone formation in the liver and gallbladder.

"It is proposed that fructose- and purine-rich foods that have in common the raising of uric acid may have a role in the epidemic of

---

[61] To dissolve uric acid crystals and improve gout, see *The Kidney Cleanse* in Chapter 5

metabolic syndrome and renal disease that is occurring throughout the world," according to the abstract of a study conducted by the University of Florida, titled "Uric Acid, the Metabolic Syndrome, and Renal Disease[62]."

Besides increasing the risk for diabetes, high blood pressure, cardiovascular health, gout, kidney disease and obesity, high levels of uric acid can worsen almost every other kind of disease condition.

Disorders of the Reproductive System

Female and male reproductive systems both depend largely on the smooth functioning of the liver.

Gallstones in the liver obstruct the passage of bile through the bile ducts, which impairs digestion and distorts the structural framework of liver lobules. This diminishes the liver's production of both serum albumin and clotting factors. Serum albumin is the most common and abundant protein in the blood, responsible for maintaining plasma osmotic pressure at its normal level of 25mmHg. Clotting factors are essential for the coagulation of blood. Insufficient osmotic pressure cuts down the supply of nutrients to the cells, including those of the reproductive organs.

Poor cell nourishment affects cell metabolism and interferes with efficient lymph drainage. Inadequate lymph drainage from the reproductive organs can cause fluid retention and edema filled with metabolic waste and cell debris. All of this may result in the gradual impairment of sexual functions.

Most diseases of the reproductive system result from improper lymph drainage. The thoracic duct (see Chapter 1, *Disorders of the Circulatory System*) drains lymph fluid from all organs of the digestive system, including the liver, spleen, pancreas, stomach, and intestines. This large duct often becomes severely congested when gallstones in the liver impair proper digestion and absorption of food. It is obvious, yet hardly recognized in mainstream medicine, that congestion in the thoracic duct affects the organs of the reproductive system. These organs, like most others in the body, need to release their millions of turned-over cells and metabolic waste matter into the thoracic duct.

Impaired lymphatic drainage from the female pelvic area is responsible for suppressed immunity, unbalanced hormone levels, menstrual problems,

---

[62] J Am Soc Nephrol 17: 165-168, 2006

premenstrual stress (PMS), menopausal symptoms, pelvic inflammatory disease (PID), cervicitis, all uterine diseases, vulvar dystrophies with growth of fibrous tissue, ovarian cysts and tumors, cell destruction, low libido, infertility, and genetic mutations of cells leading to cancer growth.

Thoracic blockage may also lead to lymph congestion in the left breast, thereby leaving toxins and waste products behind that can cause inflammation, swelling, lump formation, milk duct blockage, and cancerous tumors. If the right lymphatic duct, which drains lymph from the right half of the thorax, head, neck, and right arm, becomes congested, waste accumulates in the right breast, leading to similar problems there.

A continuous restriction of lymph drainage from the male pelvic area sets off benign and malignant prostate enlargement as well as inflammation of the testes, penis, and urethra. Impotence is a likely consequence of this development.

The consistent increase of gallstones in the liver, a common factor among middle-aged men in affluent societies, is one of the major reasons for lymph blockage in this important part of the body.

Venereal diseases occur when the affected parts of the body reach a high level of toxicity and lose their ability to ward off microbes. Microbial infection is typically preceded by major lymph congestion. The collapsing capacity of the lymphatic system (which includes the circulating immune system) to repel invading microorganisms is the true reason for most reproductive and sexual disorders.

When all gallstones from the liver are removed and a healthy diet and lifestyle are maintained, lymphatic activity can return to normal. The reproductive tissue receives improved nourishment and becomes more resistant. Infections subside; cysts, fibrous tissue, and tumors are broken down and removed; and sexual functions are restored. Numerous women, unable to conceive a baby for many years, have reported that cleaning out their liver helped them become pregnant.

Disorders of the Skin

Nearly all skin diseases such as eczema, acne, and psoriasis have one factor in common: gallstones in the liver. Almost every person with a skin disease also has intestinal problems and impure blood, in particular. An over-reactive immune system and allergies may also play a role. These are mainly caused by gallstones and the harmful effects they have on the body as a whole, and also by an unbalanced diet and lifestyle.

Gallstones can trigger numerous protective events throughout the body - particularly in the digestive, circulatory, and urinary systems. What we call skin disease - an annoyance at best - is actually the body trying to save itself. In its attempt to eliminate what the colon, kidneys, lungs, liver, and lymphatic system are unable to remove or detoxify, the lower layers of the skin become flooded and overburdened with acidic waste. Although the skin is the largest organ of elimination in the body, it eventually succumbs to the acid assault generated from inside the body.

The toxic material is deposited first in the connective tissue underneath the dermis. When this *waste depot* is filled up, the skin begins to malfunction and erupt in some way or another.

The skin cells and the immune system located in the skin may react differently to each type of toxin or antigen it is exposed to. Since in today's world there are tens of thousands of different chemical toxins entering the body through vaccination shots, inhaling polluted air, eating processed foods, drinking fluoridated and chlorinated water, using chemical makeup and body care products, etc., there can be literally thousands of different types of abnormal skin conditions. The immune system needs to react differently to each encountered toxin or antigen, which means one person's skin problem can never be identical to anyone else's, just like one person's cancer or diabetes can never be the same as someone else's cancer or diabetes. In other words, eczema, acne, or dermatitis is unique to the person who suffers from it. Usually, though, almost all diseases of the skin include irritation, swelling, inflammation and some form of discoloration.

Excessive amounts of noxious, acidic substances, cell debris, microbes from different sources (such as gallstones), and various antigens from improperly digested foods congest the lymphatic system and inhibit proper lymph drainage from the various living layers of the skin. The toxins and putrefying protein from damaged or destroyed skin cells attract microbes and become a source of constant irritation and inflammation of the skin. Skin cells begin to suffer malnourishment, which may greatly reduce their normal turnover, which occurs about once every 4-6 weeks. This may also cause extensive damage to skin nerves (see **Figure 14** of a young woman in Germany who suffered from neurodermatitis and completely healed after just 6 liver and gallbladder flushes).

Chronic dermatitis is a skin disorder which is extremely difficult to cure, and for which allopathic medicine can only offer temporary relief. This young woman mentioned to me that her first few flushes released so many stones and toxins that the skin condition temporality *worsened* before clearing up completely. This is to be expected and part of the healing process of almost every chronic health condition.

When I requested her permission to publish this picture, she asked me to include the following explanation: "The time between taking these 2 photos was 5 months... I took the first picture myself and the second one was taken by a professional photographer with a better light. I used only mascara, eye shadow and lip gloss. No other makeup was used in either of the two pictures. You can see that the rash healed without leaving any scars, although I am not yet completely through with the flushes..."

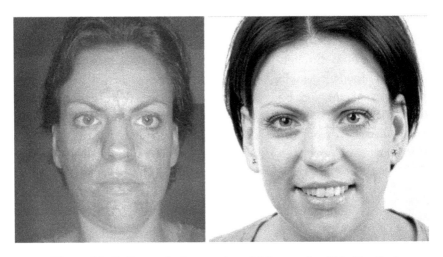

Figure 14: Before and after a series of 6 liver and gallbladder flushes

If the sebaceous glands, which pour their secretion, sebum, into the hair follicles, become nutrient deficient, hair growth becomes abnormal and, in particular, scalp hair may fall out. When the body's *melanin* supply becomes deficient, the hair turns gray prematurely. Sebum deficiency alters the healthy texture of the hair and makes it look dull and unattractive. On the skin, sebum naturally acts as a bactericidal and fungicidal agent, preventing the invasion of microbes. It also prevents drying and cracking of the skin, especially when exposed to sunshine and hot, dry air.

A genetic predisposition toward developing baldness or any other skin disorder may play a role but is *not* a major causative factor in hair loss, as is often assumed. Healthy skin functions are often completely restored and hair growth, particularly among women, is returned to normal, once all gallstones are removed and the colon and kidneys/bladder are kept clean.

Hypothyroidism, which often causes excessive hair loss (alopecia), also responds well to cleaning out these important organs of elimination[63].

Risks of Treating Diseases

Gallstones are a major cause of illness in the body. They impair the functioning of one of the more complex, active, and influential organs of the body - the liver. Nobody has ever devised an artificial liver, because it is so complex. Second only to the brain in complexity, the liver masterminds the most intricate processes of digestion and metabolism, thereby affecting the life and health of every cell in the body. The disorders described in this chapter only reflect a fraction of imbalances directly or indirectly related to gallstones.

There are at least 6,000 rare diseases and over 12,000 disease categories listed on the WHO website. Scientists have identified over 44,000 disease symptoms. In truth, there are just a few diseases, all of which share one or both of two causes: *deficiency* and *toxicity*.

We simply cannot consider a disease to be a disease of the individual part. For example, the symptom of high blood sugar is not the cause of diabetes but rather its effect. Likewise, osteoporosis is not a disease of low calcium and heart disease is not a disease of high cholesterol. A disease cannot be caused by its symptomatic expressions but by a corruption of the most basic processes in the body.

Often fatal consequences arise when we treat the symptoms of disease instead of its causes. Consider this example of a recent research study published in the *British Medical Journal*[64]. The study's researchers found that men and women over 40 who take calcium supplements increase their risk of heart attack by a whopping 30 percent, compared to people who don't take the supplements.

---

[63]For details on colonic irrigation and kidney cleansing, refer to my book *Timeless Secrets of Health and Rejuvenation*

[64]Effect of calcium supplements on risk of myocardial infarction and cardiovascular events: meta-analysis: *BMJ 2010;341doi: 10.1136/bmj.c3691(Published 29 July 2010)*

To this day, ill-informed doctors still tell their patients to take calcium supplements to ward off osteoporosis. Blindly trusting in their doctor's advice, these patients may indivertibly cause their own heart attack and still not prevent bone fractures. Calcium supplements cause vascular calcifications, kidney stones, gallstones, cancers of the breast, and numerous other disorders while only having marginal benefits for osteoporosis.

Indeed, there is a solid body of research indicating that higher bone density, which can be artificially achieved by taking calcium supplements, may actually increase the risk of malignant breast cancer by 300 percent or more[65]! Letting your doctor treat the symptoms of disease, or rather what she considers to be a disease, is more often a trap than it is a remedy. As I point out in my book, *Timeless Secrets of Health and Rejuvenation*, the Vata body type has a naturally and significantly lower bone density than the Kapha body type. Given the misdiagnosed *low bone density* in a Vata person, a calcium supplement is akin to committing murder.

The neurotic fixation ingrained on the psyche of medical practitioners on increasing bone density with calcium supplements is not only misplaced but responsible for increasing the overall risk of developing cancer and cardiovascular disease[66]. According to 11 clinical studies, calcium from elemental sources, which include limestone, oyster shell, and bone meal, poses the greatest risk of heart attack.

Obviously, symptom-oriented medicine is not interested in discovering or treating the principal causes of disease symptoms. To the contrary, scientists working for or benefiting from pharmaceutical companies are specialized in dreaming up names of new diseases and lists of symptoms every day of the year.

Pharmaceutical industries also have no intention of finding cures for diseases. They are in the business of creating an ever-increasing number of new diseases to generate an ever-increasing number of vaccines and other drugs to treat the ever-increasing number of side effects that their toxic products produce.

The single most common cause of death and injury today is prescription drugs. In the US, nearly 784,000 people die each year as a result of medical treatments, according to the statistical research by Dr. Gary

---

[65]High bone density increases the risk of malignant breast cancer by 300 percent:http://www.greenmedinfo.com/anti-therapeutic-action/high-bone-density
[66]Effect of calcium supplements on risk of myocardial infarction and cardiovascular events: meta-analysis.BMJ 2010; 341 doi: 10.1136/bmj.c3691

Null et al[67]. Who reaps the greatest benefits from sickness? Those large corporations which produce drugs and medical procedures that can effectively suppress symptoms of disease, thereby giving the impression they benefit those who receive them. Being public, for-profit companies, these pharmaceutical giants are only accountable to their stockholders, even if they are well aware that their products actually kill people.

For example, although the breast cancer drug Avastin has never been proven to be more effective for breast cancer than a placebo, it has been kept on the market for many years to treat breast cancer at a cost of nearly $90,000 per year of treatment, in spite of all the serious side effects it produces (such as severe high blood pressure, hemorrhaging, and death). Although the US Federal Drug Administration (FDA) has known about the drug's uselessness for many years and only recently banned it for use in breast cancer, it continues to be sold for other cancers.

Even if Avastin were to have any benefits (which has not been shown to be the case), and you were taking this drug for whatever type of cancer, there is still no guarantee that you will get the actual drug or its fake version. A 2012 article published in the *Inquisitr*, titled "Avastin Maker Warns That Counterfeit Versions of the Drug Are Circulating[68]," reveals the sinister scandals involving this and similar cancer drugs. The author of the article, Kim LaCapria, states: "Now Avastin's maker Genentech is warning that counterfeit Avastin has been found in hospitals and healthcare centers in the US - and the origin of the fake medication is not known. What they do know about the high profit drug copies (Avastin generates a whopping $6 billion in revenue for Genentech each year) is that it does not contain the active ingredient in Avastin."

Of course, without its active ingredient, a drug is ineffective and useless (unless you count the possible placebo effect it may produce). However, the main scandal is not about the fact that doctors give a $90,000 snake oil to their patients, but that they continue giving it to their patients even when they must have noticed that the drug is completely useless. Is it for the vast sums of money that they are prescribing the drug, or is it because of their blind trust in chemical medicine?

I have written extensively about the trap of using anti-cancer drugs in my book, *Cancer is Not A Disease - It's a Healing Mechanism*, but I

[67]Death By Medicine, Dr. Gary Null et al: http://www.webdc.com/pdfs/deathbymedicine.pdf
[68]Avastin Maker Warns That Counterfeit Versions of the Drug Are Circulating, *Inquisitr*, Kim LaCapria, Posted: February 15, 2012

would like to mention here the widely used cancer drug tamoxifen. Tamoxifen is a clear example of the deceptive and seriously flawed arguments in favor of cancer drug therapy.

Millions of high-risk women are being prescribed tamoxifen to prevent breast cancer or breast cancer recurrence, and it is usually taken for 5 years. However, research conducted in Israel found that tamoxifen can cause cancer instead. According to a 2008 study published in the March/April 2008 issue of the *International Journal of Gynecological Cancer*[69], the treatment of breast cancer with tamoxifen results in an increased risk of uterine cancer incidence and mortality among women taking this drug compared with women who are not using it.

In addition, according to researchers at the Tenovus Centre for Cancer Research at Cardiff University, while drugs such as tamoxifen may have had some success in treating breast cancer, for a significant proportion of sufferers the drugs either fail to work, or after an initial successful response, the patient relapses as the cancer acquires or possesses resistance to the drug.

In my opinion, merely substituting one cancer for another is not a treatment option that should be offered to cancer patients at all. What is worse, most *high-risk* women will never even develop cancer, but by taking tamoxifen, this chance is greatly increased.

Or check out the Avandia fraud. This is a quote taken from the FDA Press Release issued on September 23, 2011: "The US Food and Drug Administration announced that it will significantly restrict the use of the diabetes drug Avandia (rosiglitazone) to patients with type 2 diabetes who cannot control their diabetes on other medications. These new restrictions are in response to data that suggest an elevated risk of cardiovascular events, such as heart attack and stroke, in patients treated with Avandia." Since it was introduced in 1999, this best-selling blockbuster diabetes drug has killed nearly 200,000 people from heart attacks - the very disease that kills most diabetics.

The FDA, of course, has known about these risks for many years, but has chosen to ignore them and let people get sick or die without knowing why. The question is how many people in the past 15 years have died from heart attack-linked diabetes or Avandia?

---

[69]The Risk of Developing Uterine Sarcoma After Tamoxifen Use, International Journal of Gynecological Cancer, 352–356 doi:10.1111/j.1525-1438.2007.01025.x

It is becoming increasingly clear that while prescription drugs are successful in suppressing a few symptoms of disease (which almost always represent the body's attempts to heal) they do this at the expense of possibly incurring kidney failure or liver failure, or suffering a fatal heart attack or stroke.

Symptom-oriented medicine has become so popular among doctors and patients alike that even the thought of addressing the underlying causes of disease is considered weird or a waste of time and energy. Going the route of getting a quick fix seems much more attractive to most. Over 90 percent of patients never even ask their doctor about potential side effects of the treatments they receive. All they care about is to get "that damn disease" under control.

Although controlling the symptoms of a disease actually prevents its cure, patients who are left in the dark about why they have fallen ill insist on making this concession of sabotaging their health in the future in exchange for gaining some temporary relief. There are many money-hungry predators out there who take advantage of the masses and their fear-induced reluctance to pursue cause-oriented medicine in order to heal their own ailments.

Oftentimes, the discovery of just one symptom of a newly invented disease becomes an excuse for a pharmaceutical company to patent a new chemical drug to be marketed as a panacea for that targeted *disease*. For example, the repeated lowering of the number of what constitutes the new *normal* cholesterol level over the past several decades each time turned millions more healthy people with a truly normal cholesterol level into patients at risk of suffering a heart attack or stroke. From one day to the next, all of these people suddenly suffered from *high cholesterol disease*, even though high cholesterol has never shown to cause heart disease. That is why statin producers cannot claim that their product can actually reduce the risk of heart disease.

The bottom line is that more than 3 out of 4 adult Americans now have a diagnosable *chronic disease* for which the medical establishment wants them to receive treatment. Every week thousands of fairly healthy people become patients as new diseases are being invented by *scientific* research sponsored by pharmaceutical companies.

In actuality, toxicity and deficiency, which are the main causes of chronic illness, are not diseases at all. They merely require cleansing of the body and taking care of our basic needs for healthy nutrition and a balanced lifestyle.

It was in 1994 that I first began making the liver and gallbladder flush available to many people around the world. I discovered that when you remove the obstacles that prevent the liver from doing its hundreds of jobs efficiently, your body can return to a state of continuous balance and vitality.

Proper healthcare neither needs to be a struggle, nor does it need to be expensive. Hippocrates, the father of modern medicine, wisely stated: "Let your food be medicine and your medicine be food." This simple liver cleansing procedure uses some very inexpensive foods to accomplish what even the most expensive medication cannot achieve, that is, to help the body heal itself.

Chapter 2

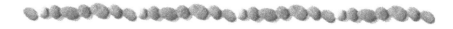

How Can I Tell I Have Gallstones?

During my research with thousands of patients suffering from almost every kind of illness, including terminal diseases, I found that each person had large numbers of gallstones in the liver and, in many cases, also in the gallbladder. When these individuals eliminated these stones through the liver and gallbladder flush and took simple health-supportive measures, they recovered from diseases that defied both conventional and alternative methods of treatment. Although this method has nothing in it to treat any particular disease, it nevertheless creates the precondition for the body to heal itself, regardless of the affliction.

What follows is a description of some of the more common markers indicating the presence of gallstones in the liver and gallbladder. If you have any of them, you will most likely derive great benefits from cleansing your liver and gallbladder.

In my practice, I have found these indications to be highly accurate. In case you are not sure whether you have stones, it may be useful to cleanse the liver anyway; it can improve your health significantly, regardless.

There is an old saying: "The proof of the pudding is in the eating." The only way to discover for yourself whether you have gallstones or not is to do the liver and gallbladder flush. You will find that when you remove all the stones that may be present, the symptoms of disease will gradually disappear, and health will return to normal.

However, I must mention at this point that the liver and gallbladder flush is not a panacea for all ills. There are other causes of ill health, such as poor nutrition, irregular sleeping habits, lack of regular sun exposure to obtain vitamin D, etc. Although most of these other causes lead to gallstone formation in the liver, they also need to be taken care of separately, otherwise liver flushing merely acts as a Band-Aid and will not significantly improve your health. (I have covered these topics in Chapters 3 and 5)

Signs and Marks

The Skin

The major function of the skin is to continuously adjust our internal body to the ever-changing external environment, which includes temperature, humidity, dryness, and light. In addition, skin covers the body to protect us against injury, microbes, and other harmful agents. Apart from having to deal with these external influences, the skin also monitors and adapts according to internal changes taking place within the body.

The skin reflects the condition of the organs and body fluids, including the blood and lymph. Any long-term abnormal functioning of the body will inevitably affect the health of the blood and lymph and show up in the skin as skin blemishes, discoloration, or changed condition, such as dryness, oiliness, wrinkles, lines, and so forth.

Almost all skin disorders have their root in an imbalanced liver condition. Gallstones lead to circulatory disorders, which reduce the nutrient supply to, and waste removal from, the skin and prevent healthy development and normal turnover cycles of skin cells. The following skin changes are particularly indicative of gallstones in the liver and gallbladder:

- **Black spots and small or large brown patches** that are the color of freckles or moles. They usually appear on the right or left side of the forehead, between the eyebrows or under the eyes. They may also show up just above the right shoulder or between the shoulder blades. Most prominent are the so-called *liver spots* or *age spots* on the back of the hands and forearms, often seen among middle-aged and elderly people.

  If gallstones, which are spontaneously excreted by the liver or gallbladder, get caught in the colon, such spots may also appear in the area where the thumb and index finger meet. These liver spots usually start fading after the majority of stones are removed from the liver, gallbladder, and intestines.

  Liver spots or dark blemishes tend to particularly appear in individuals whose skin is very thin (the Vata and Pitta body types[70])

---

[70]These are 2 of the 3 main Ayurvedic body types discussed in great detail in my book *Timeless Secrets of Health and Rejuvenation*. The Kapha type has the thickest skin among all and rarely shows any skin blemishes.

and whose liver bile ducts are congested. This may force bile to enter the blood and accumulate in certain areas of connective tissues under the skin. In time, ever-increasing amounts of bile make their way into the top layers of the skin.

The backwashed bile contains toxins which cause the skin pigment melanin to pool around them and help neutralize them, thereby protecting the skin cells from becoming damaged. The pooled mixture gives rise to the appearance of dark spots. Bile pigments also contribute to the discoloration of the skin. In extreme cases, the whole complexion and the eyes turn yellow (jaundice). If the skin turns grey and dark, it indicates the liver has very little capacity to remove toxins from the blood.

Most people assume that liver spots are due to sun damage and *normal* aging. This is a myth. Liver spots, as the name suggests, come from the liver. Sun exposure merely brings to the surface of the skin any existing toxic waste deposits combined with bile pigments and melanin. It is actually far healthier for the body to move these deposits from the underlying connective tissues to the surface layers of the skin, and sun exposure makes this possible.

- **Vertical wrinkles between the eyebrows:** There may be one deep line or two, sometimes three, lines in this region. These deep lines or wrinkles, which are *not* a part of natural aging, indicate an accumulation of many gallstones in the liver. They also show that the liver is enlarged and has hardened. The deeper and longer the wrinkles are, the more the deterioration of liver function has progressed. Fine lines showing up there after age 60 are more likely due to a loss of elasticity of the skin than any link to congestive liver problems.

A deep line near the right eyebrow also indicates congestion in the spleen and spleen enlargement. The spleen may have difficulties with effectively removing abnormal dead blood cells from the blood and also its own metabolic waste products.

Furthermore, the deep vertical lines represent a great deal of repressed frustration and anger. Anger arises when gallstones prevent proper bile flow. A bilious nature is one that keeps toxins trapped - toxins that the liver tries to eliminate via bile. Some of the toxic bile backwashes into the blood, thereby creating the emotional agitation that results in anger. Vice versa, anger can trigger gallstone formation. Anger is a powerful emotion that has long been known to disturb the bile flora (bacteria population in bile) and change the natural balance between bile components.

If white or yellow patches accompany the wrinkles, a cyst or tumor may be developing in the liver. Pimples or growth of hair between eyebrows, with or without wrinkles, indicate that the liver, gallbladder and spleen have lost some of their capacity to remove cellular debris and waste products.

- **Horizontal wrinkles/lines across the bridge of the nose:** These are a sign of pancreatic disorders due to gallstones in the liver. If a line is deep and pronounced, there may be pancreatitis or diabetes.

- **Green or dark color of the temple area at the sides of the head:** This shows that the liver, gallbladder, pancreas, and spleen are underactive because of deposits of gallstones in both the liver and gallbladder. This may be accompanied by a green or blue color on either side of the bridge of the nose, which specifically indicates impaired spleen functions.

- **Oily skin in the area of the forehead:** This reflects poor liver performance due to gallstones. The same applies to excessive perspiration in this part of the head. A yellow color of the facial skin indicates disorders of the bile functions of the liver and gallbladder, and a weakness of the pancreas, kidneys, and excretory organs.

- **Hair loss in the central region of the head:** This indicates that the liver, heart, small intestines, pancreas, and reproductive organs are becoming increasingly congested and overtaxed with toxic waste. There is a tendency to develop cardiovascular disease, chronic digestive problems, and the formation of cysts and tumors. Early graying of hair (before age 40) shows that liver and gallbladder functions are underactive.

The Nose

- **Hardening and thickening of tissue at the tip of the nose:** This indicates chronic liver weakness, resulting in hardening of the arteries and the accumulation of fat around the heart, liver, spleen, kidneys, and prostate glands. If the enlargement is excessive and blood vessels are visible, a heart attack or stroke may be imminent.

- The nose is constantly red: This condition shows an abnormal condition of the heart, with a tendency toward high blood pressure (hypertension). A purple nose indicates low blood pressure. Both conditions are largely due to imbalanced liver, digestive, and kidney functions. A high protein-diet is a major contributing factor.

- Cleft nose or indentation of the tip of the nose: This indicates irregular heartbeat and heart murmur. If one half of the cleft nose is larger than the other, this shows that one side of the heart is abnormally enlarged. Arrhythmia and panic attacks may accompany this condition. There may be severe lymphatic congestion caused by digestive disorders such as constipation, colitis, stomach ulcer, and so on. Liver functions are subdued because of large amounts of gallstones cutting off the blood supply to the liver cells. Bile secretions are insufficient. (Note: I have personally seen clefts in the nose disappear after liver flushing)

- The nose is bending toward the left: Unless caused by an accident, this asymmetric shape of the nose implies that the organs on the right side of the body are underactive. These include the liver, gallbladder, right kidney, ascending colon, right ovary or testicle, and right side of the brain. The main cause of this condition is an accumulation of gallstones in the liver and gallbladder. The nose is likely to return to center once the stones are removed.

The Eyes

- Skin color under the eyes is yellowish: This indicates that the liver and gallbladder are overactive. A dark, even black color in the same area results when the kidneys, bladder, and reproductive organs are overtaxed because of a prolonged disorder of the digestive system. A grayish, pale color occurs if the kidneys, and occasionally, the lungs are malfunctioning owing to improper lymph drainage from these organs. Also, the endocrine system may be affected.

- Water-containing bags under the lower eyelids: These are formed as a result of congestion in the digestive and excretory organs, which results in inadequate lymph drainage from the head area. If these eye bags are chronic and contain fat, this points toward the presence of inflammation, cysts and, possibly, tumors in the bladder, ovaries, fallopian tubes, uterus, or prostate.

- A white cloud covers the pupil of the eye: The cloud consists mostly of mucus and degenerate protein fragments. It indicates the development of cataracts brought about by longstanding poor liver and digestive performance.

▪ Constant redness in the white of the eye: This condition is caused by the protrusion of capillaries, indicating disorders in the circulatory and respiratory functions. White or yellow mucus patches in the white of the eye show that the body is accumulating abnormal amounts of fatty substances because the liver and gallbladder have amassed large quantities of gallstones. When this occurs, the body has a tendency to develop cysts, and both benign and malignant tumors.

▪ A thick white discoloration around the peripheral areas of the iris of the eye, particularly its lower parts: This white color, which covers up the true color of the iris, indicates the accumulation of large amounts of cholesterol in certain parts of the circulatory system. The lymphatic system also experiences major congestion and fat retention. (Note: If you wish to understand what structural and color-related changes in the iris relate to abnormal changes in different parts of the body, I recommend you study the science of eye interpretation, also known as iridology)

▪ The eyes have lost their natural luster and shininess: This signals that both the liver and kidneys are congested and unable to filter the blood properly. *Contaminated* blood, loaded with toxins and excessive waste products, is heavier and more sluggish than clean blood. The thickened blood slows circulation and reduces oxygen and nutrient supply to the cells and organs, including the eyes. If this condition persists, an increasing number of cells will deteriorate and age quickly or die off.

▪ The eye and brain cells are especially affected because the blood has to flow against gravity to reach them. Most vision problems are the direct or indirect result of reduced blood-cleansing capacity by the liver and kidneys. Clean and nutrient-rich blood from a healthy, efficient liver can flow easily and nourish the eye tissues better, thereby improving most eye problems.

Tongue, Mouth, Lips, and Teeth

- **The tongue is coated yellow or white, especially at the back**: This indicates an imbalance in the secretion of bile, which is the major cause of digestive disorders. Toxic residues of undigested and fermented or putrefied food linger in the intestinal tract. This blocks lymph flow in the thoracic duct and prevents toxins and microbes in the throat and mouth area from being broken down and removed. Especially, fermenting bacteria, such as Candida albicans, thrive and proliferate in the coated layers of excretions on the surface of the tongue. There may also be a burning sensation and increased sensitivity.

- **Teeth impressions on the sides of the tongue, often accompanied by white mucus discharge:** This indicates poor digestion and inadequate absorption of nutrients from the small intestine.

- **Pimples on the tongue:** They are indicative of a compromised intestinal flora and excessive presence of fermenting and putrefying food in both the small and large intestines.

- **Cracks on the tongue:** These are signs of long-term intestinal trouble. When food is not being mixed with a sufficient amount of bile, it remains partially undigested. Undigested foods are subjected to bacterial putrefaction and, thereby, become a source of toxicity. Constant exposure of the intestinal wall to the toxins that these bacteria produce irritates and injures it. The resulting lesions, scars, and hardening of the intestinal walls is then reflected by the cracks on the tongue. There may be little or no mucus discharge on the tongue.

- **Repeated mucus discharge into the throat and mouth:** Intestinal congestion may cause bile, toxins and bacteria to back up into the stomach, thereby irritating its protective lining and triggering the secretion of excessive amounts of mucus. Some of this sticky material may reach the mouth area. This can create a bad (bitter) taste in the mouth and give rise to frequent attempts at clearing the throat, which sometimes involve coughing. Mucus discharge without this bitter taste results when food is not digested properly, and toxins are generated. The mucus helps to trap and neutralize some of these toxins, but as a side effect, it may lead to congestion in the chest, throat, sinuses and ears; and possibly, infections.

▪ **Bad breath and frequent burping:** Both these conditions point toward the presence of undigested, fermenting, or putrefying food in the gastrointestinal (GI) tract. Bacteria acting on the waste material produce gases, which can be very toxic at times, hence the bad odor emanating from the breath. Chronic congestion in the upper respiratory tract and tooth decay may also play a role.

▪ **Crust formations at the corners of the mouth:** This indicates the presence of duodenal ulcers, caused by regurgitation of bile into the stomach, or by other reasons discussed earlier. Ulcers in various parts of the mouth or on the tongue show that inflammation or ulceration is occurring in the corresponding parts of the GI tract. For example, a mouth ulcer on the outside of your lower lip points to the presence of ulcerous lesions in the large intestine. Herpes (cold sores) on the lip corresponds to more severe inflammation and ulceration of the intestinal wall.

▪ **Dark spots or patches on the lips:** These marks occur when obstructions in the liver, gallbladder, and kidneys have resulted in slowness and stagnation of blood circulation and lymph drainage throughout the body. There may be advanced, abnormal constriction of blood capillaries. If the color of the lips is reddish (dark) or purple, this indicates that heart, lung, and respiratory functions are subdued.

▪ **Swollen or enlarged lips:** This condition indicates intestinal disorders. If the lower lip is swollen, the colon suffers constipation, diarrhea, or both, alternating between them. Toxic gases are formed from improperly digested foods, which give rise to bloating and abdominal discomfort. A swollen or enlarged upper lip indicates stomach problems, including indigestion, frequently accompanied by heartburn.

▪ A tightly closed mouth shows that a person suffers from disorders of the liver, gallbladder, and, possibly, the kidneys. If the lower lip is dry, peels, and splits easily, there may either be chronic constipation or diarrhea, with large amounts of toxic acids prevalent in the colon. This condition is accompanied by advanced dehydration of the colon cells.

▪ **Swollen, sensitive, or bleeding gums:** Any one of these symptoms occurs when lymph drainage from the mouth area is inefficient as a result of intestinal lymph congestion. The blood is dumping excessive acid waste compounds, which the liver is not able to remove, into the tissues, including the gums.

- **Inflammation deep in the throat**, with or without swelling of the tonsils, is also caused by lymphatic blockage. Tonsillitis, which often occurs among children, is a sign of constant retention of toxins contained in the lymph fluids and back-flushing of waste from the GI tract into the tonsils. Tonsils act as important blood filters to protect the brain and sensory organs. Commercial sugar and other junk foods greatly increase the risk of tonsillitis.

- **Tooth problems** are generally caused by nutritional imbalance. Poor digestion and overconsumption of refined, processed, and highly acid-forming foods, such as sugar, chocolate, meat, cheese, coffee, soda, and so forth, deplete the body of minerals and vitamins. Adults usually have 32 teeth. Each tooth corresponds to a vertebra of the spine, and each vertebra is connected to a major organ or gland. If any of the 4 canines are decaying, for example, it indicates the presence of gallstones in the liver and gallbladder. A yellow color of the teeth, and of the canines in particular, indicates the presence of toxins in the organs located in the mid-abdominal region i.e. the liver, gallbladder, stomach, pancreas, and spleen.

Bacteria are *not* the cause of tooth decay. They only attack tooth tissue that already has a highly unbalanced acid/alkaline ratio and contains a large amount of toxins. Proper saliva secretions also play a major role in the protection of the teeth.

Truly healthy teeth last a lifetime and are maintained by a healthy digestive system and a balanced vegetarian diet. For example, at age 58, I still have all my teeth intact, including all my wisdom teeth, with only one small filling for damage that was caused by crunching on a small, hard stone contained in a bean dish. I also don't develop any plaque and never need to have my teeth cleaned.

Hands, Nails, and Feet

- **White, fatty skin on the fingertips** is a sign of dysfunctional digestive and lymphatic systems. In addition, the liver and kidneys may be forming cysts and tumors. An excessive discharge of fats may occur, seen as oiliness on the skin, especially on the forehead.

- **Dark-red fingernails** point toward an excessively high content of cholesterol, fatty acids, and minerals in the blood. The liver, gallbladder, and spleen are congested and underactive, and all excretory functions are overburdened with waste products.

- **Whitish nails** indicate the accumulation of fat and mucus in and around the heart, liver, pancreas, prostate, or ovaries. This condition is accompanied by poor blood circulation and low hemoglobin levels (anemia).

- **Vertical ridges in the fingernails** generally indicate poor absorption of food and the disruption of important digestive, liver, and kidney functions. There may be general fatigue. Strong vertical ridges on the thumbnails, possibly with split ends, show that a person's testicles and prostate or ovaries are not functioning properly. This is caused by the ineffectiveness of the digestive and circulatory systems.

- **Horizontal indentations in the nails** show unusual or drastic changes in dietary habits. The changes can either mean there is a correction of an existing imbalance or a generation of a new imbalance.

- **White dots on the nails** appear when the body eliminates large amounts of calcium and/or zinc in response to excessive consumption of sugar or sugar-containing foods and beverages. Sugar has highly acid-forming properties and leaches out these minerals from the bones and teeth. Eating too many fruits or drinking fruit juices can have the same effect.

- **A hard protrusion at the ball of the foot:** This condition shows progressive hardening of the organs located in the middle of the body, including the liver, stomach, pancreas, and spleen. It points to the accumulation of numerous gallstones in the liver and gallbladder.

- **A yellow color of the feet** indicates the accumulation of many gallstones in the liver and gallbladder. If the color of any part of the feet is green, then spleen and lymph functions are severely disrupted. This may lead to cysts and benign or malignant tumors.

- **Hardness at the tip of the fourth toe or a callus in the area under the fourth toe** shows that gallbladder functions are stagnant. General rigidity, a bent condition, and pain in the fourth toe imply a long history of gallstones in the gallbladder and liver.

- **Curving of the first toe:** If the large toe curves inward toward the second toe, it shows that liver functions are subdued owing to the presence of gallstones in the liver bile ducts. At the same time, spleen and lymphatic functions are overactive because of the accumulation of toxic residues from inadequately digested foods, metabolic waste, and cellular debris.

▪ **White color and rugged surfaces on the fourth and fifth toenails** indicates poor performance of the liver and gallbladder, as well as of the kidneys and urinary bladder.

The Constitution of Fecal Matter

▪ **The stool or fecal matter emits a sharp, sour, or penetrative odor:** This indicates that food is not being digested properly, or the consumed foods are inappropriate for the body. Fermented and putrefied food and the presence of large quantities of *unfriendly* bacteria in the feces give rise to an unpleasant odor and sticky fecal texture.

▪ Normal stool is coated with a thin mucus lining, which prevents the anus from being soiled. Having to use toilet paper to clean it indicates an ineffective digestive system. Just like healthy animals in the wild, healthy humans have no need for toilet paper following defecation.

▪ **Dry and hard stools** are an indication of constipation, mostly due to inadequate secretion of bile by the liver and gallbladder, and so are sticky stools. Diarrhea is yet another sign of weak performance of the digestive system and of the liver, in particular.

▪ **Feces look pale white, gray or clay-colored:** This is still another indication of poor liver performance and insufficient bile secretion (bile pigments in bile give the stool its natural brown color).

▪ **Floating stool** contains large amounts of undigested fats, making it lighter than water. In the absence of bile, fats, oils and protein foods (which normally contain fats) become indigestible and are instead excreted in feces, a condition called steatorrhea.

▪ Steatorrhea, which is also recognized by frothy, foul-smelling stools, can lead to malabsorption of essential fatty acids and fat-soluble vitamins. Undigested fats in the large intestine turn rancid, thereby causing toxicity and incurring serious damage to the intestinal wall.

Conclusion

There may be many more signs and symptoms indicating the presence of gallstones in the liver and gallbladder than those listed above. Pain in the right shoulder, tennis elbow, frozen shoulder, numbness in the legs, and sciatica, for example, may have no obvious relation to gallstones in the liver. Yet when the gallstones are removed, these conditions usually disappear.

The body is an intricate network of information and communication, and every part influences and communicates with every other part. Seemingly insignificant marks on the skin, in the eyes, or on a toe may be the harbingers of serious health issues. When you recognize them and flush your liver and gallbladder, in concert with adopting a healthy regimen of diet and lifestyle, you will find that the signs of wellness and vitality begin to reappear. To prevent illness and make permanent good health a practical reality in your life, it is important to understand what actually causes gallstones in the first place.

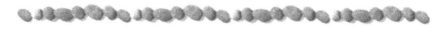

Chapter 3

The Most Common Causes of Gallstones (and Diseases)

B ile consists of water, mucus, bile pigments (such as bilirubin), bile salts, fats and cholesterol, as well as enzymes and beneficial bacteria. Liver cells secrete this dark-green to yellowish-brown fluid into tiny canals, known as bile canaliculi. The bile canaliculi join up to form larger canals that, in turn, connect with the right and left hepatic ducts. The two hepatic ducts combine and form the common bile duct, which drains bile from the liver and supplies the gallbladder with the right amount of bile required to make the digestive process smooth and efficient.

Besides aiding in the digestion of fats, the alkaline bile also has the function of neutralizing any excess stomach acid before it enters the final section of the small intestine (ileum).Bile salts also act as natural bactericides, destroying microbes contained in ingested food.

Any abnormal change in the composition of bile affects the solubility of its constituents and, thereby, causes gallstones. For the purpose of simplicity, I have categorized gallstones into two basic types: cholesterol stones and pigment stones. There are also mixed stones, meaning, they have various compositions of bile constituents.

Some cholesterol stones are composed of at least 80 percent cholesterol by weight and are oval, 2 to 3 cm in length, often having a tiny dark central spot. They vary in color from light-yellow to dark-green or brown, and are typically rock-hard. Most stones with a lesser content of cholesterol have a bright pea-green or beige-green color and are initially very soft, like putty. If they occur in the gallbladder, they may eventually become hard and calcified. If they occur in the liver bile ducts, they remain soft and waxy.

Some stones may contain organic, fatty material.

Pigment stones are brown, red, or black stones, owing to their high content of colored pigment (bilirubin). The percentage of calcium salts they contain determines their degree of hardness. They contain less than 20 percent of cholesterol.

Unlike the soft, non-calcified cholesterol stones, calcified cholesterol stones and pigment stones are radiographically (x-ray) or sonographically (ultrasound) visible. They tend to develop only in the gallbladder.

An abnormal alteration of the components of bile can occur in a number of ways. The dissolving action of bile salts and, of course, copious amounts of water, normally keep cholesterol in liquid form. An increased amount of cholesterol in the bile (normally at only 0.3 percent) overwhelms the dissolving capacity of the bile salts, thereby promoting the formation of cholesterol stones. Similarly, a decrease in the amount of bile salts being produced in the liver also leads to cholesterol stone formation. In addition, due to insufficient water intake, the fluidity of bile decreases, and much of the cholesterol is not dissolved properly; instead it reconstitutes into small cholesterol pebbles. In time, these small pebbles grow into larger ones.

Pigment stones form when the bile pigment, bilirubin, a waste product of the breakdown of red blood cells, increases in the bile. People with excessive amounts of soft cholesterol stones in the liver are at risk for developing liver cirrhosis, sickle-cell anemia, or other blood diseases. Any of these complications can produce high concentrations of bilirubin pigment in the bile. Abnormally elevated bilirubin levels lead to the formation of pigment stones (see **Figure 14**) in the liver and gallbladder.

When the composition of bile in the liver is no longer balanced, small cholesterol crystals begin to combine with other bile components to accrete into tiny lumps in the liver's bile ducts. These tiny bile clots can easily obstruct the even tinier bile canaliculi. This slows the bile flow further, causing more and more bile to attach itself to these existing clots. Eventually, the clots become large enough to be called stones.

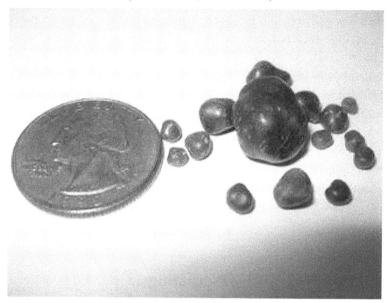

Figure 14: Red bilirubin stones

Some of these stones may pass into the larger bile ducts and cluster together with other stones. They may also grow to larger-sized stones themselves. The result is that bile flow becomes increasingly obstructed in the larger bile ducts as well. Once several of the larger bile ducts are clogged, hundreds of smaller ducts are similarly affected, which closes the vicious cycle.

Eventually, the hepatic ducts are so severely clogged with intrahepatic stones (those that occur inside the liver) that the amount of bile available for the digestive process is drastically reduced. Since the liver continues to produce bile, more and more of it is being converted into stones while some of it ends up in the blood. Once bile has leaked into the blood, it may lead to toxicity, discoloration of the skin (yellow or gray), and skin blemishes, such as liver spots.

Sluggish bile flow in the liver alters the composition of bile still further, which, in turn, affects the gallbladder. A small clot of bile in the gallbladder may take as long as 8 years to grow large enough to be noticeable and become a serious health threat. It is known that 1 in 10 Americans has gallstones in the gallbladder. This amounts to 31 million American having this condition. Of these, 500,000 opt for gallbladder surgery each year. Very few physicians and patients, however, are aware of the fact that almost every person with any kind of persistent health problem has gallstones in the *liver*. In my estimation, about 95 percent of adults in industrialized nations have gallstones in the biliary system of their liver.

Gallstones in the liver can cause many more diseases than gallstones in the gallbladder. To prevent illness and to generate a genuine and lasting breakthrough in the understanding and treatment of disease, we need to have a clear understanding of what dehydrates the bile fluid, alters its natural flora, destroys its enzymes, and increases its cholesterol and bilirubin content. The following 4 categories shed light on the most common factors responsible for causing gallstones.

1. Dietary

Overeating

Dietary mistakes play a leading role in producing imbalanced bile composition and, consequently, gallstones. Among all dietary blunders, overeating affects health most severely. By regularly eating too much food or eating food more frequently than the body needs to nourish and sustain itself, the digestive juices (including bile and hydrochloric acid) become increasingly depleted. Since there is a natural limit to the amounts of digestive secretions the body can produce during any given meal, overeating leaves large proportions of the ingested foods incompletely digested.

Undigested food putrefies and ferments, becoming a source of harmful microbial activity. This rather unnatural method of breaking down food alters the pH (acid/alkaline balance) of the intestinal environment, turning it into a favorable environment for yeast growth and parasites. Decomposing bacteria and parasites produce powerful toxins that can interfere with digestive functions and immune health.

Cleansing of the liver and colon, and eating a balanced diet rich in fresh, alkaline-forming foods, are among the most effective approaches to prevent and treat bacterial and parasitic infestation; the killing of bacteria and parasites does not address their origins and may only have limited benefits, if any.

As more and more toxic substances begin to accumulate or linger in the intestinal tract, the lymph and blood start absorbing some of these harmful substances. This leads to progressive congestion of the lymphatic system and thickening of the blood. All of this overtaxes the liver and excretory functions.

Intestinal disorders can critically deplete bile salts in the body owing to poor reabsorption from the lower parts of the small intestine. Low levels of bile salts lead to the formation of gallstones, and gallstones lead to low levels of bile salts in bile. This reciprocal link is clearly demonstrated by the markedly increased risk of gallstones among patients suffering from Crohn's disease and other forms of irritable bowel syndrome, and those who have gallstones have an increased risk of developing intestinal disorders.

Overeating is a major cause of bacterial toxins entering the blood and lymph. An imbalanced blood and lymph condition leads to decreased blood flow in the liver lobules, thereby altering the normal balance of bile constituents and producing gallstones. Gallstones in the liver further congest the blood and lymph, which upsets the body's basic metabolism.

The more one overeats, the fewer nutrients become available to the cells of the body. In fact, constant overeating leads to cell starvation, which creates the strong urge to eat food more often than the body is able to process, without suffering from congestion and increased toxicity. The repeated desire to snack, known as food craving, is a sign of serious malnourishment and metabolic imbalance. Moreover, it indicates imbalanced liver activity and the presence of gallstones. Healthy people have no desire to snack unless they are truly hungry. They also desire only foods that their body can actually digest and use.

Eating to the point at which you feel completely full, or feel that you cannot eat any more food, is a clear signal that the stomach has reached the point of dysfunction. Digestive juices in the stomach are only able to combine with ingested food as long as the stomach is at least one-quarter empty. Two cupped handfuls of food (use your own hands to measure) equal about three-quarters the size of your stomach. This is the maximum amount of food the stomach can process at one time. Therefore, it is best to stop eating when you reach the point at which you feel you could still eat a little more. Leaving the dinner table slightly hungry greatly improves digestive functions and prevents gallstones and diseases from arising.

Eating Between Meals

Ayurveda, the most ancient of all health sciences, considers eating before the previous meal has been digested to be one of the major causes of illness. The following factors are among the more common reasons why people eat between meals:

- A stressful and hurried lifestyle
- The temptation generated by the huge variety of processed, refined, and attractively packaged foodstuffs available
- The convenience of having fast food meals (low in nutritional value) available at virtually any time of the day or night
- Lack of satisfaction and nourishment from foods eaten; hence, food cravings develop; therefore the urge to eat popcorn or junk food while watching a movie
- Emotional eating to comfort oneself and avoid dealing with fear or insecurity issues

Any or all of these may have contributed to the irregular eating habits prevalent in a large percentage of today's population. As a rule, the more processed and altered foods are, the fewer nutrients and less life energy (chi) they contain. Since the nutritional value of such foods is so low, we need to eat more in order to satisfy the daily requirements of the body.

(**Note**: taking food supplements can neither replace real food nor provide the satisfaction that arises from eating, which is what the body requires to successfully digest and process nutrients)

Irregular eating habits, which include eating between meals and snacking in the middle of the night, greatly upset the body's finely tuned biological rhythms[71]. Most of the important hormonal secretions in the body depend on regular cycles of eating, sleeping, and waking. For example, the production of bile, gastric secretions, and other digestive juices, which are necessary for breaking down foods into their basic nutrient components, naturally peaks during midday. This suggests that the biggest meal is best eaten around that time.

In contrast, the body's digestive capacity is considerably lower during the morning and evening hours. If, day after day, the lunch meal consists merely of light snacks, the gallbladder cannot squeeze *all* its contents into the intestines, so it leaves behind enough bile to form gallstones. Note that

---

[71] See more details about biological rhythms in my book *Timeless Secrets of Health and Rejuvenation*

the gallbladder is naturally programmed to release the maximum amount of bile during the midday period. If you don't use what the body produces naturally, it can turn on itself.

In addition, eating only non-substantial meals during lunchtime causes nutritional deficiencies, which most often manifest themselves as a frequent urge for foods or beverages that promise a quick energy boost. These include sweets, pastries, breads and pastas made from white flour (starches act like white sugar), chocolate, coffee, black tea, soda, energy drinks, fruit juices, and the like. For every little snack eaten, the gallbladder releases a small amount of bile. However, the secretion of just a little bile is not sufficient to completely empty the gallbladder, which increases the risk of gallstone formation.

Having a constant urge to eat between meals suggests a major imbalance of the digestive and metabolic functions. If you decide to eat something an hour or two after a meal, for example, the stomach is forced to leave the previously eaten meal half-digested and attend to the newly ingested food instead. The older food begins to ferment and putrefy, thereby becoming a source of toxins in the digestive tract. Eating between meals not only increases stomach emptying time, but also delays the colon's natural defecation schedule, resulting in constipation.

The newly ingested food, by contrast, receives inadequate amounts of digestive juices, leaving it only half-digested as well. While the body is engaged in digesting a meal, it is simply incapable of producing and delivering sufficient amounts of bile and other digestive juices to properly handle another meal at the same time. If this *stop and go* process is repeated many times, it results in the generation of ever-increasing amounts of toxins, while the body's cells receive ever-decreasing amounts of nutrients.

Both these stressful situations cause a reduction in bile salts (poor digestion of food decreases the reabsorption of bile salts) and an increase of cholesterol production by the liver in response to poor digestion of fats. The body is left with no other choice but to produce gallstones.

To escape this vicious cycle, allow yourself to go through the initial phases of food cravings with more awareness. Feel what your body is *telling* you when it signals discomfort. Ask yourself what your body *really* wants. If you crave something sweet, try eating a piece of fruit instead of a piece of chocolate or cake.

In many people, the urge to eat is actually a sign of dehydration, and all that the body really wants is water. Because hunger and thirst signals are identical, the hunger pang or discomfort may subside once you drink one or two glasses of water. At the same time, make certain that you get a substantial and nutritious meal at lunchtime.

In time, and provided you have completely cleansed your liver, your body will receive enough nutrients from your main meal at lunchtime to satisfy nearly all its daily nutritional requirements. This will effectively stop food cravings and the desire to eat between meals.

Eating Heavy Meals in the Evening

A similar eating disorder occurs when the main meal of the day is consumed in the evening. Secretions of bile and digestive enzymes are naturally reduced later in the afternoon, especially after 6 p.m. In the evening, the digestive capacity may be merely 20 percent of what it is during the midday period. For that reason, a meal consisting of heavy foods such as meat, chicken, fish, cheese, or eggs cannot be properly digested later in the day. Oily foods or those fried in butter or oil are also far too difficult for the body to digest in the evening. Instead, such a meal turns into toxic waste matter in the intestines.

Undigested foods always end up congesting the body, first in the intestinal tract, and then in the lymph and blood. This greatly affects the quality of digestion during daytime meals as well. Gradually, the digestive power, which is determined by balanced secretions of hydrochloric acid, bile, and digestive enzymes, becomes subdued, causing similar side effects to those that result from overeating. That said, eating a large meal in the evening is a major contributing factor in the development of gallstones in the liver.

Eating food before going to sleep also upsets the digestive functions, for similar reasons. Ideally, there should be at least 3 hours between eating and bedtime. The ideal time for evening meals is around 6 p.m., and the ideal bedtime is before 10 p.m.

Overeating Protein

As mentioned earlier, excessive protein consumption leads to the thickening and congestion of the basal membranes of the blood vessels (capillaries and arteries), including the liver sinusoids[72]. Protein deposits in the blood sinusoids hinder serum cholesterol from leaving the bloodstream. Therefore, the liver cells *assume* that there must be a shortage of cholesterol in the body. This perceived *shortage* stimulates the liver cells to raise cholesterol production to abnormally high levels (although much of the cholesterol is used to repair, heal, and protect injured parts of the arteries). This extra cholesterol enters the liver bile ducts to be delivered to the small intestines for absorption. However, because the membranes and openings of the sinusoids are clogged with accumulated protein fiber (collagen), most of the extra cholesterol never makes it there and, instead, is trapped in the bile ducts. Any excessive cholesterol (not combined with bile salts) forms small clumps of crystals that combine with other bile components in the liver and gallbladder. This is how cholesterol stones are made.

Interestingly, Asians generally have a low-protein but high-fat diet, and rarely have cholesterol stones in their gallbladders. On the other hand, cholesterol stones in the gallbladder are very common among Americans whose diet is rich in flesh and milk protein.

Dietary fats play only a secondary, almost insignificant, role in raising cholesterol levels in the blood. The liver cells produce most of the cholesterol the body requires on a daily basis for the normal metabolic processes. The main reason we need fats in our diet is not so much to meet our need for cholesterol, but to help digest and absorb other foods and to derive fat-soluble vitamins. The liver raises cholesterol production to abnormal levels only when the basal membranes of the sinusoids are plastered with protein deposits.

Other factors that generate excessive amounts of protein in the blood include stress, smoking, excessive alcohol, and caffeinated beverages. Smoking, for example, causes inhaled carbon monoxide to destroy red

---

[72] My book Timeless Secrets of Health and Rejuvenation explains in great detail how overconsumption of protein foods (of any origin) affects the sinusoids and other parts of the circulatory system, and how reducing proteins in our diet clears the arterial plaque obstructing blood flow to the liver, heart, kidneys, brain and other organs of the body.

blood cells, thus unleashing a large amount of protein particles into the blood. Once enough of these denatured proteins are deposited in the blood vessel walls, adequate quantities of cholesterol can no longer reach the body's cells. To meet the need for more cholesterol, the liver cells automatically increase cholesterol production. The side effect of this response is gallstone formation. Smokers have a very high risk of developing gallstones.

If you are not a vegetarian, it is best to cut out red meat, eggs and cheese first, and keep other types of animal protein, such as poultry and fish, to a minimum. According to the results of The Nurses' Health Study (Nov. 2006), which is among the largest prospective investigations into the risk factors for major chronic diseases in women, women double their risk of hormone-receptor-positive breast cancer by eating more than one and a half servings a day of beef, lamb, or pork. A serving is roughly equivalent to a single hamburger or hot dog. If such a small amount of meat can cause cancer, it can surely cause a lot of other health problems as well, including gallstones.

Although all animal-based protein has a gallstone-generating effect, white meat, including chicken, turkey, and rabbit, causes a little less damage to the liver, provided it is of free-range origin and not eaten more often than once or twice a week. However, please be aware of the fact that poultry contains the highest concentration of parasites and parasite eggs among animal products. For example, more than 80 percent of all poultry in the United States is infested with salmonella. Cadavers like meat, poultry, and fish are naturally subject to parasitic infestation.

Once your taste for meat or other animal protein begins to diminish (which usually happens when the liver gets cleaner), you can gradually switch to a balanced vegan/vegetarian diet.

It is best to avoid fried and deep-fried foods, such as French fries, as they aggravate both the gallbladder and the liver. These foods are also loaded with trans fatty acids, which are a major cause of cancer. Trans fats are so dangerous to human health that New York City recently banned them from use in restaurants.

Large portions of the world's population are still vegetarian (they eat some dairy) or vegan (they eat nothing from animals) and, therefore, they consume little or no animal protein. These population groups show almost no signs of such degenerative illnesses as heart disease, cancer, osteoporosis, arthritis, diabetes, obesity, MS, and the like.

Our Body - A Protein Factory

The body's protein requirements are actually quite small, and certainly not as high as you have been led to believe by the food and medical industries. First, about 95 percent of the body's protein is recycled. Second, the liver synthesizes new proteins from amino acids that are not necessarily derived from the foods you eat. In fact, each cell in the body makes protein.

The nucleus of each cell is constantly engaged in protein production. Brain cells produce proteins, known as neuropeptides, in response to every thought or feeling you have. Neuropeptides, also known as neurotransmitters, are the molecular language that allows mind, body, and emotions to communicate. The body makes thousands of different enzymes, all of which consist of proteins. Not eating enough protein foods does not diminish the body's ability to make proteins. On the contrary, overeating proteins can severely congest the blood and lymph and can suffocate cells, thereby diminishing their ability to manufacture proteins. In fact, most protein deficiencies result from eating too much protein.

All proteins are made of various chains of amino acids, and amino acids consist of nitrogen, carbon, hydrogen, and oxygen molecules. These atoms are ingested by the body during inhalation of air, drinking of water, and eating of foods. Carbon, oxygen, and hydrogen atoms bond to form what we call carbohydrates. If nitrogen is added to the mix, proteins are formed. Since all of these molecules readily enter the blood in one form or another, they are almost immediately made available to all cells in the body.

Analysis of the human body has revealed that it consists of 65 percent oxygen, 18 percent carbon, 10 percent hydrogen, and 3 percent nitrogen. About 4 percent of body mass consists of 37 trace minerals, all present in sea salt or a variety of foods.

I assert that breathing air is the most efficient way for the brain cells and all the other cells in the body to be self-sufficient with respect to their protein-producing requirements. Although no scientist has ever conducted research to prove that the body can make protein directly from these molecules, there is also no research to show that it can't.

Can We Still Trust In Science?

We are expected to blindly trust that science, albeit without offering us any scientific evidence, is correct about some of the most basic phenomena controlling life on earth. For example, every child is taught at school that through a process called photosynthesis, plants take up carbon dioxide from the environment and convert it into oxygen. But just because biology textbooks say so, and nearly everyone agrees with it, doesn't make it true, though.

Anyone can conduct some very simple experiments (such as the D. Enger experiments[73]) which prove that plants, flowers, and trees, *do not* produce any oxygen at all, and they also *do not* absorb carbon dioxide (CO2), as biological science claims it. Instead, it can be shown that photosynthesis is due to the plants taking up nitrate nitrogen instead. The argument that "you must be out of your mind" falls apart, of course, when you conduct the actual experiments.

The original science experiment, upon which photosynthesis, one of biology's greatest discoveries, is based, consists of slicing the stem of a plant and measuring the amount of escaped oxygen. After performing this experiment, the scientists concluded that plants and trees must be producing oxygen, although no such evidence has ever been produced to support this theory. Ever since, anyone with a *rational* mind understood that in order to produce oxygen, trees and other plants require assimilating CO_2 in order to survive. By absorbing CO_2, plants naturally release oxygen for humans and animals to breathe; why would anyone doubt this?

Slicing a human artery and then proclaiming that the human body is capable of producing oxygen because there is oxygen found in the blood, is, of course, ridiculous, but this incredulous claim is what the original biological science experiment implies.

To prove whether plants really produce oxygen, as the scientists want us to believe, we will need to alter the experiment. Instead of measuring the oxygen content of the plant's sap, it makes a lot more sense to measure the oxygen and carbon dioxide contents of the air surrounding plants. If

---

[73]D. Enger experiments,
http://translate.googleusercontent.com/translate_c?hl=de&ie=UTF8&langpair=de
percent7Cen&oe=UTF8&prev=/language_tools&rurl=translate.google.com&twu=1&u=http://www.cts-
systems.de/fehler/videos.php&usg=ALkJrhjSSUgvxhPS0jPu3eDwNYBNRBUTuA

plants truly release oxygen and take up carbon dioxide, as claimed, we would find an increased concentration of oxygen and decreased concentration of CO_2 in the air surrounding plants, right? This would be so easy to prove, or disprove, and you don't even need to be a scientist to do it.

1. Place a small well-watered potted plant into a resealable cello bag that prevents air from moving in or out.

2. Place a digital analyzer that measures oxygen levels inside the bag, and close it.

3. Point two 150 watt lamps toward the bag (all plants need light for photosynthesis to take place).

Instead of increasing it, within the first six minutes of the experiment the oxygen content of the air inside the bag actually drops by 0.2 percent. After three days, the percentage of oxygen in the air will have gone from 20.9 to 15.4., and if you also measured CO_2 content, carbon dioxide will have increased from 0.00 to 6.4 percent. At this stage, the plant will be dead; oxygen-starved and suffocated by carbon-dioxide.

You can repeat this experiment a thousand times and you will get the same results each time: the oxygen content in air of the closed system becomes depleted and the carbon dioxide levels become highly concentrated. It's an undeniable fact that plants use oxygen and release carbon-dioxide, just like humans and animals do.

The theory that greenhouse gases are responsible for climate changes are based on the unproven idea that combustion engines, animals, and humans release large amounts of carbon dioxide into the environment. However, this is not true either. Take your device that measures CO2 emissions and hold it in the air near a busy highway, and you will find zero CO_2 in it.

Or if you prefer, place your CO_2 analyzer into an empty plastic bag; then take a deep breath and blow into it. You will find zero CO_2 in the bag, but you will also notice that the oxygen content has increased from the normal 17 percent of oxygen in exhaled air back to the 21 percent of oxygen normally contained in the air around you. This is quite unexpected, and not explained by science.

Both these experiments show that CO_2 breaks down into carbon and oxygen the moment it is being released. Plants absorb oxygen and produce carbon dioxide, like we do. The released carbon dioxide breaks down into usable carbon and oxygen. This makes plants, humans and animals indirectly responsible for oxygen generation on the planet.

The invention of the greenhouse gas theory only benefits a multi-billion dollar industry, but is not based on true science.

Can we continue relying on a man-made science that is so flawed and corrupted that it cannot even admit having made some of the most monumental errors ever made in the history of human life on earth? About what other important issues has science been misleading humankind?

Is Eating Protein Essential?

We know that a good number of individuals, whose bodies have adjusted themselves to living on water or air only (breatharians), suffer no protein deficiency at all. When I was a child (between 8 and 14 years), during every summer I abstained from food for 6 weeks for health reasons, and I only drank herbal tea and water while also detoxifying the body through intestinal cleanses, sunbathing, exercising, abdominal herbal packs, and moor baths. While the first three days of fasting always felt very uncomfortable, the complete lack or protein intake in no way led to a protein deficiency or stunted the growth of my body.

In addition, for the past 40 years, with the exception of butter, I have been eating a purely vegan diet. Unless you count vegetables, avocadoes, and a few nuts to be high protein foods, according to the mainstream medical theories I should have died 4 decades ago. Yet, at age 58 (in 2012), I am more healthy than ever.

I personally know people who have not eaten any food for several years, and they are extremely healthy, too. Clearly, there must be a mechanism in the body that permits these individuals to make the billions of bits of proteins required each day to maintain all the basic processes responsible for maintaining the human physiology. However, the current medical theories are not able to explain this phenomenon.

If there is a mechanism at work in some individuals which allows them to take in a large number of atoms (carbon, oxygen, hydrogen and nitrogen) from the air and convert them into nutrients, like plants do it, we should take this seriously and not debunk it as pseudoscience. Although we all are breatharians to some extent, I don't recommend anyone to become a full breatharian (one who lives without food) at this time in human history, for there are great risks involved when the body is toxic or not in optimal health.

If you are still concerned about not getting enough protein in your diet, did you know that one half cup of beans contains as much protein as a 3 oz. steak? Besides beans, nuts and seeds, collard greens, kale and avocado are rich in usable proteins. Cauliflower and broccoli both consist of a whopping 40 percent protein. Other common vegetables contain no less than 30 percent. Grains, such as wheat, barley, oats, and rice are very rich in protein, too. The grain quinoa actually contains complete protein. The same is true for chia seeds. Even fruits have around 5 percent protein.

In fact, all plant foods contain protein. It is protein that gives them their cell structure. Plant proteins contain the same 22 amino acids as animal proteins, and they are relatively easily digested. Although most plant-based foods like legumes, nuts, seeds, whole grains, vegetables, and fruits may not contain complete protein by themselves, the body forms an amino acid pool from the different kinds of plant foods eaten throughout the day. In other words, when a vegan consumes a variety of foods eaten at breakfast, lunch, and dinner, the body can easily combine these amino acids to make complete protein.

Flesh Food Health Risks

Besides causing gallstones, eating animal proteins can have other, more serious consequences. It is far too complicated, inefficient, and laborious for the body to convert degenerated cadaver-proteins from killed animals into wholesome, usable proteins. Heating fish, eggs, meat, and poultry almost completely destroys (coagulates and denatures) these proteins, making it difficult for human cells to make use of them. If any of these harmful protein fragments make their way into the blood, which is highly likely, they inflame blood vessels. This can have grave consequences for the heart, brain, and kidneys and all other parts of the body.

Unlike carnivorous animals, such as cats, dogs, and wolves, humans simply don't have the right physiological makeup needed to make use of flesh foods without the risk of being harmed. The concentration of hydrochloric acid (HCl) produced in the stomach of a young person is merely capable of digesting up to 20 percent of a 6 oz. steak. At least 80 percent of the consumed meat becomes subject to putrefaction and, therefore, a source of toxification. Nitrites in the stomach can react with food proteins to form N-nitro compounds (carcinogenic nitrosamines); these highly toxic compounds can also be produced when meat containing nitrites or nitrates is heated.

The concentration of gastric juice is a clear determinant of a species' natural diet. No wild animal is inclined to eat foods it cannot also successfully digest. The only reason wild cats can eat flesh without a problem is because their stomach secretions consisting of HCl and the protein-splitting enzyme pepsinogen have concentrations 1100 percent greater than those produced by humans, sufficient to dissolve even the hardest of bones.

These extremely acid juices also serve to prevent putrefaction while the flesh undergoes digestion. In contrast, the comparatively small amount and weak concentration of acid secreted by the human stomach does neither allow for complete digestion of flesh nor does it curtail the bacterial decomposition of flesh.

For meat to not cause harm in carnivores, it must leave their stomach very quickly. However, the human stomach is oblong and consists of a series of expandable folds, called rugae, which serve to retain food for unduly long periods.

Normally, predigested food in the stomach chemically stimulates the release of gastrin from G cells located in the last portion of the stomach. Gastrin is a peptide hormone that stimulates secretion of HCl by stomach cells and aids in gastric motility. However, meat, poultry and fish may not even combine with HCl for several hours after ingesting them. In some cases, they must remain there for as many as 6-8 hours before they are released into the intestinal tract. Consequently, these foods begin to rot while still in the stomach. By contrast, most vegetarian foods leave the stomach within less than 3 hours. Most fruits pass through the stomach within 20 minutes.

These are not the only problems that occur in meat-eating humans. Whereas meat moves quickly through the carnivore's relatively short digestive tract and is quickly expelled, in the human's lengthy intestine low-fiber foods such as meat, poultry, eggs, fish, and dairy move very slowly. Inevitably, these animal foods decrease the motility of the human intestine, resulting in putrefaction and the release of powerful carcinogenic toxins, such as nitrosamines, putrescines and cadaverines. This also explains the high incidence of colon cancers among flesh eaters.

Regular consumption of animal protein also damages the kidneys and the liver. The sizes of the liver and kidneys in carnivores are relatively massive when compared to ours. A lion's kidney, for example is not much smaller than an elephant's kidney. The lion needs such a large kidney to handle the large amounts of nitrogenous waste products resulting from the digestion of flesh.

Our relatively small kidneys are not designed to process all the nitrogenous waste resulting from the digestion of meat, including the highly toxic ammonia which requires much water to flush it from the body. The waste product uric acid is less toxic but also requires a lot of water to remove it; otherwise, kidney stones are formed. It is rare, though, for regular meat eaters to drink the 2-3 liters of water a day necessary to prevent these waste products from accumulating in the kidneys, blood, and tissues.

Numerous research studies have shown that a high-protein diet can lead to or worsen hypertrophy of kidney mass, bone loss, kidney stones, diabetic nephropathy, idiopathic hypercalciuria, calcium nephrolithiasis, and reduced creatinine clearance[74]. Abnormally high levels of creatinine particularly warn of possible malfunction or failure of the kidneys.

In addition to enlarging and damaging the kidneys, regular meat consumption also places a heavy strain on the relatively small liver and gallbladder of humans, impairing these organs' functions over a long period of time. A lion's liver is very large, capable of breaking down enormous amounts of proteins and removing large amounts of nitrogenous waste from the blood; its gallbladder holds three times the amount of bile of the human gallbladder, just enough to digest all the proteins and fats contained in flesh food.

The human liver is not designed to do the work of a carnivorous animal and cannot completely detoxify the poisonous products inherent within animal foods such as ammonia and uric acid. Excessive uric acid in the blood alone is responsible for injuring blood vessels throughout the body, a major cause of degenerative disease.

If the human body depended on eating a high-protein diet on a regular basis, most people in the developing world who do not eat these foods would either be deathly ill or dead by now. However, this has not happened. On the contrary, in countries like Mauritius where an increase in prosperity among the population replaced their traditional plant-based diet with a meat-based diet, heart health declined very rapidly. Statistics provided by the World Health Organization (WHO) show that in the 1940s, only 2 percent of the population in Mauritius died from heart disease. By 1980, this number had increased to an incredible 45 percent.

---

[74] Kidney Disease studies, http://ecologos.org/kidney.htm

Backed by numerous scientific studies, a detailed report in 1991 released by the WHO stated that a diet rich in animal products *promotes* heart disease, cancer, and several other diseases. The report linked diets rich in sugar, meat and other animal products, saturated fat, and dietary cholesterol with increases in chronic diseases, and made this ominous prediction: "If such trends continue, the end of this century will see cardiovascular disease and cancer established as major health problems in every country in the world." As we now know, its predictions have become reality.

In 1995, the Physicians Committee for Responsible Medicine (PCRM) - a highly-respected group of 5,000 doctors - confirmed the lower rates of disease among vegetarians and urged the government to recommend a vegetarian diet to US citizens. Before this, the US Dietary Guidelines had never even commented on the important role of vegetarianism in promoting good health. However, in 1996, PCRM issued the following statement: "...vegetarians enjoy excellent health. Vegetarian diets are consistent with the Dietary Guidelines and can meet Recommended Daily Allowances for nutrients. Protein is not limited in vegetarian diets ..."

The PCRM report reviewed over 100 pieces of published research and subsequently issued clear recommendations about what we should be eating: "The scientific literature supports the use of vegetables, fruits, legumes (peas, beans, chick peas) and grains as staples. Meats, dairy products, and added vegetable oils should be considered optional." While science overwhelmingly backs a balanced vegetarian diet, it considers animal proteins to be non-essential foods for humans.

Unless people are chronically dehydrated or suffer from malnutrition due to famines, you will hardly find anyone in the developing world with a protein deficiency. On the contrary, the unhealthiest people on the planet live in the United States and other industrialized nations where protein is considered a *necessary* food.

Health conditions directly linked with overeating of protein include acid reflux, obesity, lymph edema, gout, and arthritis, excessive calcium leaching from the bones, osteoporosis, plaque buildup in the arteries, high blood pressure, increased risk of stroke, high cholesterol, high blood pressure, kidney damage, kidney stones, diabetes, foul-smelling breath, cancers, especially colon cancer, and of course, gallstones, which can lead to many other conditions.

The common assumption that you need to eat protein-rich food daily is not only misleading but also highly unscientific and potentially harmful. People on a balanced vegan diet rarely suffer from a chronic illness. A recent study showed that a vegan diet may even reverse diabetes. On the other hand, eating meat on a regular basis increases one's risk of dying from all causes, including diabetes, heart disease, cancer, and osteoporosis.

A federal study by the National Cancer Institute looked at the records of more than half a million men and women aged 50 to 71, following their diet and other health habits for 10 years. Between 1995 and 2005, 47,976 men and 23,276 women died. The study was featured in *Archives of Internal Medicine*, March 24, 2009[75].

The researchers divided the volunteers into 5 groups or *quintiles*. All other major factors were accounted for - eating fresh fruits and vegetables, smoking, exercise, obesity, etc. People eating the most meat consumed about 160 g of red or processed meat per day - approximately a 6 oz. steak.

Women who ate large amounts of red meat had a 20 percent higher risk of dying of cancer and a 50 percent higher risk of dying of heart disease than women who ate less. Men had a 22 percent higher risk of dying of cancer and a 27 percent higher risk of dying of heart disease. That's compared to those who ate the least red meat, just 5 oz. per week, or 25 g per day - approximately a small rasher of bacon.

The study also included data on white meat and found that a higher intake was associated with a slightly reduced risk of death over the same period. However, high white meat consumption still posed a major risk of dying. If meat consumption can kill so many people, it can be safely assumed that it can make many more people sick.

Former American Cancer Society doctor and nationally known surgeon, author, and professional speaker, Christine Horner, M.D., admitted to being brainwashed during the 10 years she worked with this powerful organization. Dr. Horner spearheaded legislation in the 1990s that made it mandatory for insurance companies to pay for breast reconstruction following mastectomy. She says that she was taught to tell patients: "We don't know what causes breast cancer, we don't have any known cure for it, so the best thing women can do is get mammograms and breast exams in an effort to catch it early and save lives." Of course, she

---

[75]Meat Intake and Mortality. Rashmi Sinha et al, *Arch Intern Med*. 2009; 169(6):562-571.

now knows that it is well-known what causes breast cancer, and she tours the country and the world to inform the people about it.

For example, there are numerous epidemiological studies to show that breast cancer rates are much higher in American women versus Asian women; and Asian women who move to the United States experience a drastic risk increase. In fact, according to scientific research, women who consume the most red meat have a 400 percent greater risk for developing breast cancer! Even within Japan, affluent women who consume meat daily have an astounding 850 percent higher risk of breast cancer than poorer women who rarely or never eat meat[76].

Further, large studies in England and Germany showed that vegetarians were about 40 percent less likely to develop cancer compared to meat eaters[77].

In a prospective analysis by Harvard researchers of 90,655 premenopausal women, ages 26 to 46, showed that intake of animal fat, especially from red meat and high-fat dairy products, during premenopausal years is associated with an increased risk of breast cancer[78]. Vegetable fats did not increase risk.

In a National Institutes of Health (NIH)-AARP Diet and Health Study, researchers Genkinger and Koushik from the US National Cancer Institute examined the health data of 494,000 participants. In this 8-year study[79], the researchers compared the rate of cancer occurrence among the 20 percent of participants who ate the most red and processed meat[80] with the data on the 20 percent who ate the least.

The results of the study were dramatic. Participants who consumed the most red meat had a 25 percent higher risk of developing colorectal cancer compared with those who ate the least, and a 20 percent higher risk of developing lung cancer[81]. The risk of esophageal and liver cancer was

[76]Hirayama T. Epidemiology of breast cancer with special reference to the role of diet. Prev Med 1978;7:173-95

[77] 1. Thorogood M, Mann J, Appleby P, McPherson K. Risk of death from cancer and ischaemic heart disease in meat and non-meat eaters. Br Med J 1994; 308:1667-70
2.Chang-Claude J, Frentzel-Beyme R, Eilber U. Mortality patterns of German vegetarians after 11 years of follow-up. Epidemiology 1992;3:395-401
3. Chang-Claude J, Frentzel-Beyme R. Dietary and lifestyle determinants of mortality among German vegetarians. Int J Epidemiol 1993;22:228-36

[78] Cho E, Spiegelman D, Hunter DJ, et al. Premenopausal fat intake and risk of breast cancer. J Natl Cancer Inst 2003;95:1079-85

[79]Published in *PLoS Med*. 2007 December; 4(12): e345, and online 2007 Dec. 11. doi:10.1371/journal.pmed.0040345

[80]Meat originating from a mammal, beef, lamb, pork, and veal; and meats preserved by salting, smoking, or curing

[81]Lung and colorectal cancers are the first and second leading causes of cancer death, respectively

increased by between 20 and 60 percent. Higher meat intake also correlated with an increased risk of pancreatic cancer in men. In recent meta-analyses of colorectal cancer that included studies published up to 2005, summary associations indicated that red meat intakes were associated with 28-35 percent increased risks while processed meats were associated with elevated risks of 20-49 percent.

The researchers indicated that 1 in 10 cases of lung or colorectal cancer could be averted by limiting red meat intake. According to the China study and other cancer research considered during the past 60 years, cancer could actually become a rare illness if animal proteins were avoided altogether.

Other studies have found associations between meat intake and the risk of bladder, breast, cervical, endometrial, esophageal, glioma, kidney, liver, lung, mouth, ovarian, pancreatic, and prostate cancers. On the other hand, there are plenty of studies that point to the cancer-preventing effects of a fruit and vegetable diet[82], including recent studies published in 2007 in the *American Journal of Epidemiology* and in *Archives of Internal Medicine*[83].

It is more than obvious that The American Cancer Society is blatantly lying to the unsuspecting population when it claims: "We don't know what causes cancer." There are literally thousands of scientific studies and references that point to the various causes of cancer.

That said, above and beyond having the lowest risk of developing cancer, life-long vegans also have the lowest incidence of gallstones and heart disease[84].

Besides the cancer risks, there are additional risks that arise from eating contaminated meat. A review of Just *The Current And Active Recalls* posted on the US Department of Agriculture's (USDA) Food Safety and Inspection Service (FSIS) website shows that more than 60 million pounds of beef, pork, chicken, and turkey products were recalled in 2011 for contamination with listeria, E. coli, and salmonella - a total of 60 million pounds[85].

Food poisoning resulting from eating contaminated meat products is a major cause of debilitating illness and death. Flesh (cadaver) is naturally

---

[82]For detailed information, see my book *Cancer is Not a Disease - It's a Healing Mechanism*
[83]American Journal of Epidemiology and in 2007 Jul 15; 166(2):170-80. Epub 2007 May 7 and Archives of Internal Medicine 2007 Dec 10; 167(22):2461-8.
[84] To learn more about vegetarianism and a wholesome vegetarian diet according to body type (Ayurvedic), refer to my book Timeless Secrets of Health and Rejuvenation
[85] Current and active recalls of meat products:
http://www.fsis.usda.gov/FSIS_Recalls/Open_Federal_Cases/index.asp

prone to bacterial infestation, and even with the greatest measures of precaution there is no guarantee of safety. About 1 in every 4 people in the US gets sick from eating contaminated food every year, according to the Centers for Disease Control and Prevention (CDC). That amounts to 76 million cases of food borne illness, or food poisoning, annually.

The most common symptoms of E. coli food poisoning include severe stomach cramps, bloody diarrhea, fever, and vomiting. Some infections may lead to hemolytic-uremic syndrome, which causes kidney failure. More than 325,000 people become hospitalized and 5,000 die in the United States each year; that's in addition to the many unnecessary deaths caused by regularly consuming the even non-contaminated meat products.

Seafood - An Unsuspected Killer

Seafood is naturally high in parasites, some of which can greatly affect human health. Swallowing live tapeworm larvae can cause a tapeworm infestation. The tapeworms may live in the human intestinal tract for several years. Symptoms can include abdominal pain, weakness, weight loss and anemia. Eating raw fish is particularly risky, given the high risk of parasitic infection.

Seafood generally is high in contaminants, such as mercury and aluminum, for fish can easily absorb them but not eliminate them again. King mackerel, tilefish, swordfish, and shark are among the most contaminated sea animals. Seafood may cause severe food poisoning. Snapper, mackerel, barracuda, and grouper can cause ciguatera food poisoning, characterized by a lower heart rate, a decrease in blood pressure, and joint and muscle pain. Farmed fish is often filled with antibiotics, chemicals, and coloring agents to make fish look healthy. For instance, sickly-looking and grayish farmed salmon is made to look pink and fresh. Researchers from the Mayo Clinic claim that antibiotics, pesticides, and other chemicals used in raising farmed fish may have harmful effects on people who eat the fish.

With regard to the purported benefit of fish or fish oil in the prevention of arteriosclerosis, the evidence to that effect is not conclusive. On the other hand, a paper by Michael R. Zimmerman, M.D., Ph.D., Assistant Professor of Pathology University of Pennsylvania School of Medicine, provided the oldest available evidence (1,600 years to be exact), that a fish diet can actually cause arteriosclerosis.

The results of a complete autopsy performed on the frozen body of an Eskimo woman who died over 1,600 years ago found significant atherosclerotic plaques affecting the coronary arteries. The autopsy also found osteoporosis affecting her bones in spite of the Eskimo's calcium-rich diet. Today, we know, of course, that consumption of excessive animal protein causes calcium to be leached from the bones to counteract the strong acidity of animal protein.

The Inuit population subsisting on a traditional marine diet had an approximate life expectancy (excluding infant mortality) of 43.5 years. Most deaths occurred between the ages 25 and 45, according to a mortality table from the records of a Russian mission in Alaska which recorded the ages of death of a traditionally-living Inuit population during the years 1822 to 1836 (compiled by Veniaminov, taken from *Cancer, Disease of Civilization*)[86]. Their immune systems were particularly weak and acute infection was the commonest cause of death.

Vitamin B12 deficiency

If eating animal protein is such a strong risk factor for a large number of diseases and even death, it is highly likely that meat-eaters are also more prone to anemia owing to a deficiency in vitamin B_{12} than vegan/vegetarians.

In fact, I see far more anemic meat-eaters than anemic vegan/vegetarians. I personally suffered years of childhood anemia while on animal proteins, but completely recovered from it after several weeks on a vegan diet.

Foods high in protein lack dietary fiber; low fiber foods tend to slow bowel functions, thereby leading to chronic intestinal congestion. Accumulated or trapped waste material in the large intestine may consist of impacted feces, hardened mucus, dead cellular tissue, gallstones that were released from the gallbladder, dead and living bacteria, parasites, worms[87], metals, and other noxious substances. Intestinal congestion greatly undermines the colon's important role in absorbing essential minerals and some bacteria-produced vitamins, including the all-important vitamin B_{12}. Parts of the waste matter may enter the lymph and blood systems, which can make you feel tired, sluggish, or ill.

---

[86]Mortality and Lifespan of Inuit   http://wholehealthsource.blogspot.com/2008/07/mortality-and-lifespan-of-inuit.html
[87] All meat eaters have a relatively large number of worms and parasites in their intestinal tract

The statement that cobalamins or B$_{12}$ vitamins can only be found in animal foods, such as meat, fish, eggs, cheese, etc., is plain false. B$_{12}$ is found in fermented plant foods and algae, and of course, in a healthy mouth and digestive tract. A deficiency of this vitamin is thought to cause pernicious anemia and degeneration of nerve fibers of the spinal cord responsible for neuropathy and dementia.

The argument that people who don't consume any animal foods must also be B$_{12}$ deficient and thereby endanger their health is unscientific, unfounded and misleading. Apart from producing vitamins K, B$_1$, and B$_2$, as well as energy-providing short-chain fatty acids, the billions of beneficial bacteria residing in our intestines and mouth can produce more than enough vitamin B$_{12}$ to guarantee good health. And you don't need much of it. The amount of vitamin B$_{12}$ a healthy person will require throughout his lifetime is about the size of half the nail of your little finger.

In addition, the liver can store B$_{12}$ for many years and knows how to recycle this vitamin. This may explain why *vegans* (those who don't eat any type of animal products) eating a balanced diet almost never suffer from B$_{12}$ deficiencies (contrary to public opinion).

If the body for some reason required more of this vitamin, it would instinctively desire foods (versus craving them) that would meet the increased demand. However, if the liver and intestines are congested, and one's natural instinct becomes subdued, a B$_{12}$ deficiency may eventually develop, regardless of whether a person is a meat-eater, vegetarian, or vegan.

To make B$_{12}$ vitamins available to the body, the stomach must make enough intrinsic factor, contained in gastric juice. Without enough intrinsic factor, B$_{12}$ cannot be properly absorbed later in the small intestine. A lack in stomach acid is not only a major cause of GERD (acid reflux disease), but it is also the main reason for B$_{12}$ deficiency.

Balanced secretion of gastric juice normally keeps the sphincter of the esophagus closed. Combining meat protein and starch foods (like potatoes, rice, or bread) in the same meal renders much of the gastric juice ineffective. This may cause the sphincter of the esophagus to remain open, which allows acid stomach contents to back up into the esophagus. Since most meat eaters also eat starches like potatoes or rice along with their animal proteins, they are far more likely to suffer acid reflux and B$_{12}$ deficiencies than vegans.

Bariatric surgery is another cause of B_{12} deficiency and development of pernicious anemia. Other risk factors contributing to these conditions include excessive consumption of alcohol, stomach tumors, gastric ulcers, Crohn's disease, tapeworm infection as a result of eating seafood, surgery that removes the part of the small intestine where vitamin B_{12} is absorbed, and intestinal malabsorption disorders. The most common cause of poor digestion and absorption is lack of bile secretion as a result of gallstones in the bile ducts of the liver and gallbladder. It is also responsible for decreased gastric secretions, especially common among older people.

In addition, drugs such as antacids and metformin (used for treatment of diabetes) interfere with gastric secretion and, therefore, with adequate absorption of vitamin B_{12}. Taking antibiotics quickly destroys beneficial bacteria, which inevitably leads to an overgrowth of destructive bacteria in parts of the small intestine and in our mouths. A disturbed intestinal flora is the most common cause of B_{12} deficiency. Many pharmaceutical drugs interfere with gastric secretions and can, therefore, be held responsible for B_{12} deficiency.

Low vitamin D alone, due to lack of sun exposure, can reduce gastric secretions and thus contribute to B_{12} deficiency. And according to British research, thoroughly washing one's organically grown, naturally fertilized vegetables can also cause it. Food fertilized with cow dung, for example, leaves plenty of B_{12} on the skins of fruits and vegetables.

So before jumping to the conclusion that a vegan diet must be behind a B_{12} deficiency, one first needs to take a closer look at all these other, more likely, reasons. Remember, just one course of antibiotics can dramatically reduce the liver's ability to store and release B_{12}, while also destroying the B_{12} generating gut bacteria for an entire lifetime!

Humans Designed to Eat Low Protein Diet

The often-cited *scientific* fact that we need to combine certain foods (such as beans and rice) in order to get complete proteins is plain misinformation, too. The body does not depend on food proteins to produce the proteins it requires to be healthy.

The strongest animals like the elephant, wild horse, orangutan, and bull do not have to eat animal proteins either. Like us, their vegan foods, the air they breathe, the sunlight they are exposed to, and the water they drink, provide them with the necessary molecules to make their own proteins and strong muscles. By giving them animal protein-based feeds, they actually become sick or die, just like many humans (as confirmed by the already mentioned research).

Some people have argued that chimpanzees, whose genetic makeup is almost identical to that of humans, eat meat, i.e. flesh food and so accordingly, it must be in *our* genes to eat meat, too. However, chimps don't eat other animals. The amount of *animal protein* they may eat is about the size of half a pea a day and it consists of small insects, not animals. The hands and nails, teeth, and digestive tract of a chimpanzee are those of a predominately vegan animal, or fruitarian, not those of a carnivorous beast that hunts down, tears apart and devours other animals.

The ultimate determinant of whether an animal is required to eat foods high in protein is the composition of its mother's milk. The milk produced by primates, to which the human species belongs, is very low in protein. Among all primates, the milk produced by humans has the lowest amount of protein, at 0.8 to 0.9 percent. It also contains 4.5 percent fat, 7.1 percent carbohydrates, and 0.2 percent ash (minerals)[88]. This still leaves protein at less than 1 g/100ml whereas cow's milk is 3.5g/100ml.

Breast milk of primates like chimpanzee, baboon, rhesus monkey, and gorilla has a protein content of only 0.85 to 1.2 percent.

Now compare the tiny percentage of protein in human milk and other primates with the large percentage of protein in the milk of a carnivorous animal, such as a cheetah. The nutrient content of cheetah milk is 99.6 g protein, 64.8 g fat, and 40.21 g lactose per kg milk[89]. That amounts to 9.96 percent protein, over 10 times the amount found in human milk. Also, can anyone give an explanation as to why our protein requirement would change so drastically from 5 percent during infancy to 10-20 percent range for adulthood?

Human breast milk is a newborn child's most important and balanced food. For a newborn's cells to divide and multiply and for its body to grow, it needs a lot of protein, or so it seems. Yet right from the beginning of life, the growing baby is naturally prevented from ingesting a concentrated protein food. This is where science fails to explain the true workings of the human body.

In reality, there is no need for a high protein food anyway since whatever the baby receives from the mother's milk, air and sunlight, the infant has everything it needs to jump-start protein synthesis by the cells

---

[88]Belitz, H Food Chemistry, 4th Edition, p.501 table 10.5
[89]Comp Biochem Physiol B Biochem Mol Biol. 2006 Nov-Dec; 145(3-4):265-9. Epub 2006 Oct5

and triple its body weight within the first 16 months of its life. Once the biggest growth spurt in a child's life has occurred, it has an even lesser need for concentrated protein foods than during the first 16 months. In fact, after breast feeding for one year, the protein content in mother's milk drops even further. This simple fact defies the very principle of *nutritional science,* which claims we need to eat a large amount of protein each day to survive.

When the body reaches adulthood and stops growing altogether, eating such foods may not only be unnecessary but can actually interfere with its most important functions. It makes no sense at all that we need less than 1 percent protein in our food when we grow the most, but 10-20 percent (as recommended by nutritionists) when we stop growing altogether.

The high concentrations of carbohydrates and fats in breast milk gives us further clues as to what our natural diet should consist of during adulthood. Fruits, vegetables, grains, etc. are rich in carbohydrates. Besides eating olives, nuts, seeds, and avocado, we can easily use such oils as olive oil and coconut oil to satisfy our naturally high requirement for fats.

Besides cleaning out the liver and gallbladder, I recommend that you check for any existing abnormal health conditions that could be due to a high-protein diet. Sometimes, just avoiding these foods for a couple of days may already bring you the desired relief.

Foods and Beverages That Trigger a Gallstone Attack

Eggs, pork, greasy food, onions, fowl, pasteurized milk, ice cream, coffee, chocolate, citrus fruits, corn, beans, and nuts - in that order - are known to bring on gallbladder attacks in patients suffering from gallbladder disease.

In a 1968 research study, an entire group of patients with gallbladder disease was free of symptoms while on a diet that excluded all these foods. Adding eggs to their diet brought on gallbladder attacks in 93 percent of the patients.

A gallbladder attack may be recognized by the following symptoms:
- Chest pain in the right side, usually under the rib cage
- Nausea or queasiness
- Vomiting, gas, and possibly, diarrhea
- Constant belching or burping

- The liver/gallbladder area is very tender to touch
- Unable to walk without bending over
- Difficulty in breathing caused by sharp pain (triggered by spasms)
- Pain radiates through to the right shoulder blade
- Pain between the shoulder blades

Pains may be sharp, excruciating or dull. They may be most pronounced during the night, and you cannot find any comfortable position to get some sleep. In my case, most of the 40 gallbladder attacks I had endured before I cleaned out my liver and gallbladder lasted up to 3 days and nights, or longer.

In most cases, the pain results from a stone passing through the cystic duct or travelling down the common bile duct. An infected gallbladder that becomes inflamed (cholecystitis) may also cause strong pain. In some cases, though, it can be due to backed up bile in the gallbladder, which causes it to become severely enlarged.

Although some attacks are triggered by lifting heavy objects, or severe stress, avoiding foods that can bring on an attack is certainly a good idea. The same foods that trigger gallbladder attacks may also be responsible for producing the gallstones that cause most of such attacks in the first place.

Some researchers believe that the ingestion of substances that cause allergies makes the bile ducts swell up, which, in turn, impedes the discharge of bile from the gallbladder - the main reason for developing gallstones in the gallbladder. This assumption, however, is only partially true. From the Ayurveda point of view, gallstone formation is a Pitta disorder, affecting mostly the Pitta body type, although any body type can suffer a Pitta disorder and produce gallstones.

In the ancient language of Sanskrit, Pitta literally means bile. People of this body type naturally secrete bile in large amounts. However, bile secretions become erratic, excessive, or irregular when the Pitta type eats Pitta-increasing foods in large amounts or on a regular basis. Bile's constituent parts become imbalanced, which predisposes it to hardening. This does not mean, though, that Pitta types are naturally prone to gallbladder disease; rather, it means that the digestive system of these individuals is not designed to digest specific foods that are not conducive to their body's growth and sustenance.

The Pitta body type is known to have only limited ability to digest, absorb and utilize certain foods and beverages, of which the most prominent are sour dairy products, including cheese, yogurt, and sour cream; egg yolks; salty butter; all nuts except a small amount of almonds, pecans, and walnuts; hot spices, as well as ketchup, mustard, pickles, and refined or processed salt; cooked tomatoes; salad dressings that contain vinegar; spicy condiments (sauces); citrus fruit and juices; all sour and unripe fruits; brown sugar; whole (non-ground) grains, such as those contained in many whole wheat breads; brown rice; lentils; excessive alcohol; tobacco; excessive coffee and regular tea; colas and other soft drinks; artificial sweeteners, preservatives, and colorings; most pharmaceutical drugs and narcotics; chocolate and cocoa (unless they are dark, unprocessed); left-over, frozen, and microwaved foods; all iced beverages.

Although the Pitta type is the most prone to develop gallstones, other body types are also at risk if they regularly eat foods that clash with their natural constitutional requirements[90]. For example, the Vata type, who is the most likely to suffer from constipation when he does not consume enough fats/oils, salt and sour foods, is also more prone to developing gallstones.

Medical professionals have long known that slow intestinal transit contributes to the formation of gallstones in women of normal weight.

In addition, manufactured and preserved foods and beverages disturb liver functions in any body type.

A study performed at the University Hospital of Riyadh, Saudi Arabia, showed that the incidence of gallbladder surgery surged there by 600 percent because the population had replaced a more nomadic existence and traditional diet with a more sedentary lifestyle that included eating fast foods and junk foods typically consumed in countries of the Western Hemisphere.

Artificial Sweeteners

Sweet Temptations - Bitter Rewards

Foods that contain artificial sweeteners, such as aspartame, neotame, Splenda, or saccharine severely upset the liver, gallbladder, and pancreas and drastically increase a person's chance of having a stroke or heart attack.

Earlier in 2011, according to research presented at the American Stroke Association's International Stroke Conference, people who drank diet soda

---

[90] For more information on diets according to body types, refer to my book *Timeless Secrets of Health and Rejuvenation*

daily had a 61 percent increased risk of cardiovascular events compared to those who drank no soda, even when accounting for smoking, physical activity, alcohol consumption and calories consumed per day[91].

According to ASA national spokesperson Dr. Larry Goldstein (Duke University Stroke Center, Durham, NC), previous studies have suggested a link between diet-soda consumption and the risk of metabolic syndrome and diabetes. The authors of the new study concluded: "This study suggests that diet soda is not an optimal substitute for sugar-sweetened beverages, and may be associated with a greater risk of stroke, myocardial infarction, or vascular death than regular soda."

Additionally, artificial sweeteners and food dyes in diet sodas and processed foods have also been linked to brain cell damage. Monsanto's newest artificial sweetener, neotame, is potentially far more brain damaging than even aspartame has ever been. Monsanto has had to produce a different synthetic sweetener because their patent on aspartame just ran out.

Like aspartame, neotame is linked to severe neurotoxic and immunotoxic damage because it metabolizes into toxic formaldehyde and other toxic substances. The FDA approved neotame, which is a synthetic sweet-tasting drug, without so much as a single conclusive, independent study proving its safety for human consumption. What's worse, neotame is unlabeled. Food manufactures can add it to any food or beverage and the conscious consumer won't have a clue if what they're eating or drinking has neotame in it or not. Remember, you are on your own when it comes to protecting your health and that of your family. To be on the safe side, I strongly recommend avoiding most processed foods and beverages, including chewing gums, tabletop sweeteners, flavored water products, sugar-free foods and beverages, diet sodas, drink flavoring products, cooking sauces, children's medicines, yogurts, and cereals.

A recent Danish study found that diet soda fattens up your organs, which may render them dysfunctional. Researchers found that this sweet beverage increases the more dangerous hidden fats, as found in the liver and even in the skeleton. Regular soda-drinkers also experience an 11 percent increase in cholesterol compared to the other groups.

In pregnant women, artificial sweeteners disrupt fetal development by aborting it or inducing defects. They can seriously damage the DNA,

---

[91] American Stroke Association International Stroke Conference. Abstract # P55. News conference February 9, 2011

which can affect the health of future generations as well. A wealth of independent research has confirmed that aspartame alone is linked to causing autism spectrum disorders, neurological problems, birth defects, gastrointestinal problems, and obesity, among other serious health conditions[92].

My book, *Timeless Secrets of Health and Rejuvenation*, discusses in great detail how artificial sweeteners cause serious damage to the cardiovascular system, pancreas, liver, kidneys, and the brain.

Drinking excessive amounts of alcohol (more than one drink a day) has a long-term dehydrating effect on both the bile and the blood, causing fat deposits in the liver. Eating foods that contain a lot of sugar has the same effect, especially soda beverages and processed fruit juices that are loaded with sugar.

While in the year 1700, the average person consumed about 4 pounds of sugar per year, in 2009, more than 50 percent of all Americans consumed a whopping 180 pounds of sugar per year. Most of the sugar is hidden in soft drinks, fruit juices, sports drinks, and in almost all processed foods, including breakfast cereals, ice cream, puddings, breads, pastries, sausages, and canned foods. Now even most infant formula contains the sugar equivalent of one can of soda. The sugar is only added to baby foods to cause sugar addiction in children and turn them into lifelong consumers of junk food and sodas.

Over 117 scientific studies have shown that processed and refined sugar, when consumed on a regular basis, can cause at least 76 different diseases or conditions[93]. Heart disease is still the biggest cause of death, and according to a new study published in the medical journal *Circulation*, drinking just one soda a day can bring on a heart attack.

A 12-oz. soda contains no less than 10 teaspoons of sugar. Such high concentrations of sugar "appears to be an independent risk factor for heart disease," says the study's lead author Frank Hu, M.D., Professor of Nutrition and Epidemiology at the Harvard School of Public Health (HSPH), in Boston. The study, which tracked 42,833 men over 22 years, found that men who drank a single 12-oz. soda per day increased their risk of heart attack by a whopping 20 percent. Two sodas increase the risk by 42 percent and three sodas by 69 percent! By comparison, people who

---

[92] Aspartame causes migraines, memory loss, depression, seizures, obesity, pain, infertility, etc. - 92 FDA-listed symptoms including death. http://www.dorway.com
[93] http://articles.mercola.com/sites/articles/archive/2010/04/20/sugar-dangers.aspx

smoke a pack of cigarettes a day have more than twice the risk of heart attack than non-smokers.

"Continually subjecting our bodies to high amounts of glucose, to high blood sugar levels that trigger large secretions of insulin results in stresses that in the long run show up as high risk of heart disease and diabetes," the study's co-author, Dr. Walter Willett, told CBS News[94].

With the exception of artificial sweeteners, there is probably no other manufactured food that can cause as many diseases as sugar. The beet, cane, or corn sugars added to thousands of different foods are highly toxic, processed, refined, unnatural products[95] that alter the body's biochemistry and metabolism.

Below is a short compilation of some of the most serious consequences of eating sugar:

Sugar can suppress the immune system; cause mineral deficiencies; lead to a rapid rise of adrenaline, hyperactivity, anxiety, difficulty concentrating, and crankiness in children; significantly raise triglycerides and LDL cholesterol, and lower HDL cholesterol; feed cancer cells and increase especially the risk of developing cancer of the breast, ovaries, prostate, rectum, pancreas, biliary tract, lung, gallbladder and stomach; cause atherosclerosis and cardiovascular disease; weaken eyesight; cause an acidic digestive tract, indigestion and increase one's risk of Crohn's disease and ulcerative colitis; lead to alcoholism; cause tooth decay and periodontal disease; cause autoimmune diseases such as arthritis, asthma, and multiple sclerosis; lead to Candida overgrowth and yeast infections; cause hemorrhoids and other types of varicose veins; damage the structure of the DNA and alter the way proteins act in the body; interfere with your absorption of food protein; cause food allergies; contribute to eczema in children; cause toxemia during pregnancy; cause heart disease; change the structure of collagen, causing loss of elasticity and luster; cause cataracts and nearsightedness; enlarge the kidneys and contribute to kidney stones and kidney disease; lead to emphysema and other lung diseases; damage your pancreas; interfere with bowel movements; cause headaches or migraines; increase your risk of Alzheimer's disease; be intoxicating and addictive, just like alcohol; cause epileptic seizures; induce cell death and kill a person; increase the size of your liver by making your liver cells

---

[94] Soda a day may lead to heart attacks in men, CBSnews.com, March 12, 2012
[95] http://sweetscam.com/how-its-made/

divide abnormally; and increase the amount of fat in your liver, leading to fatty liver disease.

Lastly, sugar consumption has been shown to cause gallstones[96]. The massive consumption of sugar by children today may explain why such a high percentage of the younger generation has already accumulated gallstones in the liver. Children normally don't develop gallstones at such an early age. I have personally met many sick children who have done liver flushes and released hundreds of gallstones, and subsequently regained their health. Children between the ages of 10 and 16 can do liver flushes at half the adult dosage (see Chapter 4 for details).

Children rarely produce gallstones if they eat a balanced, vegetarian diet that is rich in vegetables, fruits, and complex carbohydrates.

The Dangers of Genetically Modified Foods

Since I have already written about this important subject in my book *Timeless Secrets of Health and Rejuvenation*, I will merely make a few points here.

With increasing usage of genetically engineered plants, we will be faced with the following global scenario:

1. Loss of thousands of species of plants
2. All small farmers have to give up their farming businesses
3. Creation of Frankenstein foods that our bodies won't know how to handle
4. Super weeds resistant to all herbicides
5. Plants resistant to pesticides
6. Permanent damage to the reproductive capability of the human race
7. New viruses and diseases for which there won't be a cure

Already, 60 percent of processed foods now contain at least one genetically modified food item. Millions of people now consume chips with the firefly gene, potato chips with a chicken gene, or salsa with tomato containing a flounder gene. Cream of broccoli soup can have a bacteria gene in it, and salad dressing is most likely made with canola oil, vegetable oil or soybean oil (all genetically engineered). The tobacco gene is now used in lettuce and cucumbers and the petunia gene is used in

---

[96] Heaton, K. The Sweet Road to Gallstones. British Medical Journal. Apr 14, 1984; 288:00:00 1103_1104. Misciagna, G., et al. American Journal of Clinical Nutrition. 1999;69:120-126

soybeans and carrots. If you have celiac disease, you may need to avoid walnuts because they can have the barley gene in them. Even strawberries are not harmless anymore; they can now have undisclosed genes in them, so you will never know what else you are getting when you treat yourself to this delicious fruit. Cheese contains genetically engineered bacterial rennet. Many brands of apple juice contain the silkworm gene, and grapes can contain a virus gene. Trout, salmon, catfish, bass and even shrimp, are also genetically *enriched*.

The most troubling side effect of consuming genetically modified foods (GM), especially corn and soy, is that they have been linked to infertility in a number of studies. This is largely due to their significant concentrations of the herbicide glyphosate (the active ingredient in Roundup, the world's most widely used popular weed killer, a product of Monsanto).

It is my recommendation to stick to eating mostly unprocessed foods and foods from local sources, ideally organically grown.

Hidden Risks of Refined Salt

Natural sea salts or crystal/rock salts are the ultimate mineral supplements. Natural salt contains at least 72 mineral elements, whereas refined salt (with toxic additives) contains only 2 basic elements, sodium (Na) and chlorine (Cl).

Of the 84 mineral elements found in the human body, 72 need to be supplied through a natural diet. Unrefined salt contains these 72 mineral elements in perfect proportions and ionic form. Ionic minerals are easily digested and absorbed, and they can readily be used by the body to help conduct or support hundreds of essential processes.

When cells suffer a dietary deficiency of trace minerals, they lose their ability to control their ions. This has dire consequences on the human body. Even if ion equilibrium is lost for just one minute, cells in the body begin to burst. This can lead to nervous disorders, brain damage, or muscle spasms, as well as a breakdown of the cell-regenerating process.

When ingested, natural sea salt (reconstituted seawater) allows liquids to freely cross body membranes, blood vessels walls, and glomeruli (filter units) of the kidneys. Whenever the natural salt concentration rises in the blood, the salt will readily combine with the fluids in the neighboring tissues. This, in turn, will allow the cells to derive more nourishment from the enriched intracellular fluid. In addition, healthy kidneys are able to remove these natural saline fluids, without a problem. This activity is essential for keeping the fluid concentration in the body balanced.

Refined salt, on the other hand, also called table salt, may disrupt this free crossing of liquids and minerals (see the reasons for this below), thereby causing fluids to accumulate and stagnate in the joints, lymphatic ducts and lymph nodes, and kidneys. Thus, refined salt may not be readily removed from the body and thereby cause swelling, edema, and cellulite. Just 1 oz. of accumulated salt holds 3 quarts of water or 6 pounds of excess bodily water and fluids. Holding on to fluid in the body causes congestion and leads to dehydration of organs and tissues.

The dehydrating effect of commercial salt can lead to gallstone formation, kidney stones, weight gain, high blood pressure, and other health problems. However, there is no scientific evidence to date that shows sodium chloride can directly cause high blood pressure, even when most doctors recommend a low sodium diet to their hypertensive and obese patients. Such *advice* can, in fact, have serious consequences.

In fact, if the body is not getting sufficient amounts of sodium through the diet, it must retain it. To maintain the normal concentration of sodium in the blood it will retain extra amounts of water in the blood vessels. This raises blood pressure and cause hypertension. In other words, take your doctor's advice to cut back on sodium *with a grain of salt* (pun intended).

The body also requires salt to properly digest carbohydrates. In the presence of natural salt, saliva and gastric secretions are able to break down the fibrous parts of carbohydrate foods. In its dissolved and ionized form, salt facilitates the digestive process and sanitizes the GI tract.

Commercially produced table salt has just the opposite effect. To make salt resist the reabsorption of moisture and, thereby, be more convenient for the consumer, salt manufacturers add chemicals such as desiccants, as well as different bleaches, to the final salt formula. Additives may include aluminum hydroxide, sodium ferrocyanide, calcium phosphate, stearic acid and others. Depending on one's degree of chemical sensitivity, some of these chemicals may or may not act as toxins in the body. Most table salt also has added iodine, which, unless it is detoxified, can cause damage to the thyroid.

Regardless, after undergoing processing, table salt can no longer properly blend or combine with human body fluids. This invariably undermines the most basic chemical and metabolic processes in the body.

The chemical additives combined with sodium chloride may even prevent enough sodium from becoming available to the cells.

Refined salt is still being added to thousands of different manufactured foods. Almost half of the American population suffers from water retention (a leading cause of weight gain and obesity). The consumption of large amounts of refined salt is much to blame for that.

Before salt was commercially produced, versus harvested naturally, it was considered the most precious commodity on earth, even more precious than gold. During the Celtic era, salt was used to treat major physical and mental disturbances, severe burns, and other ailments. Research has shown that seawater removes hydroelectrolytic imbalance, a disorder that causes a loss of the immune response, allergies, and numerous other health problems (for more details, see the section *Eat Unrefined Sea Salt* in Chapter 5).

In recent years, salt has earned a bad reputation, and people have learned to fear it, in the same way they fear cholesterol and sunlight. Many doctors warn their patients to stay away from sodium and sodium-rich foods. Although their warnings are actually appropriate with regard to table salt (mostly because of the anti-caking effects of certain chemical additives), a low-sodium or salt-free diet means that you may be at an increased risk of developing mineral and trace mineral deficiencies. While mineral deficiency can contribute to numerous health conditions, including an increased risk of having a heart attack and stroke, not having enough sodium poses a far greater health risk.

Research conducted at McMaster University in Hamilton, Ontario, reviewed data of sodium consumption in 30,000 individuals who already had heart disease or diabetes. The researchers found that eating too little salt is doing harm instead of good. Those patients who consumed between 4,000 and 6,000 milligrams of sodium per day - more than double the current recommendations - were at the least risk of stroke, heart attack, other hospitalizations and deaths.

A 2011 analysis of existing studies, published in the *Journal of the American Medical Association*[97], clearly shows that current US guidelines with regard to safe salt intake are quite dangerous and significantly increase risk of hospitalization and death. They recommend we should

---

[97]Fatal and Nonfatal Outcomes, Incidence of Hypertension, and Blood Pressure Changes in Relation to Urinary Sodium Excretion, Journal of the American Medical Association, 2011: 305(17); 1777-1785, Katarzyna Stolarz-Skrzypek, MD, et al.

consume less than 2,300 milligrams of sodium daily and less than 1,500 mg if we are at extra risk for high blood pressure or heart disease. As difficult this may be to believe, lower sodium intake (between 2,000 and 3,000 mg per day) increased risk of cardiovascular-related death as well as hospitalization for congestive heart by 20 percent!

A meta-analysis by the *Cochrane Review* involving a total of 6,250 subjects did not reveal that cutting salt intake reduces the risk for heart attacks, strokes, or death[98]. On the contrary, a study published last year found that lower salt consumption actually *increased* your risk of death from heart disease.

While eating too much salt (in the range of 8,000 mg of sodium or more per day) may just be as risky or even more risky as eating too little salt, we should leave it to the body to decide how much salt we should eat. Unless you eat an unnatural diet consisting of highly processed foods (in which the salty taste is masked by sweeteners), it is actually impossible to overdose on sodium without feeling sick. This is especially true for unrefined salt which has at least 50 percent less sodium in it than table salt.

Eating unrefined salt fulfills the body's need for sodium chloride and other minerals without upsetting the hydroelectrolytic balance (of electrolytes). If your diet consists of a reasonable amount of potassium in natural form, you should have no concern about being harmed by the relatively small amount of sodium in unrefined salt.

Foods that are particularly high in potassium are bananas, apricots, avocados, chard, coconut, coconut water, pumpkin seeds, Lima beans, potatoes, winter squash, spinach and many other vegetables. However, if potassium levels in the body drop below normal, sodium (even in natural salt) can become a source of imbalance.

To be safe with regard to maintaining healthy potassium levels, I recommend avoiding or reducing foods that deplete potassium. These include sugar, high-fructose corn syrup, potato and vegetable chips, salty cheese snacks, pretzels, canned foods, foods that contain monosodium glutamate (MSG), soda beverages, more than one cup of coffee or tea a day (caffeine can deplete potassium through frequent urination), and excessive use of alcohol (given its strong diuretic effects).

---

[98]Reduced Dietary Salt for the Prevention of Cardiovascular Disease: A Meta-Analysis of Randomized Controlled Trials (Cochrane Review), American Journal of Hypertension, August 2011: 24(8); 843-53, R. S. Taylor, et al.

Celtic ocean salt (grayish in color) is a very good salt to eat because it is naturally extracted through sun drying. However, make sure it is certified free of toxic metals and chemicals (ocean water can be polluted). Other great salts are sold at whole food stores or co-ops. Some salts are multicolored, such as the brand, 'Real Salt'; others have a pink color. Himalayan crystal salt is considered the best and most nutritious of all.

Ayurvedic medicine recommends black salt because it relieves heartburn, constipation and intestinal gas. It also acts as a digestive aid. Its lower sodium content makes it more suitable for those who are sodium sensitive.

If taken dissolved in water or added to the water in which foods are cooking, these salts have many beneficial effects at the cellular level. They also help to cleanse and detoxify the gastrointestinal tract, and keep pathogens at bay.

Note: Epsom salt does not contain sodium chloride. It consists of magnesium sulfate, which may actually lower blood pressure, an action of magnesium. People who have hypertension and take medication for it need to be careful with magnesium because it can act like a blood pressure-lowering drug. On the other hand, magnesium is required to keep blood pressure at normal levels (see *Product Information - Magnesium*).

Dehydration

Many people suffer from dehydration without being aware of it. Dehydration is a condition in which body cells do not receive enough water for basic metabolic processes. The cells may run dry for any of the following reasons:

- Lack of water intake (anything less than six glasses of pure water per day)
- Regular or excessive consumption of beverages that have diuretic effects, such as coffee, tea (black), most soda beverages, and alcohol, including beer and wine. (Herbal teas such as green tea, peppermint tea, and the like, have no diuretic effects; decaffeinated coffee and tea are extremely acidic and more harmful than in their caffeinated form)
- Regular consumption of stimulating foods or substances, such as meat, hot spices, very salty foods, chocolate (except small amounts of dark chocolate), sugar, nicotine, narcotic drugs, soda, energy drinks, and artificial sweeteners

- Stress
- Most pharmacological drugs
- Excessive exercise
- Overeating and excessive weight gain
- Watching television for several hours in a row
- Sitting for many hours in one place without occasionally standing up and moving about

Any of these factors has a blood-thickening after-effect and, thereby, forces cells to give up water. The cell water is used to restore blood thinness. However, to avoid self-destruction, the cells have to start holding on to water. They do this by increasing the thickness of their membranes.

Cholesterol, which is a clay-like substance, attaches itself to the cell walls, thereby preventing the loss of cellular water. Although this emergency measure may preserve water and save the cell for the time being, it also reduces the cell's ability to absorb new water, as well as much-needed nutrients.

Some of the unabsorbed water and nutrients accumulate in the connective tissues surrounding the cells, causing swelling of the body and water retention in the feet, thighs, abdomen, kidneys, face, chin, eyes, and arms. This may lead to considerable weight gain. At the same time, the blood plasma and lymph fluids become thickened and begin to congest the lymphatic vessels and lymph nodes. Dehydration also affects the natural fluidity of bile and, thereby, promotes the formation of gallstones.

Tea, coffee, and most soda beverages share the same nerve toxin (stimulant), caffeine. If taken in excess, caffeine, which is readily released into the blood, triggers a powerful immune response that helps the body to counteract and eliminate this irritant. The toxic irritant stimulates the adrenal to secrete the stress hormones adrenaline and cortisol into the bloodstream.

The resultant sudden surge in energy is commonly referred to as the *fight-or-flight* response to enable the body to fight off a threatening situation or run away from it. If consumption of stimulants continues regularly, however, this natural defense or survival response of the body becomes overused and ineffective. The almost constant secretion of stress hormones, which are highly toxic compounds in and of themselves, alters the blood chemistry and causes damage to the immune, endocrine, and nervous systems. Future defense responses are weakened, and the body becomes increasingly susceptible to infections and other ailments.

The boost in energy experienced after drinking a strong cup of coffee is not a direct result of the caffeine it contains, but rather of the immune system's attempt to get rid of the caffeine. An overexcited and suppressed immune system fails to provide the energizing adrenaline and cortisol boosts needed to free the body from the acidic nerve toxin, caffeine. At this stage, people say that they are used to a stimulant, such as coffee. So they tend to increase their intake of it to feel the benefits. The often-heard expression "I am dying for a cup of coffee" reflects the true peril of this situation.

Since the body cells have to sacrifice some of their own water for the removal of the nerve toxin caffeine, the regular consumption of coffee, tea, or colas causes them to become dehydrated. For every cup of tea or coffee you drink, the body has to mobilize 2 to 3 cups of water just to remove the stimulants, a luxury it cannot afford. In Mediterranean countries like Greece, Turkey, and Cyprus, coffee shops traditionally serve a glass of water along with each cup of coffee, to help prevent the dehydrating effects of caffeine. If you would like to enjoy a nice cup of coffee, I recommend that you also drink enough water, either before or afterwards.

This also applies to soft drinks, medicinal drugs, or any other stimulants, including watching TV for many hours (see section on *Miscellaneous Causes* in this chapter). As a general rule, all stimulants have a strong, dehydrating effect on the bile, blood, and digestive secretions.

Having said that, caffeine is really only toxic when the liver is unable to detoxify it properly. This usually happens either when the liver is congested or when there is just too much caffeine coming in at once. For example, in my book, *Timeless Secrets of Health and Rejuvenation*, I describe the great benefits of green tea and compare it to black tea. Green tea contains much of the fiber of tea, which when ingested, releases the caffeine over a period of 6-8 hours. When tea is fermented, though, it becomes black tea, which releases all the caffeine at once. This over-stimulates the body, raises blood pressure and blood sugar levels, and increases the mentioned stress hormone secretions. Drinking too much tea or coffee within a short period of time can have these and other adverse effects.

In addition, if someone uses caffeine when tired, it can be harmful; but when taken when the body is already energized or energetic, it does very little or no harm at all. For instance, when a tired person uses coffee as a pick-me-up, it over-stimulates the body and uses up even more of the body's already depleted energy reserves, but when a person who feels vital and strong drinks a cup of coffee, the energy-depleting effect is absent. A clean, energized liver is very capable of dealing with caffeine.

Heavy Metal Contamination

The liver can easily be overtaxed through overexposure to toxic metals, including aluminum, arsenic, barium, beryllium, cadmium, lead, and mercury. Indoor and outdoor pollution, metal fillings in teeth, sea food, food additives, coal mining, chemtrails dumping large amounts of aluminum oxide and barium into the soil and drinking water, etc., are just a few examples of common sources of heavy metal contamination.

To check if you have accumulated excessive amounts of heavy metals, you may have a hair analysis done by a laboratory specializing in this area. However, while such a test can easily determine that your body has been exposed to such metals and is actually eliminating them with growing hair to some degree, it is not able to tell you how much metal has actually accumulated in the tissues, or is still there.

(**Note**: A hair analysis test may not be the most reliable method to determine a true mineral deficiency either. If excess minerals show up in hair, this may not necessarily be due to a mineral deficiency but can also result when the body has a surplus of minerals that it needs to remove. During stress, there may also a temporary discharge of minerals, followed by a lull once the stress reaction has passed) In other words, there is a factor of unpredictability involved in trying to measure whether a heavy metal contamination or mineral deficiency truly exists.

By doing a series of liver and gallbladder flushes, you will be able to eliminate many metals by naturally increasing the liver's ability to remove them from the blood[99]. Chelation therapy may be useful in removing metallic minerals, but it does not increase the liver's ability to prevent new metals from accumulating. So unless you clean out the liver and avoid all future exposure to heavy metals as much as possible, chelation therapy may have to be repeated over and over again. I have seen many patients who kept undergoing chelation therapy without achieving any long-term improvements, but who were able to forgo this invasive procedure after they cleaned out their liver.

---

[99] See http://www.agirsante.fr/profits.html for a case study

In the case that heavy metal accumulation is an issue for you, in addition to liver flushing, I recommend zeolite, a special type of volcanic mineral composite[100]. Zeolite helps to break down and remove heavy metals and toxic chemicals.

Zeolites are natural volcanic minerals that are mined in certain parts of the world. When volcanoes erupt, molten lava and thick ash pour out. Because many volcanoes are located on an island or near an ocean, this lava and ash often flows into the sea. Thanks to a chemical reaction between the ash from the volcano and the salt from the sea, amazing minerals like zeolites are formed in the hardened lava over thousands of years.

What makes zeolites so amazing is the fact that they are not only some of the few negatively-charged minerals found in nature, but they also have very unique structures. Zeolites have large, vacant spaces (or cages) that allow space for large, positively charged ions to be attracted to them, and then to be trapped and eliminated from the body.

Thanks to its honeycomb-like structure, a zeolite works at the cellular level to trap allergens, heavy metals and harmful toxins. In fact, because it is one of the few negatively charged minerals in nature, a zeolite acts as a magnet, drawing toxins to it, capturing them in its cage, and removing them safely and naturally from the body. This unique ability to remove dangerous toxins is well documented; it was used by the Russian government to absorb radioactive chemicals and other harmful toxins after the Chernobyl disaster. It has also been used by many individuals to remove contamination following the more recent nuclear disaster in Japan.

For centuries, the powdered forms of specific zeolites have been used as traditional remedies throughout Asia to promote overall health and well-being. I found zeolite in powder form to be far more effective in removing toxic metals and chemicals than liquid extracts.

Removing heavy metals from the body always boosts the immune system, which can benefit numerous health conditions.

Rapid Weight Loss

Overweight people are at greater risk for developing gallstones than people of average weight. It is an undisputed fact that significant health

---

[100] Pure Zeolite in powder form: http://www.ener-chi.com/wellness-products/zeolite/

benefits are gained from losing excess pounds. Weight loss, for example, can normalize high blood pressure, blood sugar, and cholesterol levels.

However, achieving rapid weight loss through diet programs that advise a very low intake of calories each day increases a person's risk of developing gallstones, in both the liver and the gallbladder. Most low-calorie diets don't contain enough fat to enable the gallbladder to contract sufficiently to empty its bile. A meal or snack containing approximately 10 grams (one-third of an ounce) of fat is necessary for the gallbladder to contract normally. If this does not happen, the gallbladder retains some of its bile, which subsequently leads to stone formation.

Obesity is associated with increased cholesterol secretion into the bile ducts, which raises the risk of developing cholesterol stones. When obese individuals undergo rapid or substantial weight loss by following an unbalanced diet program or using diet pills, the congested and, therefore, undernourished body seeks to utilize nutrient and fat components from reserve deposits. This quickly raises blood fats and further increases the risk of gallstone formation. The sudden formation of gallstones among people following rapid weight loss programs appears to be a result of increased cholesterol and decreased bile salts in the bile.

Gallstones are also common among obese patients who lose weight rapidly after gastric bypass surgery. In gastric bypass surgery, the size of the stomach is reduced, preventing the person from overeating. One study found that more than 71 percent of patients who had gastric bypass surgery developed gallstones within three months of the surgery[101].

Because gallstones are a common complication of the rapid weight loss following any type of bariatric surgery, some surgeons now also remove the gallbladder as a *precaution*. However, neither the bariatric surgery nor the removal of the gallbladder has any long-term benefit at all, but may lead to even more serious health conditions than obesity.

People who have had gastric bypass surgery or other bariatric weight loss surgery also have an even higher increased risk of brittle bones than previously found[102]. A full analysis, published in the *Endocrine Society* in June 2011, showed that patients who had bariatric surgery have 2.3 times

[101]"Follow-up of Nutritional and Metabolic Problems After Bariatric Surgery", DIABETES CARE, Journal of the American Diabetes Association, January 2012, 35 (1), http://care.diabetesjournals.org/content/28/2/481.full
[102]The Endocrine Society (2011, June 4). Bariatric surgery linked to increased fracture risk. *Science Daily*. Retrieved December 30, 2011

the chance of fractures compared with the general population, as opposed to the 1.8-fold increased risk found initially.

Other problems caused by this surgical procedure are severe hair loss, kidney disease, liver disease, nutritional deficiencies concerning vitamins B_{12}, K, A, D, and E, iron (leading to ulcers), as well as unusual body odors. Patients will also have to endure the inconveniences of having frequent bowel movements (over 10 times a day) and the foul-smelling stool that malabsorption of fat causes.

Chronic dehydration, which is one of the most serious conditions causing hundreds of different diseases, is also very common among bariatric patients. This is due to the fact that a surgically created gastric pouch has less than 50 ml holding capacity, and patients can no longer hold more than a few small sips worth of water at a time. Unless they sip small amounts of water throughout day (and night), their body becomes often severely dehydrated.

I would like to make the point that the aforementioned research findings, which refer to an increased risk of gallstones following bariatric surgery, only relate to gallstones in the gallbladder. The damage done to the liver itself through this procedure is likely to be far greater than the negative effects that organ suffers as a result of a few gallstones accumulating in the gallbladder. Liver damage is a serious side effect that can lead to cancer, heart disease, diabetes, or premature death.

If substantial or rapid weight loss increases the risk of developing gallstones, the obvious way to reduce this risk is to lose weight safely and more gradually. In fact, this problem is solved when toxic waste deposits, including gallstones in the liver and gallbladder, are removed from the body and a balanced lifestyle and appropriate diet are implemented[103]. In such a case, weight loss does not *increase* the risk of gallbladder disease, but *reduces* it.

By eliminating all stones from the liver and gallbladder and keeping the intestines clean, an obese person can drastically improve digestive functions and gain a renewed state of vitality. Such an approach cuts out the harmful side effects that may be associated with sudden weight loss and mostly unnecessary surgical procedures, such as bariatric bypass and gallbladder removal.

---

[103] For in-depth details, see my books Timeless Secrets of Health and Rejuvenation and Feel Great, Lose Weight

Low-Fat Blunders

The promotion of a low-fat diet as the *healthiest diet* can be held partly responsible for the continuous increase in liver and gallbladder disease among the populations of the developed nations. Whereas foods high in protein are still heralded as being crucial for the development of physical strength and vitality, fats, have been branded as a culprit for causing many of today's chronic diseases, including coronary heart disease.

At the beginning of the twentieth century, heart attacks were extremely rare anywhere in the world. Since that time, fat consumption, per capita, has remained almost the same. Yet, since World War II, the consumption of protein has risen most dramatically in the more affluent population groups of the world.

The overconsumption of protein foods in industrialized nations has caused an unprecedented number of circulatory diseases, as well as fatalities resulting from heart attacks. In comparison, these health problems occur only rarely among ethnic groups that consume mostly vegetarian foods. In fact, a report issued by the American Medical Association stated that a vegetarian diet could prevent 97 percent of all cases of thrombosis leading to heart attacks.

Although a balanced vegetarian diet may contain large amounts of fats, they do not seem to have any detrimental effects on the circulatory system (unless, of course, they are contaminated by harmful trans fatty acids). By contrast, overeating proteins of animal origin congests the liver's blood vessels (sinusoids), which leads to gallstone formation in the bile ducts (see *Overeating Protein* in this chapter).

The presence of gallstones in the liver's bile ducts reduces bile production in the liver. Diminished bile secretions undermine the body's ability to digest fats. Because of subsequent indigestion, possible weight gain, and other discomforts arising from such a condition, doctors tell their affected patients to cut down on dietary fats. But this well-intended advice only further restricts the gallbladder in trying to empty its bile contents. This leads to gallstones in the gallbladder and, consequently, to ever-increasing problems with fat digestion. Eventually, the body will run short of useful essential fats and fat-soluble vitamins. This prompts the liver to increase cholesterol production, causing even more gallstones to be formed.

The less fat the body receives with the food, the worse the situation becomes. However, since fats cannot be digested properly anymore, the body's basic functions undergo a vicious cycle, which in most cases can only be stopped by removing *all* gallstones from the liver and gallbladder and then gradually increasing fat intake to normal levels.

Milk Fat Lies

Low-fat milk is one of the culprits that could start such a vicious cycle. In its natural state, full-fat milk contains the right amount of the fats required to digest milk proteins. Without milk fats, the milk protein remains undigested. When much of the milk fat is removed from the milk, the gallbladder is not stimulated enough to release the right amounts of bile necessary to help digest both the milk proteins and the remaining milk fats. Hence, milk proteins and remaining fats are passed into the GI tract without being digested properly. Much of the protein putrefies, and the fats turn rancid.

All this leads to severe lymphatic congestion, as is often seen in the bloated stomachs of formula-fed babies[104]. The babies suffer from intestinal colic. Instead of being lean, their faces are moon-like, and their arms, legs, and stomach are puffy and bloated. These babies are susceptible to colds and other infections, have sleeping problems, and tend to cry a lot. The undigested cow's milk or milk formula may be responsible for the development of gallstones in the livers of very young children. Even the whole-fat milk offered in food stores today has a reduced fat content, making milk indigestible for most people[105].

Think milk? Think twice! There are other concerns you need to be aware if still you consider milk to be a healthy food.

First, according to a Harvard Magazine article by Jonathan Shaw (May-June 2007)[106], today's milk may no longer be nature's perfect food. The article titled "Modern Milk" discusses the implications of research conducted by Ganmaa Davaasambuu, M.D., Ph.D., who is a physician, scientist and research fellow at the Harvard School of Public Health.

---

[104] Such congestion is also seen in women who are told they need to drink milk to keep their bones strong
[105] For further details about the dangers involved in eating low-fat or *light* foods, as well as milk, see my book *Timeless Secrets of Health and Rejuvenation*
[106] Modern Milk: http://harvardmagazine.com/2007/05/modern-milk.html

"In a 2002 study of cancer and diet in 42 countries, Ganmaa and colleagues found that countries with the highest consumption of dairy products suffered the highest rates of prostatic and testicular cancer. A similar study Ganmaa did in 2005 showed much the same results for breast, ovarian, and uterine cancers," writes Shaw. Estrogens and other growth factors have been implicated in the development of these hormone-dependent cancers.

Ganmaa discovered that while the levels of hormones found in commercially produced cow's milk may be harmful to human health, in naturally produced cow's milk the hormone levels are too low to have the same effect. Apparently, the seasonal milking practices still used in Mongolia and some other developing countries - the same as those used in Westernized countries until the 1920s - ensured that "cows produce milk only during the first three months of a new pregnancy, when hormone levels are low," writes Shaw. For instance, their raw milk contains only one-tenth the progesterone that Ganmaa and her colleagues found in commercially produced milk in Japan.

Ganmaa says modern dairies milk cows well into their next pregnancy, which is the main reason why their milk contains much higher levels of biologically active hormones. Of course, modern dairy farms try to get as much milk out of their cows as possible, and for as long periods as possible, and they don't care much about what this does to the health of the cows or to the unsuspecting consumer of their products.

If you prefer not to ingest a cocktail of prescription drugs when you drink a glass of commercially produced milk, it's best to keep this altered product far away from yourself and your family. In a recent study published in the *Journal of Agricultural and Food Chemistry*[107], researchers reported that one single glass of milk can contain as many as 20 different kinds of antibiotics, lipid regulators, beta-blockers, anti-epileptics, painkillers, and hormones.

According to the study's researchers, these pharmaceutical residues, now found in cow, goat, and human breast milk, originate from a variety of medical drugs used to treat animal and human illnesses.

---

[107]Simultaneous Determination of 20 Pharmacologically Active Substances in Cow's Milk, Goat's Milk, and Human Breast Milk by Gas Chromatography–Mass Spectrometry
J. Agric. Food Chem., 2011, 59 (9), pp 5125–5132

Previous research showed that milk also contains numerous herbicides, pesticides, up to 200 times the safe levels of dioxins, blood, pus, feces, and plenty of viruses and infectious bacteria.

Dioxins, particularly, are some of the most toxic substances known to man, and the WHO admits that approximately 90 percent of the dioxins entering the human body come from dairy products, meat, fish and shellfish. Dioxins have been shown to cause serious reproductive and developmental problems, damage the immune system, interfere with hormones, and also cause cancer.

In spite of the grave harm that dioxins in foods have proven to cause to the human body, have you ever heard any regulatory health agency, such as the FDA and CDC, warn parents about feeding their kids cancer-causing chemicals when they put milk in their cereals, cheese in their sandwich, bacon on their eggs, or a hamburger on their dinner plate?

Since the all-powerful dairy and meat lobbyists still control government policies, you are on your own when it comes to protecting your children and yourself against this *legalized drug pushing* effort by the food industry. They know what's in their food, and they hate it when you find out that their products can make you sick.

Fortunately, some of the most learned members of our society are beginning to stand up for the rest of us. "I had hoped that USDA [United States Department of Agriculture] would be able to give Americans the clear advice about diet that they deserve," stated Dr. Walter Willett - Fredrick John Stare Professor of Epidemiology and Nutrition, and chair of the Department of Nutrition at Harvard School of Public Health. "However, the continued failure to highlight the need to cut back on red meat and limit most dairy products suggests that 'Big Beef' and 'Big Dairy' retain their strong influence within this department."

Dr. Willet rightly asked this rhetoric question: "Might it be time for the USDA to recuse itself because of conflicts of interest and get out of the business of dietary advice?" USDA officials were (allegedly) influenced by "powerful food-industry groups - the Grocery Manufacturers Association, the Sugar Association, the National Milk Producers Federation and the National Cattleman's Beef Association - among others," according to Dr Willet.

In September 2011, the Harvard School of Public Health sent a strong message to the USDA and the people of the United States with the release of its 'Healthy Eating Plate' food guide. The university was responding to the USDA's new MyPlate guide for healthy eating, which replaced the outdated and misguided food pyramid.

Harvard's nutrition experts declared that the university's food guide was based on sound nutrition research and unlike the MyPlate guide, not influenced by food industry lobbyists. Harvard's food guide shows an absence of dairy products based on Harvard's assessment that "...high intake can increase the risk of prostate cancer and possibly ovarian cancer[108]."

2. Pharmacological Drugs

First of all, there is no synthetic medication that is safe. All pharmaceutical drugs are designed to manipulate (suppress or stimulate) some natural functions or processes in the body, and therefore will cause either short-term or long-term side effects.

For example, a fever-reducing drug like acetaminophen (Tylenol, Tempra) or ibuprofen (Motrin, Advil) interferes with the body's natural healing system (immune system) which consists of producing specialized immune cells and antibodies in order to counteract a particular toxin or pathogen.

Not allowing the body to complete its own healing process, which may involve infection and inflammation, fever to produce more immune cells, excessive perspiration, loss of appetite and stamina to save energy and direct it toward healing, etc., can have serious consequences, such as liver damage and death. Since these drugs are available in numerous dosage forms and strengths, and doctors can never exactly know which dosage is right for the patient, dosing errors are bound to happen. It is just not possible for anyone to determine how quickly or efficiently a patient's body absorbs, metabolizes, or responds to the active ingredients of a particular drug. That is why dosing errors are a major cause of death.

Second, almost all medical drugs only target the symptoms of a disease, not the disease itself. Suppressing or alleviating the symptoms of disease leaves the underlying causes intact, which furthers a person's chances of developing a chronic illness and a dependency on using the medication, and possibly, taking other drugs to counteract the side effects created by the original medication.

---

[108]Harvard Declares Dairy NOT Part of Healthy Diet   ,http://www.care2.com/

The magnitude of this ever-escalating dilemma can be far-reaching but it is also unpredictable. Every person responds differently. A person with a stronger constitution may not notice the undercurrents of disturbance in the body for quite some time, whereas a person of a weaker constitution or an existing health history may more likely feel unwell and succumb to the impact of the medically-induced interference.

Regardless of the constitutional fortitude, or lack thereof, all synthetic drugs must be broken and detoxified by the liver. However, the liver is not designed to handle man-made chemicals. When exposed to them on a regular basis, it will suffer the consequences of their toxic effects. The liver can only remove noxious, harmful substances via its bile ducts, but this alters the natural flora and balance of bile constituents. This makes synthetic drugs to be a major reason for gallstones to develop in both the biliary tree of the liver and the gallbladder.

The wonder drugs Tylenol and Advil are only wonderful with regard to blocking pain, which plays an important part in the body's healing attempt, but they are also known for their ability to destroy one of the most powerful organs in the body. They may give you the blessing of temporary pain relief, but they also put you on the path of permanent debility, sickness, and possibly, death.

Dangerous "Drug Safety" Protocols

There is another major problem with pharmaceuticals drugs. In spite of repeated assurances by the Federal Drug Administration (FDA), claiming strict regulatory protocols ensure America's pharmaceutical drugs among the safest in the world, the exact opposite is true. It is a fact that 80 percent of US pharmaceuticals are made with overseas ingredients, nearly half of which are produced in foreign facilities never inspected by the FDA.

According to a 2009 report in *The New York Times*, titled "Drug Making's Move Abroad Stirs Concerns", most of the ingredients used for manufacturing critical drugs like antibiotics, allergy medicines, diabetes medications, and high blood pressure medications, are now almost exclusively produced in either China or India[109]. "The lack of regulation around outsourcing is a blind spot that leaves room for supply disruptions, counterfeit medicines, even bioterrorism," said Senator Sherrod Brown, Democrat of Ohio.

---

[109]Drug Making's Move Abroad Stirs Concerns, The New York Times, January 19, 2009

According to the *New York Times* report, "Of the 1,154 pharmaceutical plants mentioned in generic drug applications to the FDA in 2007, only 13 percent were in the United States, 43 percent were in China, and 39 percent were in India." Since half of all Americans take a prescription medicine every day, the number of additional injuries caused by possibly counterfeit, tainted, or otherwise altered drugs, is simply unimaginable. I doubt that the extent of harm done by tainted drugs can ever be measured, given the already high degree of normally occurring side effects that even *safe* drugs produce in the human body.

What's most disturbing about this trend is that very little is being done to address this problem. In 2008, for example, at least 81 people in the US died from a tainted heparin drug (a common blood thinning medication) produced in India. The drug contained an active ingredient that was produced in China. It is now becomingly increasingly difficult to trace drug ingredients to their source. Since even a *safe* version of heparin can cause debilitating side effects such as hemorrhaging to death, liver damage, neuropathy and osteoporosis, just imagine what a *lesser than safe* heparin can do to a patient!

The corrupt FDA protects the pharmaceutical industry at any cost and it prefers to use its financial resources to shut down companies that sell harmless food supplements (made in the US) or harass and prosecute farmers who sell raw milk to members of raw food clubs.

The *New York Times* article noted "One federal database lists nearly 3,000 overseas drug plants that export to the United States; the other lists 6,800 plants. Nobody knows which is right." According to this report, "Drug labels often claim that the pills are manufactured in the United States, but the listed plants are often the sites where foreign-made drug powders are pounded into pills and packaged."

In other words, drug safety regulation is between completely obscure to minimally existent. If you are taking a medical drug, you may be playing Russian roulette with your life. You cannot even determine whether the drug-caused injury you experience is due to the normal toxicity of the drug or because it is contaminated with mold, toxic metals, viruses, common allergens, or other harmful substances.

Nightmares of Medicinal Addiction

Despite the fact that most major causes of preventable death are now on the decline (due to improved hygiene and sanitary conditions, heightened health awareness, more exercise, balanced diet, etc.), deaths from prescription drug use are on the increase, and growing almost exponentially. This has been revealed by a *Los Angeles Times* analysis of recently released data from the US Centers for Disease Control and Prevention (CDC).

Prescription drugs are now killing far more people than illegal drugs or traffic accidents, according to the *Los Angeles Times* analysis of 2009 death statistics. In that year, 37,485 people died from prescription drugs and 36,284 from traffic accidents. Apparently, it's more life-endangering to take a prescription drug than to drive a car.

Further, abuse of popular prescription drugs like Xanax, Vicodin, OxyContin, and Soma is now responsible for more deaths than heroin and cocaine combined.

What is most disconcerting about this analysis is that not only is the death toll highest among people in their 40s, but also teenagers and older people are affected by this new health crisis. In the April 10, 2010 issue of the *Baltimore Sun,* Dr. Nancy Rosen-Cohenin wrote a sobering piece on this subject: "The Quiet Epidemic, Prescription Drug Abuse Destroys Millions Of Lives," in which she writes, "The dangers of prescription drug abuse are growing at an exponential rate. Between 1992 and 2002, the number of prescriptions written increased by 61 percent, but the number of prescriptions written for opiates increased by almost 400 percent. Opiates reflect three-quarters of all prescription drugs abused. Actor Heath Ledger had Vicodin (hydrocodone), OxyContin (oxycodone), Valium (diazepam), and Xanax (alprazolam) in his bloodstream when he died. All are legal opiates."

This unsettling trend was confirmed by recently published CDC data, which shows that hospitalizations for poisoning by prescription opioids, sedatives and tranquilizers jumped 65 percent from 1999 to 2006. According to the report, one-third of new addicts admit that their first drug experience was with prescription drugs.

At a time when medical treatment is causing more harm than good, we are being challenged to take responsibility for our own health. Treating away the symptoms of an illness with magic bullets (medical drugs) and disregarding the body's natural response to it are at the root of a medical catastrophe unfolding before us. I don't know anyone who doesn't know someone in their circle of their relatives or friends who does not suffer from some kind of debilitating illness or another, and who does not also take at least one prescription drug. It is almost considered *normal* now to suffer from one ailment or another.

Just removing the symptoms of an illness while disregarding what causes them, is certainly very tempting, but achieving such temporary relief can also become the source of an incurable drug addiction. Since all drugs alter the body's biochemistry, including that of the brain, drug addiction may actually start right from the first day of birth.

Children's vaccines contain a cocktail of up to 63 toxic chemicals, preservatives and drugs, such as the carcinogenic formaldehyde, antibiotics, metals, anti-freeze agents[110], etc. By the time these children become teenagers, many of them will feel restless, confused, or disoriented. Their brain's pleasure centers are no longer able to secrete balanced amounts of pleasure drugs or pain/tension-relieving drugs (such as dopamine, serotonin, endorphins, etc.) and they start craving happiness, peace of mind, and bliss. These can be temporarily increased through the action of externally delivered drugs, such as heroin and cocaine, or synthetic drugs that contain the same or similar addictive substances.

All painkillers, antidepressants, antipsychotics, anxiolytics, antiemetics, and antimigraine drugs, as well as the psychedelic drugs and empathogens disrupt complex and normally well-balanced regulatory systems in the human brain. A recent study published in the *British Medical Journal* has found that antipsychotic drugs are responsible for killing at least 1,800 dementia patients in US nursing homes a year. Antipsychotics are not typically administered to dementia patients, but an increasing number of doctors and nursing home personnel are now prescribing them for dementia, anyway.

"For a minority of people with dementia, antipsychotics should be used, but then only for up to 12 weeks, and under the correct circumstances," said Dr. Anne Corbett, research manager at the Alzheimer's Society, commenting on the research. "For the majority (of patients), they do far more harm than good." Of course, the study only looked at dementia patients. Atypical antipsychotic drugs are given to

---

[110]For details, see my book <u>Vaccine-nation: Poisoning the Population, One Shot at a Time</u>

millions of people, mostly for schizophrenia; they serve as killing machines to get rid of tens of thousands of *useless* members of society, or at least to make them more sick and reap the financial benefits from treating the horrendous side effects these drugs cause. Many antipsychotic drugs do not work, cause other diseases, and increase health costs, according to a 2011 Stanford University School of Medicine and University of Chicago study[111]. The researchers show that in 2008, nearly 17 million Americans received antipsychotic drug treatment, at the staggering cost of $10 billion. It is unimaginable how hundreds of thousands of people died or fell seriously ill because of being abused this way. This FDA-sanctioned genocide of the psychologically or otherwise mentally challenged members of our society reminds me of Hitler's approach of exterminating *undesirable parasites* from Nazi Germany.

Taking mind-altering drugs, such as antipsychotics like Abilify and Zyprexa and antidepressants like Prozac, not only endangers one's own life, but that of others, too. Since every person is unique, it is impossible for anyone to predict what behavioral changes may occur in a person whose brain chemicals and personality traits are being altered by severely toxic drugs.

A study published in 2010 in the prestigious medical journal PLoS ONE titled, "Prescription Drugs Associated with Reports of Violence Towards Others" found that acts of violence towards others are a genuine and serious adverse drug event associated with the use of antidepressants with serotonergic effects, and with other drugs that increase the availability of dopamine[112]. The most dangerous drugs implicated with causing suicide and homicide, for example, in school shootings, include: varenicline (Chantix), fluoxetine (Prozac), paroxetine (Paxil), amphetamines: (various), mefoquine (Lariam), atomoxetine (Strattera), triazolam (Halcion), fluvoxamine (Luvox), venlafaxine (Effexor), and desvenlafaxine (Pristiq).

Usually, a person who takes a hallucinogenic or prescription drug feels motivated or tempted to do so because he wants to feel more pleasure or relieve depression or stress. Repeated drug use disrupts the brain chemistry to the degree that the original motivation behind it is replaced with an all-consuming desire to take the drug. The reward for taking the drug lies in a

---

[111]Evidence lacking for widespread use of costly antipsychotic drugs, says researcher, Stanford University School of Medicine Jan 7, 2011
[112]Prescription Drugs Associated with Reports of Violence Towards Others, Moore TJ, Glenmullen J, Furberg CD (2010). PLoS ONE 5(12): e15337. doi:10.1371/journal.pone.0015337

surge of pleasure that results from the secretion of dopamine, the body's main pleasure hormone. The person remembers the pleasure surge and wants it repeated. Soon, all that matters is the drive to seek and use the drug, which of course, may have devastating consequences in that person's life, and affect his job, family, and relationships.

The first few times a person uses one of these drugs, he will experience very large and rapid dopamine surges (highs). However, since the brain responds to this imbalance by reducing normal dopamine activity, these periods of euphoria are soon followed by feelings of emptiness and depression (lows).

All repeated drug use leads to a reduction of dopamine activity. But since our ability to experience pleasure depends on our brain's ability to produce and release dopamine, the brain's dopamine system (which now lowers dopamine when triggered by the drug) no longer allows the addicted person to feel any pleasure even if he increases the drug's dosage or frequency of using it.

The prescription drug dilemma is wide-spread. Dr. Rosen-Cohenin says, "According to the White House Office of National Drug Control Policy, prescription drugs are second to marijuana as the drug of choice for today's teens. In fact, 7 of the top 10 drugs used by 12th graders were prescription drugs. More than 40 percent of high school seniors reported that painkillers are *fairly* or *very* easy to get. They also reported that they believed that if they were to get caught, there was less shame attached to the use of prescription drugs than to street drugs. This mirrors the perceptions of their parents, who when queried said that they felt prescription drugs were a safer alternative to drugs typically sold by a drug dealer."

Antidepressants have recently come under fire because of a Harvard study that shows placebos work no less effectively for depression than antidepressants, but without the accompanying horrendous side effects. A CBS segment that aired on February 19, 2012 on *60 Minutes Overtime*, titled, "Treating Depression: Is There A Placebo Effect?" revealed the scam tactics that the Big Pharma and the FDA have used to put millions of people on dangerous antidepressant medications without any more benefits than what harmless placebo pills can accomplish just as well.

I strongly recommend every person who either personally takes antidepressants, or who knows someone who does, to watch this short video[113]. According to the Harvard research, it is not the drugs used for treating depression that makes people feel better, it is the placebo effect.

Modern Medicine - Mankind's Greatest Killing Machine

Overall, over 20 million Americans have experimented with prescription drugs for reasons other than medicinal. But addiction-causing drug use (leading to abuse) is not the only problem created by widespread use of pharmaceutical drugs. Adverse drug reactions (ADRs) are responsible for 106,000 deaths each year in US hospitals alone, and the total number of people having in-hospital adverse drug reactions each year are more than 2.2 million, according to a 2003 review study of existing research data[114]. The review study found that the average number of yearly iatrogenic (doctor-caused) deaths is 783,936. The total cost of just the adverse drug reactions to society are more than $136 billion annually - far greater than the total cost of cardiovascular or diabetic care.

In 1998, the *Journal of the American Medical Association* released its own study and admitted this in the study conclusion: "The incidence of serious and fatal ADRs in US hospitals was found to be extremely high[115]." Yet not much has changed since this catastrophic problem was first officially acknowledged and studied. According to a more recent 2010 analysis by the *New England Journal of Medicine*[116], researchers found that despite efforts to improve patient safety in the past few years, the healthcare system is still as injurious and life-endangering as before.

None of the mentioned data actually include the counts of ADRs and deaths reported by general practitioners. In addition, the FDA admits that medical doctors only report between 1 and 10 percent of all drug reactions. The true numbers of iatrogenic disease and death may therefore be much higher than those recorded.

According to the US Census Bureau, approximately 2.5 million people die each year in the US from all causes, including deaths from accidents,

[113]Treating Depression: Is there a placebo effect? CBS 60 Minutes; to view, go to www.cbsnews.com and copy/paste this title into their search window.
[114]Death By Medicine: http://articles.mercola.com/sites/articles/archive/2003/11/26/death-by-medicine-part-one.aspx
[115]Incidence of adverse drug reactions in hospitalized patients: a meta-analysis of prospective studies, JAMA. 1998 Apr 15;279(15):1200-5
[116]Temporal trends in rates of patient harm resulting from medical care. N Engl J Med. 2010 Nov 25;363(22):2124-34

medical treatments, and old age. The medical system, though, is clearly the single most leading cause of injury and death.

Each year, an ever-increasing number of people become sick because of short-term and long-term adverse drug reactions, especially children. A comprehensive study published in the *Journal of Pediatrics* (16 September 2011), titled, "The Growing Impact of Pediatric Pharmaceutical Poisoning" pointed out the seriousness of this medical predicament.

The authors of this study evaluated 453,559 children for ingestion of a single pharmaceutical product. The researchers found that child self-exposure (of medication) was responsible for 95 percent of hospital visits. Child self-exposure to prescription products dominated the healthcare impact with 248,023 of the visits (55 percent), 41,847 admissions (76 percent), and 18,191 significant injuries (71 percent). According to the stated results of the study, the greatest resource use and morbidity followed self-ingestion of prescription products, particularly opioids, sedative-hypnotics, and cardiovascular agents. The authors concluded that prevention efforts have proved to be inadequate in the face of rising availability of prescription medications, particularly the more dangerous medications.

According to the National Institute of Drug Abuse (NIDA), in 2009, there were nearly 4.6 million drug-related ER visits nationwide[117]. Almost half of these visits were attributed to adverse reactions to pharmaceuticals taken as prescribed.

In a revealing article titled, "The Problem with Medicine: We Don't Know If Most of It Works[118]", published online in *Discover Magazine* (February 11, 2011), authors Jeanne Lenzer and Shannon Brownlee aptly describe the current medical deception:

"In a recent poll conducted by the Campaign for Effective Patient Care, a nonprofit advocacy group based in California, 65 percent of the 800 California voters surveyed said they thought that most or nearly all of the healthcare they receive is based on scientific evidence. The reality would probably shock them. A panel of experts convened in 2007 by the prestigious Institute of Medicine estimated that well below half of the procedures doctors perform and the decisions they make about surgeries, drugs, and tests have been adequately investigated and shown to be

---

[117]Highlights from the 2009 Drug Abuse Warning Network InfoFacts: Drug-Related Hospital Emergency Room Visits, http://www.nida.nih.gov/infofacts/hospitalvisits.html
[118]The Problem With Medicine: We Don't Know If Most of It Works, November 2010 issue; published online February 11, 2011 (www.discovermagazine.com)

effective. The rest are based on a combination of guesswork, theory, and tradition, with a strong dose of marketing by drug and device companies. Doctors are often as much in the dark as their patients when they implant new devices... perform surgery, or write prescriptions. ... Many widely adopted surgeries, devices, tests, and drugs also rest on surprisingly thin data..."

"...According to an Agency for Healthcare Research and Quality report published in 2001[119], more than 770,000 Americans are injured or die each year from drug complications, including unexpected side effects, some of which might have been avoided if somebody had conducted the proper research," write Lenzer and Brownlee.

Believe it or not, you can find this report on the website of the US Department of Health & Human Services. Not every health agency is determined to cover up the grave dangers to life caused by modern medicine.

The lesson we can learn from all this is that there can be no science-backed guarantee that the prescription medication you may be taking is not going to seriously harm you or even kill you - regardless of the *safety* assurances your doctor may be giving you. When millions of people end up in the emergency room after taking an aspirin, an antibiotic, a blood sugar drug or a painkiller, it is crystal clear that there is no real objective science behind the advertised benefits of pharmaceutical drugs. Every person responds to the chemical suppression of symptoms of disease in different and unpredictable ways. As it turns out, the bypassing or blocking of the body's own natural healing mechanisms can be very risky.

Cancer Drugs Make Tumors More Deadly

For the past 20 years, I have been making the so-called *outrageous* claim that common cancer treatments, including chemotherapy medications, radiation therapy, and angiogenesis inhibitors used for shrinking cancerous tumors are largely responsible for making them more aggressive and develop in other parts of the body (erroneously called *metastases*) as well[120]. Over the years I have received a fair amount of ridicule, defamatory comments, and outright death threats for publishing my unrelenting stance on the subject.

[119]Reducing and Preventing Adverse Drug Events To Decrease Hospital Costs. **Research in Action,** Issue 1. AHRQ Publication Number 01-0020, March 2001
[120]For details, see my book Cancer is Not a Disease - It's Healing Mechanism

The National Cancer Institute states on its website: "Angiogenesis inhibitors are unique cancer-fighting agents because they tend to inhibit the growth of blood vessels rather than tumor cells. In some cancers, angiogenesis inhibitors are most effective when combined with additional therapies, especially chemotherapy." However, a 2012 study which was supported by the National Institutes of Health (NIH) sheds new light on why this *effectiveness* of these cancer-fighting drugs is actually short-lived and can turn into a frightening scenario with possibly fatal consequences. The new research shows that aggressive treatment (used for shrinking or removing even relatively small, slow-growing or encapsulated, harmless tumors) may create a situation where the entire body is riddled with highly aggressive cancers.

This study, published in the January 17, 2012 issue of *Cancer Cell*[121], finds that a group of little-explored cells that are part of every primary cancerous tumor may serve as important gatekeepers against cancer progression and metastasis. A relatively new class of anti-cancer drugs - angiogenic inhibitors - diminishes or destroys these cells, called pericytes, by cutting off the blood supply to the tumors.

Scientists and oncologists from around the world made the shortsighted assumption that by cutting off a tumor's life support system consisting of a tumor's blood vessels they could achieve a successful and permanent tumor regression. Little did they know that this would open a Pandora's box and create a cancer nightmare.

Cancer's Wisdom in Action

Seen from a holistic and truly scientific perspective, the above assumption is critically flawed. I have frequently made the argument that cancer is one of the body's final healing attempts to return to a balanced condition (homeostasis), and this new research clearly illustrates that cancer constitutes one of the body's most highly evolved and sophisticated protective mechanisms.

The study found that therapies - which shrink cancer by cutting off tumors' blood supply - may be inadvertently making tumors more aggressive and likely to spread. Said differently, to help prevent a cancer from getting out of control and invading other parts of the body, the body

---

[121]Pericyte Depletion Results in Hypoxia-Associated Epithelial-to-Mesenchymal Transition and Metastasis Mediated by Met Signaling Pathway. Cancer Cell, Volume 21, Issue 1, 66-81, 17 January 2012 (http://www.cell.com/cancer-cell/retrieve/pii/S1535610811004478)

tenaciously and purposefully grows extra blood vessels. "Why would the body do such a thing?" you might ask.

Well, all cancer cells are normal cells that have turned anaerobic, meaning, they are so oxygen-deprived (due to congestion-caused oxygen deficiency) that they must mutate in order to survive and produce energy without having to use oxygen. To increase the oxygen supply to these congested cells and to support the action by pericytes to prevent cancer progression and metastasis, the body *needs* to grow new blood vessels. The currently applied medical approach of destroying these blood vessels is therefore counterproductive and must be considered dangerous. It destroys the very system the body uses to make sure a particular cancerous tumor remains an isolated and curable event and does not escalate into a widespread, uncontrollable, and self-perpetuating disease process.

To make this very clear, cancer drugs don't just destroy cancer cells but also cancer-protective cells and blood vessels transporting oxygen to both cancer cells and normal cells. Ionizing radiation and cancer drugs are outright carcinogenic, and thus, they can cause new cancer cells to develop almost anywhere in the body. With over 450 different cancer drugs on the market (mostly bestselling), all of which are extremely toxic to the human body, you can only imagine the vast number of new cancers that this must causing.

Controlling Tumor Growth Makes Cancer Spread

There is no doubt that chemotherapy drugs, angiogenic drugs, or radiation therapy can achieve significant tumor regression, but not without paying the hefty price of producing a multitude of new cancers. Besides the billions of corpses of dead cancer cells and pericytes this biological genocide leaves behind, there are also billions of inflamed or otherwise damaged cells and blood vessels that greatly increase the chances of developing any number of new, aggressive, deadly cancers.

Most of these cancers are too small, though, to be detected right away by diagnostic instruments, and doctors can get away with the proud expression, "We got it all," at least for a while. But when a year or two later, these cancers have grown larger and therefore are detectable, the same doctors tell their patients, "Unfortunately, your cancer has come back and it has now metastasized to other parts of your body as well."

The above study provides us with the unexpected finding that may actually prove current cancer treatments, including chemotherapy, angiogenic therapy, and radiation therapy, to be the greatest contributors to developing aggressive, terminal cancers and significantly lowering one's chances of survival.

In this investigation, senior author Raghu Kalluri, M.D., Ph.D., Chief of the Division of Matrix Biology at Beth Israel Deaconess Medical Center (BIDMC) and Professor of Medicine at Harvard Medical School (HMS), had actually intended to find out if targeting of pericytes could inhibit tumor growth in the same way that other drugs inhibiting blood vessel growth to tumors can. After all, pericytes are an important part of tissue vasculature[122], covering blood vessels and supporting their growth. What Kalluri and his team stumbled upon instead was both startling and extremely disturbing.

In an article titled, "Study Shows How A Group of Tumor Cells Prevent Cancer Spread - Paradoxical Discovery Finds That Pericyte Cells Help Prevent Metastasis[123]", Bonnie Prescott at Beth Israel Deaconess Medical Center, Harvard Medical School, describes the dire implications of the study in some greater detail.

When applied to breast cancer, "Kalluri and his colleagues found that by depleting pericyte numbers by 60 percent in breast cancer tumors they saw a 30 percent decrease in tumor volumes over 25 days," writes Prescott.

Since such significant tumor shrinkage will prevent or slow the growth of the targeted cancer; conventional medical wisdom dictates that this would be a favorable effect, and oncologists have hailed this approach to be a breakthrough in cancer treatment. However, the researchers also discovered that by destroying pericytes by 60-70 percent the number of secondary lung tumors increased threefold, indicating that the tumors had metastasized.

"If you just looked at tumor growth, the results were good," says Kalluri, "but when you looked at the whole picture, inhibiting tumor vessels was not controlling cancer progression. The cancer was, in fact, spreading."

"We showed that a big tumor with good pericyte coverage is less metastatic than a smaller tumor of the same type with less pericyte coverage," says Kalluri, who corroborated these findings in multiple types

---

[122]The vessels and tissue that carry or circulate fluids such as blood or lymph through the body
[123]Study Shows How A Group of Tumor Cells Prevent Cancer Spread(http://www.bidmc.org/News/InResearch/2012/January/Kalluri_Cancer.aspx)

of cancer by repeating these same experiments with implanted renal cell carcinoma and melanoma tumors, writes Prescott.

All this questions the very argument pushed on unsuspecting cancer patients by medical professionals that treatment-caused tumor regression is a desirable objective. Just imagine that you were diagnosed with a cancerous tumor and your doctor told you that his proposed treatment could reduce the size of your tumor by 30 percent but at the same time increase your chances of developing secondary tumors by a whopping 300 percent!

Beware of Conventional Cancer Treatments

The history of conventional anti-cancer therapies is replete with cases where the treatment turned out to be far more devastating than the disease itself. This single piece of research provides us with the understanding that the body isn't reckless or irresponsible when it actually builds new blood vessels to support tumor growth. On the contrary, it is well equipped with the superb wisdom and physical means to pursue the best possible routes of survival, regardless of the circumstances such as toxicity, congestion, and emotional stress.

Attacking the body's tumor cells is still an attack on the body which is exacerbated when doctor and patient perceive cancer cells to be evil monsters that must be destroyed at any cost. Cancer diagnosis and treatment are severely stressful, violent acts against the body that will evoke a powerful fight-or-flight response that affects every part of the body. The death fright triggers continuous releases of stress hormones into the blood - powerful enough to shut down the digestive and immune system, and to constrict important blood vessels, including those that support the cancer-protective pericytes.

As this new study has demonstrated, the destruction of pericytes goes hand in hand with a dramatic increase in the number of secondary tumors in other parts of the body. The body is not a machine but a living being, and it responds with emotions and biochemical changes to everything you think, feel, and expose yourself to. Threatening the body on any level jeopardizes its healing abilities.

Cancer has a deeper meaning or purpose which I have elaborated on in my book *Cancer is Not a Disease, It's a Survival Mechanism.* Ignorance about the true purpose of cancer is at the root of these misdirected cancer treatments. The body uses its own built-in survival and healing programs to keep cancer under control and to let it (the cancer) do its job of mopping up accumulated toxins and waste products and to keep itself from spreading or showing up in other parts of the body.

After examining 130 breast cancer tumor samples of varying cancer stages and tumor sizes and comparing pericyte levels with prognosis, the scientists found that samples with low numbers of pericytes in tumors correlated with the most deeply invasive cancers, distant metastasis and 5- and 10-year survival rates lower than 20 percent.

To understand the exact mechanism behind the drastically increased risk of metastasis that follows drug treatment, I recommend you check their study, which I consider to be one of the most important pieces of cancer research ever done. I am certainly not the only one to share this belief.

"These results are quite provocative and will influence clinical programs designed to target tumor angiogenesis," says Ronald A. DePinho, president of the University of Texas MD Anderson Cancer Center. And for Kalluri and his team, the new discoveries suggest that certain assumptions about cancer must be revisited. "We must go back and audit the tumor and find out which cells play a protective role versus which cells promote growth and aggression," says Kalluri. "Not everything is black and white. There are some cells inside a tumor that are actually good in certain contexts."

One of the infamous drugs used to target the blood vessel supporting tumor is Avastin, which has already been proven to be worthless, and potentially deadly to the patient. As mentioned before, this is the same expensive drug for which there exists a commonly used counterfeit version that has its active ingredient missing.

Lessons That Cancer Teaches Us

To me, it makes no sense at all to use cancer-causing drugs and ionizing radiation to shrink malignant tumors in the short-term while causing existing cancers to become deeply invasive and deadly, and new cancers to show up in parts of the body distant to the original tumor.

With regard to chemotherapy drugs, scientists at the University of Alabama at Birmingham (UAB) Comprehensive Cancer Center and UAB Department of Chemistry are currently (in 2012) investigating the suspected possibility that dead cancer cells left over after chemotherapy become the trigger for cancer to spread to other parts of the body (metastasis). "What if by killing cancer cells with chemotherapy, we inadvertently induce DNA structures that make surviving cancers cells more invasive? The idea is tough to stomach," Katri Selander, M.D., Ph.D., an assistant professor in the UAB Division of Hematology and Oncology and co-principal researcher on the grant, said in a statement to the media.

Dead cancer cells have already been found to activate a pathway in the body mediated as a protein dubbed *toll-like receptor 9*, or TLR9, which is present in the immune system and in many kinds of cancer.

"If TLR9 boosts metastasis, then researchers will work on finding targeted therapies that block or regulate this molecular pathway," Dr. Selander stated. While angiogenic therapy has already been implicated with causing deadly metastasis, chemotherapy is almost certainly following in the same track for the same and additional reasons.

A few years ago, a leading oncologist in the US contacted me and asked me if liver flushes could help his wife who suffered from terminal lung cancer. He told me that during the past 6 years he had tried all of the most advanced chemo drugs, but to no avail. After each round of chemotherapy, more and more malignant tumors developed in the lungs and had spread to her liver and bones (now we know why). I told him that at that advanced stage, she had nothing to lose, but could turn the situation around by ridding the liver, blood and tissues of accumulated toxins. This would make tumor growth unnecessary.

The oncologist personally monitored and recorded the results of his wife's first liver flush. He reported back to me, saying that she had released an astonishing amount of at least 2,500 gallstones which kept pouring out of her over a period of three days (something that is almost unheard of).

Four weeks later, this oncologist informed me that the tumors in his wife's liver and bones had completely vanished and there was only one tiny tumor left in her left lung. I recommended that she continued doing the liver flushes until all the stones were gone. He also told me that she had become like a new person. A life-long constipation problem was gone, and her skin looked rejuvenated and was no longer pale and grayish-looking. He said she had regained the energy she used to have 20 years ago and the deep depression she had suffered from since her first cancer diagnosis had completely lifted.

Hormone Replacement and Contraception Drugs

The risk of developing gallstones is 4 times higher among women than among men. It is especially pronounced among women who have used or use birth control pills and hormone replacement therapy (HRT). According to research published in the *American Journal of Obstetrics & Gynecology,* oral contraceptives and other estrogens double a woman's chance of developing gallstones[124]. The female hormone, estrogen, which is contained in contraceptive pills and hormone replacements, increases bile cholesterol and decreases gallbladder contraction. Therefore, this estrogen-effect may be responsible for not only causing gallstones in the liver and gallbladder, but also for many other diseases that arise from diminished liver and gallbladder functions.

Several other large studies have shown that HRT doubles or triples the risk for gallstones or gallbladder surgery. A 2005 *Journal of the American Medical Association* study found that while all types of HRT raise the risks, estrogen alone has higher risks than combined estrogen and progesterone therapy. Excessive estrogen can impair liver functions and raise triglycerides, a fatty acid that increases the risk for cholesterol stones.

Recent studies on HRT reporting negative effects on the heart and increased risks for breast cancer are also making this treatment a less attractive option for most postmenopausal women. Earlier medical research also implicated progestogens such as Medroxy progesterone acetate (MPA, Depo Provera) contained in HRT drugs in the development of gallstones[125].

Contraceptive drugs containing drospirenone are potentially life-endangering drugs. After it completed its review of two 2011 studies that evaluated the risk of blood clots (venous thromboembolism) for women who use drospirenone-containing birth control pills, the FDA recently posted this warning on its website: "Women currently taking a drospirenone-containing birth control pill should be informed of the potential risk for blood clots[126]." Of course, blood clots can kill.

---

[124]Oral contraceptives and other estrogens, American Journal of Obstetrics & Gynecology (Ob Gyn, 1994; 83: 5-11)

[125]Medroxy progesterone acetate (MPA, Depo Provera) causes gallstone development Res Comm in Chem Path & Pharm, 1992; 75 [1]: 69-84

[126]FDA Drug Safety Podcast for Healthcare Professionals: Safety review update on the possible increased risk of blood clots with birth control pills containing drospirenone, Federal Drug Administration, http://www.fda.gov

Regardless of the evidence that women taking these commonly prescribed birth control pills are 150 percent more likely to develop deadly blood clots than women not using them, many conventional doctors continue prescribing them.

Synthetic drospirenone is an imitation progesterone found in Bayer's Yasmin, Safyral, Yaz, Angeliq, and Beyaz birth control drugs. These drugs have been shown to significantly increase risk of high blood potassium (hyperkalemia); blood clots in the legs indicated by pain in the calf, leg cramps, leg and foot swelling; blood clots in the lungs indicated by shortness of breath, sharp chest pain, and coughing up blood; chest pain and heaviness which may indicate a heart attack; sudden loss of vision or vision changes due to a blood clot in the eye; stroke as indicated by vision or speech changes, weakness or numbness in the arm or leg or severe headache; liver damage as indicated by jaundice, dark urine, and upper-right abdominal pain; other side effects include depression, migraines, breast lumps and breast pain, unusual vaginal bleeding, high blood pressure, acne, allergy, and endocrine disruption.

Although the highly corrupt FDA knew about these risks for many years, it decided to not make the risks public. Tragically, the drugs have been killing the women who take them. But then we cannot expect otherwise from a federal agency that has ties with drug manufactures and is sponsored by the same to protect the people from killer drugs, according to some of the FDA's own whistle-blowing scientists.

On November 23, 2004, on PBS Online News, Dr. David Graham, Associate Director for Science and Medicine in the Office of Drug Safety at the FDA, made this stunning admission: "I would argue that the FDA as currently configured is incapable of protecting America against another Vioxx. Simply put, FDA and the Center for Drug Evaluation Research (CDER) are broken. "For details of a more recent interview with Dr. Graham, see the NaturalNews.com article titled, "The FDA Exposed: An Interview with Dr. David Graham, the Vioxx Whistleblower[127]."

All hormone replacement drugs (both HRT and contraception pills) produce gallstones and disrupt liver functions. If you have used either of these in the past, I strongly recommend you clean out your liver and gallbladder.

---

[127]The FDA Exposed: An Interview With Dr. David Graham, the Vioxx Whistleblower, stunning interview with Dr. David Graham, Associate Director for Science and Medicine in the Office of Drug Safety, FDA (NaturalNews.com)

In addition, women who are going through menopause can find great relief from menopausal symptoms by doing a series of liver flushes. Improved liver performance and an increased production of bile, in particular, can prevent and reverse osteoporosis and other bone/joint problems, provided diet and lifestyle are also balanced.

Other Pharmaceutical Drugs

Sleeping Pills

If you don't want to increase your risk of dying by at least 35 percent, you are strongly advised to stay away from any common sleeping pills, even if you only take 18 or less pills a year. This is the important message we can all take to bed from a recent, carefully controlled study published in the *British Medical Journal Open*[128]. Researchers from the Daniel Kripke Viterbi Family Sleep Center, Scripps Institution in San Diego, USA, found that sleeping medications increase the risk of dying 4 times and the risk of cancer 3.5 times. What's more, people taking more than 132 sleeping pills per year are 5 times more likely to die than those not taking any hypnotics. According to the study's estimates, these drugs may have been responsible for an additional 320,000 to 507,000 deaths in the US in 2010.

Subjects (mean age 54 years) in the study were 10,529 patients who received hypnotic prescriptions and 23,676 matched controls with no hypnotic prescriptions, followed for an average of 2.5 years between January 2002 and January 2007. All other disease and mortality risk factors were excluded in the study.

Heart disease, cancer and, possibly, accidents were found to be among the most serious side effects. In the US, between 6 and 10 percent of the adult population take sleep medication, and in some parts of Europe, that percentage is even higher.

The big surprise in this study was that even a short-term, low dosage intake can have serious health risks. The researchers warned that no amount can be considered safe. The examined hypnotics included zolpidem, temazepam, eszopiclone, zaleplon, other benzodiazepines, barbiturates and sedative antihistamines. Most people are more familiar with the drug names: Ambien, Intermezzo, Lunesta, and Sonata.

---

[128]Hypnotics' association with mortality or cancer: a matched cohort study, BMJ Open 2012;2:e000850doi:10.1136/bmjopen-2012-000850

"We are not certain. But it looks like sleeping pills could be as risky as smoking cigarettes," study author Dr. Daniel F. Kripke, professor of psychiatry at the University of California, San Diego, told WebMD.

The problem with studies like the above is that hardly anyone takes notice of them. Most doctors continue dispensing sleeping pills to their patients who insist on taking an effective hypnotic drug, even if it can kill them or give them cancer.

Avoid Taking These Dangerous Drugs

Some of the world's bestselling drugs are also the most dangerous ones that are best avoided. While leaving the root causes intact, they merely replace one relatively minor health issue with a potentially life-endangering one. For example, proton pump inhibitors like Nexium and Prilosec for acid reflux disease (GERD) are now believed to increase the risk of bone fractures by about 30 percent, according to a recent study titled, "Use of Acid-Suppressive Drugs and Risk of Fracture: A Meta-analysis of Observational Studies." Bone fractures are not to be taken lightly, especially if they occur in the elderly. In fact, they are a leading cause of death among this age group. Of course, most people taking these drugs are unaware of the risks.

Prescription medications used to lower the level of fats (lipids) in the blood, including clofibrate (Atromid-S) or similar cholesterol-lowering drugs, actually increase cholesterol concentrations in the bile and, thereby, lead to an increased risk of gallstones. These drugs successfully lower blood fats, which they are designed to do. However, having high blood fats actually implies a shortage of fats. Fats become trapped in the blood when they are unable to cross capillary membranes and are, therefore, lacking in the cells. By lowering blood fats with drugs, the body's cells are starved of fats. This can lead to serious cell degeneration.

Octretide, one of the new generations of statin drugs, prevents the gallbladder from emptying itself after a fatty meal, leaving plenty of bile behind to form stones. The dangers involved in such a method of medical intervention are obvious; they are certainly more serious than having raised levels of blood fats. (Contrary to common belief, there is no scientific evidence, to date, that shows high blood fats are responsible for causing heart disease)

According to several studies published in various medical journals[129], such as the *Lancet*[130], certain antibiotics also cause gallstones. One of these is ceftriaxone, used for treating lower respiratory tract infections, skin and urinary tract infections, pelvic inflammatory disease, and bone and joint infections, as well as pneumonia and meningitis. Children are increasingly likely to develop gallstones and have their gallbladder removed, and antibiotic drugs - those given for infection and added to vaccines - are culprits in this disturbing trend.

While gallbladder disease is still relatively rare among children, with 1.3 pediatric cases occurring per every 1,000 adult cases, pediatric patients undergo 4 percent of all gallbladder surgeries (cholecystectomies). Gallbladder disease affects as many as 25 million American adults, resulting in 500,000-700,000 cholecystectomies per year.

Antirejection or immune-suppressive drugs, such as cyclosporine, given to kidney and heart transplant patients also increase the likelihood of gallstone formation[131].

Thiazides, which are water pills used to control high blood pressure, may also bring on acute gallbladder disease in patients with gallstones[132].

As mentioned before, Clofibrate and other cholesterol lowering drugs, such as ocreotide, also cause gallstones.

Furthermore, children taking furosemide (Lasix), used for treating hypertension and edema, are likely to develop gallstones, according to research published in the *Journal of Perinatology*[133]. The drugs Edecrin and Indapamide have similar side effects.

Prostaglandins, which are also used to treat high blood pressure, cause gallstones as well[134].

There are numerous drugs that raise cholesterol, thereby increasing the risk of gallstones. They include glucocorticoids such as prednisone used to suppress pain and inflammation; beta blockers such as amiodarone used for treating ventricular arrhythmias and atrial fibrillation; anabolic steroids such as testosterone; protease inhibitors used for combating human immunodeficiency virus (HIV).

---

[129]i: 165; Monatsschrift Kinderheilkunde, 1992; 140 [8]: 488-9; Schweizerische Rundschau für Medizin Praxis, 1992; 81 [33]: 966-7);
http://synapse.koreamed.org/Synapse/Data/PDFData/5037JKSS/jkss-81-423.pdf
[130]Antibiotics causing gallstones, Lancet, 1988; ii: 1411-3 and 1989; i: 165
[131]Antirejection drugs causing gallstones, J of Ped Surg, 1995; 30 [1]: 61-4
[132]Thiazides increase risk of acute cholecystitis, BMJ, 1984; 289: 654-55
[133] Furosemide (J of Perinatology, June 1992; 12 [2]: 107-111
[134]Prostaglandins (Vet & Hum Tox, Dec, 1994; 36 [6]: 514-6)

A study funded by the drug producer Boehringer Ingelheim claimed that the drug Pradaxa reduced the risk of stroke 35 percent more than the blood thinner warfarin in patients with atrial fibrillation. This sounds like good news, but the same study also found that this *miracle* drug boosts their risk of heart attack at about the same percentage when compared to warfarin. By the way, warfarin is also used as rat poison.

In spite of having had no real impact on mortality rates among these patients, this drug has been hailed as a great medical achievement. But all that the drug really does is give people a heart attack instead of letting them suffer a stroke. Of course, in spite of the absence of any real benefit of taking this drug, the researchers of the study recommended it anyway, and so does the FDA.

The FDA has already recorded over 50 cases of people who bled to death after taking Pradaxa (the real figure may be between 500 and 5,000, given that only between 1 and 10 percent of drug related deaths are actually reported to the FDA). There are plenty of other adverse effects that come with taking this heart attack-boosting medication, such as unusual bleeding from the gums, frequent nose bleeding, menstrual or vaginal bleeding that is heavier than normal, severe or uncontrollable bleeding, pink or brown urine, red or black stools that look like tar, unexplained bruises or those that get larger, coughing up blood or blood clots, vomiting blood or vomit that looks like coffee grounds.

Of course, it is expected that any rat poison-mimicking drug would have such dreadful side effects. If you are bleeding to death after taking this poison, you cannot blame your doctor for killing you. Doctors are legally obligated to administer the best available drugs even if it means they are so toxic that they will cost you your life. But human life is quite dispensable, and the business of medicine must go on.

While it is very difficult to manipulate the blood into balance at the risk of vomiting blood or dying, it is very easy to accomplish this naturally and permanently through a plant-based diet and a few liver and gallbladder flushes.

Painkillers such as aspirin and Tylenol have recently been shown to raise blood pressure by up to 34 percent, thereby damaging the liver and other organs. "People with high blood pressure don't know the risks of taking some of these painkillers," says Nieca Goldberg, M.D., a cardiologist and spokesperson for the American Heart Association. "They assume that anything you can buy over the counter is safe. But these drugs are chemicals that can cause side effects."

Women taking extra-strength Tylenol daily are twice as likely to develop high blood pressure as those who don't, suggests an older 2005 study[135].

Painkillers can raise blood pressure in both men and women, suggest new findings from Gary C. Curhan, M.D., ScD, and colleagues at Brigham and Women's Hospital and Harvard Medical School, Boston[136]. Compared with men who did not use pain relievers, the risk of high blood pressure increased by 38 percent in men who took non-steroidal anti-inflammatory drugs (NSAIDs) 6 or 7 days a week, 34 percent in men who took acetaminophen 6 or 7 days a week, and 26 percent in men who took aspirin 6 or 7 days a week.

Of course, for decades now, aspirin has been sold to an unsuspecting population as a safe drug that can prevent heart attacks. Now we know that aspirin can significantly increase one's risk of suffering a fatal heart attack by raising blood pressure. High blood pressure affects about 1 in 3 U.S. adults - an estimated 68 million, according to the CDC; and so I ask this legitimate question: "How many of these cases are actually due to daily aspirin *consumption* (many people consume it as if it were a food supplement)?"

Well, Americans consume more than 50 billion aspirin tablets and compound aspirin preparations annually. You can do the math. Given the results of the above study, that's certainly enough to create millions of new high blood pressure patients each year, many of whom may become heart disease patients. I would add here that selling so many aspirin tablets is good for business, but not good for patients.

However, besides cleaning out the liver and gallbladder and making the appropriate dietary adjustments recommended in this book, there are other natural alternatives you can use to balance an abnormal blood pressure. For instance, consider this new study by Barts and the London School of Medicine and the Peninsula Medical School, announced by BBC News online[137]. It suggests a low-cost way to treat hypertension. Drinking 500

---

[135]Tylenol raises blood pressure in women: http://www.msnbc.msn.com/id/8961817/ns/health-womens_health/t/tylenol-linked-high-blood-pressure-women/#.Twm37rKs_-J
[136]Frequency of Analgesic Use and Risk of Hypertension Among Men; Forman, J.P. *Archives of Internal Medicine*, Feb. 26, 2007; vol 167: pp 394-399
[137]http://news.bbc.co.uk/2/hi/7228420.stm

ml of beetroot juice a day can significantly reduce blood pressure, according to the study.

Hypertension has been estimated to cause around 50 percent of coronary heart disease, and approximately 75 percent of strokes. Since more than 25 percent of the world's adult population is hypertensive, an affordable, natural method like drinking beet juice is certainly a better choice than taking a potentially deadly drug.

Other serious, possibly fatal side effects of aspirin include gastrointestinal ulcers, stomach bleeding, and tinnitus, especially in higher doses. In children and adolescents, aspirin can cause Reye's syndrome, a potentially fatal disease that causes brain and liver damage, and abnormally low blood sugar.

Recently, the mass media was abuzz with new reports that daily use of aspirin can prevent cancer. However, this news flash was based on a flawed study and most likely another scam attempt by the pharma-medical industry to rescue this all-time bestselling drug from a further drop in its already declining popularity (because of its dangerous side effects).

In 2002, Professor Peter Rothwell at the Stroke Prevention Research Unit at Oxford University suggested that taking an aspirin a day could reduce your risk of cancer within 10 years after beginning the therapy. Now in 2 new studies, Dr. Rothwell claims that protective effects would be seen after just 3 years of taking the drug once daily.

However, the new claims are actually not based on any new research at all but consist of a re-analysis of about 90 previously published studies. The main flaw in this new analysis is that, for some unexplained reason, Dr. Rothwell excluded several major US trials that followed at least 61,000 men and women for 10-12 years and failed to show any cancer-protective benefit from aspirin use[138].

In addition to cherry-picking some possible protective benefits from the selected 90 previous studies, while completely ignoring the contradicting evidence, the average dose of aspirin given to the subjects in these studies far exceeded the recommended *safe* dose of 75-81 mg/day. Since no doctors would prescribe their patients a higher daily dose (because it can cause severe bleeding or stroke), Dr. Rothwell's statement, "In terms of prevention, anyone with a family history (of cancer) would be sensible to take aspirin," is simply dangerous and irresponsible.

---

[138] JAMA. 2005 Jul 6; 294(1):47-55. http://www.ncbi.nlm.nih.gov/pubmed/15998890.1

If Dr. Rothwell's recommendation were to be followed by medical practitioners, millions of more people would be put on the safe dose of aspirin (which may still cause serious side effects), in spite of the fact that it is not potent enough to have any significant cancer-protective benefits. To this day, no cancer-preventive benefit has been shown by taking the recommended daily dose of 75 mg. And even if there are some cancer-preventive effects from daily aspirin use, we need to ask the question: Is it worth the significantly increased risk of dying from gastrointestinal bleeding or hemorrhagic stroke?

Many doctors give aspirin to people right after they suffer a heart attack. Over the course of several decades I was fortunate to help many individuals get over a heart attack within 2-3 minutes simply by strongly squeezing the sides of the tips of their little fingers (where the heart and small intestinal meridians end) for about 1-2 minutes. Those individuals walked away saying they never felt this good in years. This method almost right away removes all chest pressure, and no damage occurs to the heart muscles. Another good approach is to give them a teaspoon of cayenne pepper in a cup of water to drink, if they are in the position to drink it. I have never seen the same instant results with people taking aspirin.

Once hooked to aspirin, it is difficult to get off it without risking one's life. One 2011 study published in the British Journal of Medicine[139] has shown that discontinuation of low dose aspirin increases the risk of non-fatal myocardial infarction in patients with a history of ischemic events in primary care. In other words, once you are a heart attack patient and take aspirin, by going off the drug even just for a day or two, you are two thirds more likely to suffer another attack.

It's obvious that aspirin doesn't cure anything; it just keeps you enslaved to taking this drug forever, while giving you more and more adverse effects. This is the price we pay for continuing to be fascinated with suppressing the symptoms of disease instead of addressing its root causes.

Recently, the FDA has approved the new, expensive cancer drug, Voraxaze (glucarpidase), to help treat the deadly side effects caused by the highly toxic chemotherapy drug, methotrexate. Voraxaze was designed to expel methotrexate from the body, but not without causing its own set of serious side effects.

---

[139] Discontinuation of low dose aspirin and risk of myocardial infarction, BMJ 2011;343:d4094

Methotrexate has been shown to fatally damage the liver, kidneys, and intestines. The drug tends to remain in the body because it damages these eliminative organs so severely that they cannot remove it anymore. Of course, when the person dies, the death certificate will say he died from cancer, not from drug poisoning.

All pharmaceutical drugs are toxic by nature and require detoxification by the liver. Yet, impaired liver function permits many of these toxic chemicals to enter the bile. This alters the natural balance of its constituents and leads to the development of gallstones in the liver and gallbladder. It is worth mentioning that the above findings refer only to gallstones in the gallbladder and do not reveal the severity of damage that these drugs can cause to the liver itself.

If pharmacological drugs are able to generate some gallstones in the gallbladder, we can assume that they produce hundreds, if not thousands, of stones in the liver bile ducts. I have repeatedly observed that people who have taken pharmacological drugs in the past have had considerably more gallstones than those who took none.

Treating symptoms of disease (versus its causes) always has a hefty price tag attached to it, that is, an impairment of basic liver function. It is far easier and far more beneficial for the body if we remove all gallstones, restore normal blood values, and improve digestion and waste removal than if we try to suppress the symptoms of a disease.

Symptoms are not the disease; they only indicate that the body is attempting to save and protect itself. They signal the body's need for attention, support, and care. Treating disease as if it were an enemy, when in reality it is a survival or healing attempt, actually sabotages the body's healing abilities and sows the seeds for further illness.

Fluoride Poisoning

Fluorosilicic acid, commonly referred to as fluoride, is a liquid by-product of fertilizer manufacturing. It is a highly toxic and corrosive chemical that wreaks extensive, sometimes irreversible, havoc on the body. Since the liver is unable to break down fluoride, it attempts to pass this hazardous chemical into the bile ducts (which are the only alternative way for the liver to deal with such toxins). This quickly alters bile flora and leads to bile duct congestion and numerous other ailments.

Fluoride is added to 60 percent of the drinking water in the United States and a number of other countries, supposedly to prevent tooth decay (although there is no research to show that it does). Fertilizer manufacturers, desperate to get rid of this hazardous waste product, sell it so it can be added to a wide range of products, including soy products, toothpaste, fluoride tablets, fluoride drops, fluoride chewing gum, tea, vaccines, household products, fluoridated salt or milk, anesthetics, mattresses emitting fluoride gases, Teflon, and antibiotics. It is also found in polluted air and polluted ground water.

Because of its proven high toxicity, in August 2002, Belgium became the first country in the world to prohibit fluoride supplements. Numerous counties in the US have recently banned fluoride in drinking water.

"Fluoridation … is the greatest fraud that has ever been perpetrated and it has been perpetrated on more people than any other fraud has," said Professor Albert Schatz, Ph.D. (Microbiology), Nobel Prize winner and discoverer of streptomycin. Fortunately, much of Western Europe has rejected water fluoridation. This includes Austria, Belgium, Denmark, Finland, France, Germany, Italy, Luxembourg, the Netherlands, Norway, and Sweden.

Exhaustive research has shown that tumors in laboratory animals were found to be the direct result of fluoride ingestion. Other animal studies found that fluoride accumulates in the pineal gland and interferes with its production of melatonin, a hormone that helps regulate the onset of puberty, thyroid functions, and numerous other basic physiological processes.

In humans, fluoride has been found to cause genetic damage, mottling and destruction of the teeth, arthritis, osteoporosis, hip fractures, cancer, infertility, Alzheimer's disease, immune deficiency and brain damage.

Until the 1950s, European doctors used fluoride to treat hyperthyroidism (overactive thyroid) because of its ability to block uptake of iodine by the thyroid. The daily dose of fluoride that people are now receiving in fluoridated communities far exceeds the dose of fluoride that was found to depress the thyroid gland. Because of fluoridation, millions of people suffer from severe iodine deficiency, resulting in hypothyroidism (underactive thyroid).

Lack of iodine reduces or shuts down the production of the thyroid hormone thyroxin, the hormone that regulates metabolism and numerous important mechanisms in the body. Iodine deficiency can, in turn, lead to an increased risk for cancer of the breast[140], thyroid gland, ovary, and

---

[140]Iodine and Mammary Cancer; Adv Exp Med Biol. 1977;91:293-304

prostate. By the way, brominated vegetable oil (BVO), added to some American soft drinks, such as Mountain Dew and some other citrus-flavored sodas, also causes iodine deficiency. If you live in Europe or Japan, you are safe. This chemical, first patented by chemical companies as a flame retardant, is banned there, and for a good reason.

Hypothyroidism is currently one of the more common medical problems in the United States. It is estimated that 21.6 million Americans have hypothyroidism, according to statistics by the American Association of Clinical Endocrinologists (AACE) and other medical organizations, but this condition may be grossly underdiagnosed. Some experts claim that between 10 and 40 percent of Americans suffer from suboptimal thyroid functions.

Today, over 150 symptoms can be identified in hypothyroidism. Almost all of these correlate with known symptoms of fluoride poisoning. The symptoms of hypothyroidism include depression, dizziness, fatigue, cold intolerance, weight gain, muscle and joint pain, hair loss, dry and prematurely aged skin, headaches, migraines, shortness of breath, GI problems, menstrual problems, unbalanced blood pressure, increased cholesterol levels, gallbladder disease and liver congestion, allergies, insomnia, panic attacks and moodiness, irritability, memory loss, irregular heartbeat, congestive heart failure, cancer, diabetes, and loss of libido. Basically, all the organs and systems in the body slow down, including the brain.

A large number of children and adults in India and other developing countries are crippled and their teeth are destroyed because of fluoride poisoning from industry pollution.

To avoid having to dispose this hazardous waste product of the chemical industry at huge costs, it is easier to get rid of it by dumping it into the drinking water and adding it to foods. The side effect of causing hypothyroidism in millions of men and women in the US greatly increases the number of prescriptions for thyroid medication, which is good for business; hence, the reluctance by the health agencies to speak out against fluoride.

Once diagnosed with hypothyroidism, you are a candidate for lifelong consumption of thyroid medication. We certainly cannot expect the for-profit medical industry to help us get healthier or protect us from health hazards like fluoride.

To help the body deal with fluoride-caused illnesses, including hypothyroidism, it is important to clean out the liver bile ducts, avoid fluoride-containing products, and use a water filtration system that removes fluoride (if fluoride is still added to your drinking water).Distillation and a good reverse osmosis (R/O) system are effective in removing most of the fluoride (along with other contaminants), but they also remove the water's beneficial minerals. For more ideal filtering devices, you may need to contact your local dealer for water filters. Ask for a filtration system that uses a special fluoride/arsenic reduction medium called activated alumina.

Zeolite and sulfur remove fluoride from the body (see *Product Information*). The mineral boron has been shown to do the same. Eating cilantro with your salad each day also helps remove it or keep it at bay. A decongesting diet according to body type[141], regular sleeping and eating habits, and stress-free living conditions are essential for recovery.

The form of fluoride that is actually good for you:

It should be noted that only the form of fluoride (fluorosilicic acid) that is intentionally added to the drinking water, toothpastes and other products is harmful to the human physiology. For some reason, many fluoride opponents believe that there is only one kind of fluoride, and it is dangerous to health. However, there are naturally occurring forms of fluoride that are actually very important for the thyroid, the teeth, and the rest of the body.

Fluoride makes up 0.03 percent of the earth's crust. Most natural fluorides occur in the form of the minerals cryolite (sodium fluoride) and fluorospar (calcium fluoride). These minerals are found in small amounts in many foods and natural, untreated water supplies. They are also found in unrefined salts like Himalayan salt crystals and sea salt. The amounts of fluoride present in Himalayan salt and sea salt are determined by nature to support life, not destroy it. Nature certainly didn't make a mistake when it put fluoride into water and foods, and salt, without which humans and animals could not survive.

---

[141] See my book *Timeless Secrets of Health and Rejuvenation* for details on determining your body type and choosing the corresponding foods.

Children's Medicines Coated With Brain-Damaging Chemicals

If you live in the United States, avoid giving your children medicines that contain Aluminum Lake food coloring; be aware that they contain dangerous amounts of aluminum and harmful synthetic petrochemicals. These additives are carcinogens containing petroleum, antifreeze agents and ammonia, each of which produces a whole array of adverse reactions.

Aluminum poisoning alone can lead to memory impairment, autism, epilepsy, mental retardation, and dementia, as well as increased bone fracturing and cancer of the kidneys, bladder, testes, thyroid, and adrenals. Aluminum also compromises the immune system.

You are mistaken if you believe that the FDA is protecting your child from being poisoned by aluminum or other chemicals added to children's medicines or foods. The FDA's *Regulatory Process and Historical Perspectives* contains this revealing statement: "Color additives are important components of many products, making them attractive, appealing, appetizing, and informative. Added color serves as a kind of code that allows us to identify products on sight, like candy flavors and medicine dosages."

Because coloring agents are so *appetizing and appealing*, manufacturers are putting 15 million pounds of toxic dyes in America's foods, drinks, candy, and medicine every year - a practice that is banned in Europe. On an average, children in the US will have consumed over 3 pounds of aluminum packed dye before age 12, according to research. Makes you wonder why autism rates are so high among children.

Dyes and colors are added to cough syrups, NyQuil, Tylenol, drugs, vitamins, baked goods, powdered drink mixes, manufactured beverages, candy, cereal, Cheetos, Doritos, Skittles, pet food, personal care products, cosmetics, Robitussin, Jello, gelatins, Fruity Pebbles, Maraschino cherries, sausages, Mountain Dew, chewing gum, and dozens of other food products.

American companies exporting their products to Europe are required to change their cheap chemicals food additives to more expensive natural colorings to meet the strict regulations set forth by the European Union.

Gelatin in Drugs, Vaccines, and Processed Foods

Disease can originate from an unlikely and unsuspected source, gelatin. Gelatin is a mixture of peptides and proteins produced by partial hydrolysis of collagen extracted from the skin, boiled crushed bones, connective tissues, organs and intestines of some animals such as domesticated cattle, chicken, and pigs. Most mass production farm animals are sick and filled with cancer-causing growth hormones, chemical additives, and antibiotics.

It's not surprising that over 40 percent of humans are allergic to gelatin, which is the most commonly used, yet undisclosed animal part in pharmaceutical drugs, supplements and vaccines today. Millions of people develop severe allergies each year simply because of the prescription drugs and vaccines they receive, or the vitamin supplements they swallow. In vaccines, gelatin acts as a suspension agent and heat stabilizer.

Allergic reactions include breathing difficulties, abdominal pain and cramping, and anaphylaxis (that can include itchy rash, throat swelling, low blood pressure, and even death).

Gelatin is also used for the clarification of juices, such as apple juice, and of vinegar. Isinglass, from the swim bladders of fish, is still used as a fining agent for wine and beer.

Common examples of foods that contain gelatin are gelatin desserts, trifles, aspic, marshmallows, candy corn, and confections such as Peeps, gummy bears and jelly babies. Gelatin is commonly used as a stabilizer, thickener, or texturizer in foods such as jams, yogurt, cream cheese, and margarine.

3.Vaccines - A Death Trap

The damaging effects of vaccines

For many decades we have all been led to believe that vaccines, which are powerful pharmaceutical drugs, have eradicated the most dreaded infectious diseases, including polio, although, as of now, there is no actual scientific evidence to support this theory. To this day, national health agencies, like the CDC and FDA, still refuse to conduct long-term double blind control studies to prove that vaccines are both safe and work better than the placebo effect.

On the other hand, there are hundreds of studies to prove the damaging and sometimes fatal effects of vaccines on children. A 2012 paper published in the medical journal Lupus[142] took into consideration the available experimental evidence of vaccine injuries, prompting its authors, world-renowned researchers Lucija Tomljenovic, Ph.D., and Christopher Shaw, Ph.D., to issue the following warning: "Immune challenges during early development, including those vaccine-induced, can lead to permanent detrimental alterations of the brain and immune function." Tomljenovic and Shaw are with the Neural Dynamics Research Group, University of British Columbia, in Vancouver, Canada.

The paper, titled "Mechanisms of Aluminum Adjuvant Toxicity and Autoimmunity in Pediatric Populations" points out: "The experimental evidence also shows that simultaneous administration of as little as two to three immune adjuvants can overcome genetic resistance to autoimmunity. In some developed countries (USA), by the time children are 4 to 6 years old, they will have received a total of 126 antigenic compounds along with high amounts of aluminum (Al) adjuvants through routine vaccinations."

The authors clearly point fingers at the FDA by referring to its published flimsy argument that "safety assessments for vaccines have often not included appropriate toxicity studies because vaccines have not been viewed as inherently toxic." In my opinion, this assessment by the FDA is outrageously irresponsible, since it is scientifically documented that aluminum is a powerful neurotoxin that can even cause Alzheimer's disease.

After reviewing the scientific facts on how aluminum adjuvants grossly interfere with the natural development of the human immune system, the study's authors warn that "these observations raise plausible concerns about the overall safety of current childhood vaccination programs."

"In summary, research evidence shows that increasing concerns about current vaccination practices may indeed be warranted. Because children may be most at risk of vaccine-induced complications, a rigorous evaluation of the vaccine-related adverse health impacts in the pediatric population is urgently needed," write Tomljenovic and Shaw.

---

[142]Mechanisms of aluminum adjuvant toxicity and autoimmunity in pediatric populations. Lupus. 2012; 21(2):223-30. PMID: 22235057

Almost every day, I receive anxious questions from parents who for no lesser reasons than the above are concerned about their vaccinated children's welfare. Many of them share the negative experiences their kids had with vaccines, and that's everything what's listed as side effects on the websites of vaccine makers and the US Centers for Disease Control and Prevention (CDC).

For example, the CDC admits that several severe problems have been reported following MMR vaccine, and might also happen after MMRV. These include severe allergic reactions, and problems such as deafness, long-term seizures, coma, lowered consciousness, and permanent brain damage. However, the CDC is quick to add: "Because these problems occur so rarely, we can't be sure whether they are caused by the vaccine or not."

The problem with all this is that these vaccine injuries are not so rare as the CDC wants parents to know. In fact, they are extremely common. The Federal Drug Administration (FDA), World Health Organization (WHO), and other health agencies have all stated repeatedly that vaccine side effects are grossly underreported. According to the FDA, doctors only report between 1 and 10 percent of serious side effects.

What's worse, many vaccine side effects don't occur before one or several months after vaccination. So when a child develops asthma, constant seizures or a severe allergy, the doctor will treat these as separate diseases and not list as them as vaccine-injuries. The common assumption (not a proven fact) is that vaccine side effects occur only during the first few days following vaccination. It is believed there are no long-term side effects. That's only a belief, though, because long-term vaccine safety studies were never permitted to prove or disprove this assumption.

This is what confuses the issue even further: Although the rate of Sudden Infant Death Syndrome (SIDS) is the highest in countries where children receive the most vaccines, the medical industry claims that SIDS is unexplainable. SIDS is the leading cause of death among infants 1-month to 1-year-old, and the official line is: "The cause of death cannot be explained." In the field of law, there is something called *circumstantial evidence*, and it applies to the field of medicine just as much. Healthy children don't just die suddenly without a reason.

The pharma-medical industry denies that vaccines could have anything to do with being the biggest baby killers. However, merely denying this phenomenon does nothing to diminish the circumstantial evidence supporting it. For one thing, SIDS almost never occurs in non-vaccinated children. And why do vaccinated children have 120 percent more asthma, 317 percent more ADHD, 185 percent more neurologic disorders, and 146 percent more autism than those not vaccinated?

"Linear regression analysis of unweighted mean infant mortality rates (IMRs) showed a high statistically significant correlation between increasing number of vaccine doses and increasing infant mortality rates," according to a recent study published in the *Journal of Human & Experimental Toxicology* on September 4, 2011[143]. The study is titled, "Infant Mortality Rates Regressed Against Number Of Vaccine Doses Routinely Given: Is There A Biochemical Or Synergistic Toxicity?"

Co-author of this study, Neil Z Miller, wrote in March 2011 before publication of the research that in the US more than 2,000 babies died after receiving pneumococcal and Hib vaccines and yet nothing whatsoever was done. He noted that whilst these vaccines were suspended in Japan after just 4 deaths (shortly before the Fukushima disaster), the news of over 2,000 deaths in the US was barely even reported.

How much more circumstantial evidence do we need to at least raise this important question: What is the main difference between a vaccinated and a non-vaccinated 1-year-old?

Well, in the United States, a child receives 36 vaccinations before age 5, and 1 child in 91 develops autism. What's more astounding is that only 1 in 2,000 non-vaccinated children develop autism. 8 deaths per 1,000 in children below 5 years of age are due to vaccinations. In comparison, in Iceland a child receives 11 vaccine shots while only 1 child in 11,000 develops autism, and only 4 children per 1,000 die as a result of being vaccinated.

Of course, the above number of vaccine-linked deaths doesn't include the number of deaths from SIDS, which is the most common cause of death among infants. If 8 out of 1,000 vaccinated children die because of anaphylactic shock (anaphylaxis) right after they receive a vaccine, is it so far-fetched to assume that infants could eventually succumb to the immune-destructive effects of vaccine chemicals a month or even a year later, especially if additional vaccines are administered between their first and *final* shot?

---

[143] Infant mortality rates regressed against number of vaccine doses routinely given: Is there a biochemical or synergistic toxicity? Hum Exp Toxicol *September 2011 vol. 30 no. 9 1420-1428*

Until recently, the very long-term side effects of vaccines were unknown, but a new analysis of 151 older scientific studies has demonstrated that suppressing the primary immune response through vaccination during childhood significantly increases the risk of developing cancer later in life (also see Chapter 1). So if childhood vaccination can lead to cancer 30 years later, what else can it do that hasn't been studied yet?

The government health agencies claim that severe vaccine side effects are very rare, but how do they know that, when, because of *ethical* reasons, they prohibit any double blind control study comparing vaccinated children with non-vaccinated children? As astounding as it is in this day and age, to this day, there are no long-term, double-blind vaccine safety studies. So how can the CDC claim vaccines are safe when they have never undergone such safety scrutiny? Or would they even want to know?

How can a conscientious doctor make the determination that an infant who receives his first vaccine shot on the day of his birth (Hep B) and dies a month later for no apparent reason didn't die from the long-term effects of the vaccine? The doctor cannot even make such an assumption because the government disallows clinical vaccine safety studies. According to CDC, the vaccine couldn't possibly kill a child so many days after inoculation, because *vaccines are safe* (and there is no research to actually prove this).

The CDC goes even further than that. Ten researchers from the CDC's National Centers for Immunization and Respiratory Disease (NCIRD) recently published a paper, titled "Inhibitory Effect Of Breast Milk On Infectivity Of Live Oral Rotavirus Vaccines", which suggests that women should stop breastfeeding their babies and feed them infant formula instead in order to improve the effectiveness of vaccines!

Apparently, the immune-boosting effects of breast milk interfere with the *efficacy* of vaccines. The strong immune system in breastfed babies naturally rejects and destroys harmful viruses, including those contained in vaccines.

Instead of avoiding dangerous, toxic vaccines and letting the breast milk do its natural job of establishing complete and natural immunity, the researchers recommend women should stop the breast milk to allow vaccines to do their job.

Of course vaccine *efficacy* has nothing to do with vaccine *effectiveness* - the measure of whether a vaccine has protective benefits or not. In essence, vaccine efficacy is defined by the ability to raise antibody concentration in the blood. A person can have the perfect amount of antibodies for every pathogen that exists and still become infected by each one of them.

In the real world, immunity against pathogens can only occur if the body's antibodies have an affinity with the intended pathogen, called antibody-antigen affinity. The number of antibodies plays no role in establishing antibody-antigen affinity. That's why unnaturally elevated antibody concentrations have never been shown to confer true protection.

The FDA does not require vaccine producers to demonstrate vaccine effectiveness. They only need to show that their product has a high efficacy rate as determined by elevated antibody levels, which is easily achieved by causing a hyper-reaction of the immune system through vaccine adjuvants like aluminum, mineral oil, formaldehyde, detergent stabilized squalene-in-water, pertactin, viral DNA, phosphate, etc. Proper and long-lasting antibody-antigen affinity, on the other hand, can only be generated after allowing the body's primary immune system, also called cellular immune system, to go through an either noticeable (strong) or unnoticeable (mild) infection.

Cell-mediated immune responses do not involve antibodies but rather include activation of macrophages, natural killer cells (NK), antigen-specific cytotoxic T-lymphocytes, and the release of various cytokines in response to an antigen. Cell-mediated immunity is directed primarily at microbes and is most effective in removing virus-infected cells, but also participates in defending against cancers, fungi, amoeba and other protozoans, and intracellular bacteria.

Even if antibodies alone could bestow immunity, our modern lifestyle makes it almost impossible to benefit from vaccine-induced antibody increases. Elevated exposures in children to perfluorinated compounds, which are widely used in manufacturing and food packaging, have recently been associated with lower antibody responses to routine childhood immunizations, according to a study in the January 25, 2012 issue of the *Journal of The American Medical Association* (JAMA)[144].

---

[144]Serum Vaccine Antibody Concentrations in Children Exposed to Perfluorinated Compounds. JAMA. 2012;307[4]:391-397

The study's authors admit that non-stick cookware and fluorine compounds cause vaccines to fail. "The perfluorinated compounds (PFCs) are highly persistent and cause contamination of drinking water, food, and food chains," stated the authors. "If the associations are causal, the clinical importance of our findings is therefore that PFC exposure may increase a child's risk for not being protected against diphtheria and tetanus, despite a full schedule of vaccinations."

Although the *JAMA* study only focused on serum antibody concentrations against tetanus and diphtheria toxoids at ages 5 and 7 years, it can be postulated that this finding applies to all vaccine-induced antibody complexes. This suggestion is supported by the overwhelming scientific evidence that PFCs cause immune suppression regardless of the type of antibodies involved.

The scientists' admission of chemical-induced vaccine failure must necessarily raise serious doubt about the validity of the entire vaccine theory. A 2004 US government study found these chemicals in a shocking 98 percent of blood samples taken from a large pool of Americans[145]. Since according to this recent study these chemicals inactivate vaccine potential by disabling antibodies, vaccines are practically useless for most Americans.

If vaccines were truly as protective as claimed, the contamination of almost everyone's blood with vaccine-demobilizing chemicals would have left most people unprotected and therefore led to mass breakouts of infectious diseases. But this clearly has not happened. The study actually proves that there is no real threat from disease epidemics, largely because of the high levels of hygiene, sanitation, and nutritional measures existent in modern societies.

According to current vaccine theory, vaccine *effectiveness* is determined by a certain level of antibody concentration in the blood. Even a slightly lowered antibody count can render the vaccine ineffective. Even without the chemical interference, vaccine antibodies tend to drop, hence the need for booster shots.

However, since 98 percent of people, at least those living in the US, are exposed to PFCs nearly all the time, we can safely conclude that vaccines are not only ineffective, but also unnecessary. They are only useful in the

---

[145]Implications of Early Menopause in Women Exposed to Perfluorocarbons. Journal of Clinical Endocrinology & Metabolism, online March 16, 2011

sense that they cause harmful side effects that require further medical intervention, much to the benefit of the profit-driven medical industry.

Because vaccines only extremely rarely trigger the body's primary immune system, they have never been shown to offer any significant, long-term protection against infectious diseases, anyway. To the contrary, by bypassing the body's cellular immune system and interfering with its natural, immunity-generating mechanisms, the human body stands very little chance of protecting itself from cancers, toxins and pathogens.

The bottom line is that vaccination is not immunization but a destabilization of the immune system that renders it susceptible to the very infectious agents it is supposed to protect us from. The consequences of this medical blunder are becoming increasingly apparent.

In recent years, vaccine-derived poliovirus (VDPV), also called iatrogenic (vaccine-induced) polio, has caused almost every new case of polio case and polio-outbreak recorded.

It has been reported in the *Lancet* that the incidence of Flaccid Paralysis (AFP), especially non-polio AFP, called NPAFP, has increased exponentially in India after a high potency polio vaccine was introduced[146]. A recent paper published in the *Indian Journal of Medical Ethics (IJME)* explains that clinically, NPAFP is indistinguishable from polio paralysis. However, according to the *Office of Medical & Scientific Justice (OMSJ)*, NPAFP is twice as deadly as polio paralysis. Prior to the rollout of the massive polio vaccine campaigns, NPAFP was not even an issue in India.

The research shows that the non-polio AFP rate increases in proportion to the number of polio vaccines doses received in each area. Nationally, the non-polio AFP rate is now 12 times higher than expected. "In the states of Uttar Pradesh (UP) and Bihar, which have pulse polio rounds nearly every month, the non-polio AFP rate is 25- and 35-fold higher than the international norms," the researches in this study stated.

Playing with synthetic viruses and giving them to hundreds of millions of people, as has happened in India, has serious consequences for the health and economic survival of an entire nation like India. "The Government of India finally had to fund this hugely expensive programme, which cost the country 100 times more than the value of the initial grant," the authors said. They go on to say, "The $2.5 billion spent by India must

---

[146]Puliyel J, Sathyamala C, Banerji D. Protective efficacy of a monovalent oral type 1 poliovirus vaccine. *Lancet*.2007;370:129-30

be seen against \$2 billion spent by the United States of America on world-wide polio eradication, the \$1.3 billion expended by Bill Gates, and the \$0.8 billion raised by the loudest voice for polio eradication - Rotary International - over the last 20 years."

Ruining the health of the people in a developing country under the guise of granting them *humanitarian aid,* and then making a lot of money off that is hardly anything these *sponsors* should be proud of. Interfering with nature almost always causes more serious problems than the original ones.

Rotavirus, MMR, and other vaccines don't have a better track record either. In fact, publically available statistical data have revealed that the incidence of infection in all major disease outbreaks in recorded history has dramatically declined with the implementation of improved hygiene, sanitation and nutrition, but drastically increased again with the onset of mass inoculation[147].

Any layperson would understand that injecting vaccine ingredients such as aluminum, mercury, formaldehyde, anti-freeze agents, nail polish removers, DNA fragments from animals, antibiotics, and dozens of other, equally toxic, carcinogenic chemicals into an infant's body could actually poison it and permanently damage or destroy the immune system, as well as the brain and digestive system, especially if the child was born prematurely, was delivered by Caesarian section, or wasn't breastfed (all factors that weaken the immune system).

Pumping poisons into helpless infants' bodies

Thirty-odd jabs in the first 18 months of life! That's how many times the average American infant gets vaccinated. Children in the United Kingdom are slightly better off. They get vaccinated only 25 times at this tender age. And to make sure you're well and truly on the vaccination trail early enough, it is mandatory for babies to get 9 or more different antigens (disease-causing substances) pumped into their immature immune systems almost immediately after birth, some of them cocktails of more than one vaccine.

The best part for Big Pharma is that most of these vaccinations are backed by law. Children who are not vaccinated as per the CDC's schedule cannot enter or stay within the formal education system. As if

---

[147] See my book <u>Vaccine-nation: Poisoning the Population, One Shot at a Time</u>

this arm-twisting were not enough, entire populations the world over are brainwashed into believing that they or their children will contract life-threatening diseases if they do not get vaccinated. And don't we all want the best for our children?

For many decades, leading scientists and doctors have vehemently promoted the idea that immunization of children is necessary to protect them from contracting diseases such as diphtheria, smallpox, polio, cholera, typhoid and malaria. Yet evidence is mounting, showing that immunization may not only be unnecessary but even harmful. Pouring deadly chemicals into a lake doesn't make it immune to pollutants. Likewise, injecting the live poisons contained in vaccines into the bloodstream of children hardly gives future generations a chance to lead truly healthy lives.

Fallacy and Fallout

Ever since Louis Pasteur proposed his erroneous germ theory of disease, the scientific establishment has linked a variety of bacteria, viruses and other pathogens to life-threatening illnesses against which pharmaceutical companies have devised an armor of protection in their little vials.

The problem is that despite their claims of success, certain vaccines have been consistently linked to specific symptoms and syndromes, some of which continue to baffle scientists and doctors even today. Among the various diseases that have been correlated to vaccines are chronic fatigue syndrome, autoimmune disorders, learning disabilities, encephalitis, growth inhibition, developmental disorders, and hyperactivity.

Some of these issues, such as learning disabilities, were once dismissed as simple problems of growing up. Medical researchers now recognize them as forms of encephalitis (inflammatory disease of the brain). Here's a shocking statistic: More than 20 percent of American children (1 in 5) suffer from these or related problems.

There is a mounting body of scientific research which shows that chronic diseases such as encephalitis, rheumatoid arthritis, multiple sclerosis, leukemia and other forms of cancer, and even HIV, may be provoked by vaccines administered in infancy.

For instance, rheumatoid arthritis, an inflammatory disease of the joints, was once an affliction of the elderly. Now, this crippling disease is widely prevalent among younger people and has been consistently associated with measles and rubella vaccinations.

Guillain-Barré Syndrome, a serious disease that leads to paralysis, is another syndrome which has been consistently associated with immunizations against measles, diphtheria, influenza, tetanus, and the oral polio vaccine. This is hardly surprising when one considers the high toxicity of the vaccines. It is well-known that children whose immune systems are already weak experience more serious complications than those whose constitution and immune systems are much stronger.

Now we can also add kidney disease to the list of serious vaccine side effects. In June 2011, the prestigious *New England Journal of Medicine* published a very important study titled, "Early Childhood Membranous Nephropathy Due to Cationic Bovine Serum Albumin[148]." Membranous nephropathy is a condition where the kidneys leak large amounts of protein into the urine. When ingested or injected, the foreign (invading) protein bovine serum albumin (BSA) naturally becomes attached to an antibody, forming an antibody complex. This complex can easily become deposited in the membrane of the kidney where it can inflame and break down the filter membrane barrier. While healthy, undamaged kidneys use a selective filtration process to hold back bodily proteins, including clotting factors and immune globulins, kidneys with such tears allow these proteins to leak into the urine.

This is a very serious condition, akin to uncontrolled bleeding, which can throw children or adults onto dialysis and/or a kidney transplant and will require the life-long use of immune suppressing drugs. Other, potentially life-threatening complications may occur as well.

Bovine Serum Albumin (BSA) is not only found in cow's milk, but it is added to almost every childhood vaccine, including:

- MMRV for measles, mumps, rubella, chicken pox
- Pneumococcal (Pneumovax) for pneumococcal pneumonia
- Rabies (Rab vert) for rabies
- Rotavirus (Rota Teq) for rotavirus
- Td (Decavac) for tetanus, diphtheria
- Tdap (Boostrix) for tetanus, diptheria, pertussis
- Varicella (Varivax) for chicken pox
- Zoster (Zostavax) for shingles

---

[148] Debiec, H. et al., 2011, Early Childhood Membranous Nephropathy Due to Cationic Bovine Serum Albumin, NEJM. Jun 2;364(22):2101-10

While children who drink unprocessed cow's milk may have a good chance of defending themselves against BSA, this ability is many times reduced when BSA is directly injected into the blood with vaccines. When injected with BSA, the body is left with no other choice than to produce inflammation causing antibody complexes that sooner or later can cause havoc in the kidneys and other parts of the body.

So if you decide to give your child dairy products to eat and to have her/him vaccinated and she/he suffers from kidney damage or complete kidney failure as a result, at least science can now explain nephrotic syndrome, the mysterious kidney disease that has baffled doctors and parents for many decades. While the researchers recommended that children should avoid cow's milk and be breastfed instead, they did admit that BSA is also contained in vaccines. However, they stopped short at warning parents about having their children vaccinated. After all, modern immunization is the Holy Grail of conventional medicine.

Buying Into Dangerous Myths

It is nearly impossible to estimate the damage and suffering that has been created and that will occur in future as a result of inadequate information about the dangers of modern immunization programs. Parents want to do what is best for their children and they carry a heavy burden of responsibility to keep them healthy and safe. Misinformation can create considerable conflict in parents because they don't want to neglect their children's health or cause them any harm.

Vaccine proponents argue that their chemical formulations have not just saved lives but have also prevented epidemics and all but wiped out some deadly diseases from the face of the earth! Please note that this is nothing but a myth. The truth is that the four leading childhood killer diseases - scarlet fever, pertussis or whooping cough, diphtheria, and measles - had already declined by more than 90 percent before vaccines against these diseases were introduced! The reason these diseases vanished was that living conditions such as hygiene, sanitation and standards of living had improved significantly and people increasingly had access to healthy food. According to the CDC's website, clean drinking water is more effective in preventing infectious diseases than vaccines.

Normally, I don't give much credence to a health agency that serves the pharmaceutical industry more than the people, but in this instance, their assessment is correct. But instead of helping developing countries with basic, inexpensive methods of water purification, the CDC prefers to organize expensive vaccination campaigns. It is very evident where the CDC stands with regard to preventing disease.

It is hardly surprising that the CDC was recently caught by a nonprofit organization with deliberately manipulating and covering up scientific data showing a clear, indisputable link between vaccines containing mercury and autism[149].

As mentioned before, after having gained legal access to secret CDC files through a Freedom of Information Act (FOIA) request, the Coalition for Mercury-Free Drugs (CoMeD) discovered the CDCs fraudulent manipulation of the results of a hugely important study that shows mercury in vaccines significantly increases the risk of autism.

In 2003, the journal Pediatrics published a Danish study that recorded a substantial decline in autism rates following the country's removal of thimerosal, a highly toxic mercury-based component, from vaccines. However, being a principal spokes-agency and promoter for the vaccine industry, before submitting the study to *Pediatrics*, the CDC apparently removed large amounts of data from the study that showed a decline in autism rates following the removal of thimerosal.

According to the uncovered documents, the study's original authors contacted CDC officials to let them know that the agency had incorrectly interpreted the data. They told the CDC that its figures and conclusions were false, and that corrections needed to be made.

Disregarding the authors' pleas to make the necessary corrections, the CDC proceeded with submitting the corrupted version of the study to *Pediatrics* with the request for expedited review and publication. *Pediatrics* obliged and published the tainted study, which stated that removing the thimerosal from the vaccines had actually done the complete opposite and increased the autism rates!

This left millions of concerned parents wondering why autism has been increasing at such an alarming rate ever since mercury was added to vaccines. Still, each day, many parents see their children become autistic shortly or immediately after receiving vaccine shots.

In 1999, the CDC reasoned that "despite the lack of evidence of significant harm in the use of thimerosal in vaccines, the removal of this preservative would increase the public confidence in the safety of

---

[149]Exposed: "CDC deliberately manipulated, covered up scientific data showing link between vaccines containing mercury and autism" (NaturalNews.com and Mercury-FreeDrugs.com)

vaccines." A purely political move, I might add. Thimerosal, of course, is still being added to influenza and tetanus vaccines, and to all vaccines shipped to developing countries, something the CDC doesn't really want parents to know.

The CDC strongly recommends the seasonal flu shot for babies of age 7 and older. The tetanus vaccine is given at age 6 weeks, 3 months, and 5 months with boosters at 4 years and 11 years of age. In other words, there is still plenty of mercury in vaccines to cause brain damage.

Several nations, including Australia, Finland and Sweden have already banned flu shots for babies after they have killed, maimed, or otherwise harmed hundreds and thousands of babies. "The vaccines appear to be causing a pattern of neurological disorders affecting children and teens across the planet," said a report in India's *Bharat Chronicle*. One of the commonest side effects reported by less corrupt government health agencies around the world is that the injected children develop severe flu symptoms.

The CDC has banned any clinical studies that could once and for all prove or disprove a connection between vaccines and autism or other adverse reactions, citing *ethical reasons*. The argument that "it is unethical to not vaccinate certain children..." is but a lame excuse that prevents us from getting to the bottom of the now huge autism epidemic, once and for all. Avoiding comparison studies is not really a reasonable excuse today, as many parents have already opted out of at least some, if not all, vaccines for their children, anyway. So there are many children available for such kind of research, who would wish to participate in such research.

Even though the CDC has removed any reference to the tainted Danish study from its website, it continues to argue that the scientific community does not support an association between vaccines and autism. Of course, thanks to the persistence of the CoMeD, we now know why the CDC tried to cover its tracks and so vehemently denies that vaccines can cause autism. Fortunately for parents, *an Institute of Medicine*[150] (IOM) review[151] of more than 1,000 vaccine studies found convincing evidence of 14 dangerous side effects that can be caused by the commonly administered vaccines. These adverse events were associated with vaccines for measles, mumps, rubella (MMR); varicella (chickenpox); influenza; hepatitis A;

---

[150]The Institute of Medicine (IOM) is a prestigious not-for-profit, non-governmental American organization founded in 1970, under the congressional charter of the National Academy of Sciences. The IOM is part of the United States National Academies

[151]Institute of Medicine, Adverse Effects of Vaccines: Evidence and Causality, August 25, 2011

hepatitis B; HPV; diphtheria, tetanus, acellular pertussis (DTaP); and meningococcal.

The side effects are vaccine strain varicella zoster infection, pneumonia, encephalitis, meningitis, hepatitis, measles, febrile seizures, joint pain (arthralgia) in children and women, anaphylaxis (life-threatening allergic reaction), deltoid bursitis, or shoulder inflammation, fainting (syncope), and oculo-respiratory syndrome characterized by conjunctivitis, facial swelling, and mild respiratory symptoms.

Of course, brain inflammation is a condition which we know has strong links to autism. The health agencies cannot have it both ways. On the one hand, they admit that vaccines can cause encephalitis and meningitis, and on the other hand, they deny that vaccines can cause autism. Their irrational position must therefore be considered intentionally deceptive.

A 2009 study published in *Pediatrics & Child Health*[152] revealed another highly disturbing side effect of vaccines not listed among the abovementioned adverse effects: a potentially fatal blood disease, called idiopathic thrombocytopenic purpura, or ITP. The symptoms of the disease include blood shooting out of a child's nose in the days or weeks after a vaccine shot. That condition occurs when the vaccine causes the immune system to overreact and destroy blood platelets, which are responsible for blood clotting. This results in bleeding uncontrollably under the skin and even in the brain.

The researchers stated in the study summary: "Thrombocytopenia is a rare but important adverse event following vaccination." The MMR vaccine can trigger this serious disease in babies and toddlers; in older kids it can be caused by the hepatitis A jab and Tdap (tetanus, diphtheria, and acellular pertussis) shots. For any affected child and its parents, it can be extremely unsettling.

In its report, the IOM clearly acknowledged that there is a lack of adequate scientific understanding about the way in which vaccines act in the human body, including how, when, why, and for whom they are harmful. In other words, there is no real science behind the concept of immunization through vaccines. High quality vaccine safety science is also completely missing. Then how is it possible that billions of these snake oil vaccines are administered to unsuspecting populations around the

---

[152] Do childhood vaccines cause thrombocytopenia? Paediatrics and Child Health. 2009 January; 14(1): 31–32.

world in the name of science and medical care, when even the agencies that promote vaccines have no clue as to how, why, and whether vaccines actually work at all?

What's worse, even if vaccines were somewhat effective for some unexplainable reason, immunization programs are directly responsible for spreading disease and killing millions of people each year, according to the WHO's own admission. By 2003 WHO, UNICEF, and UNFPA recommended that all immunization be provided in all countries using only auto-disable syringes because unsafe injections cause annually 21 million new cases of hepatitis B, 2 million cases of hepatitis C, 250,000 cases of HIV, and an estimated 1.3 million deaths[153].

However, the practice of administering unsafe injections has never changed in poor countries and the massacres in the name of medical progress continue unabated.

In 2006, WHO issued a revised statement titled, "Injection Safety: Misuse and Overuse of Injections Worldwide." The document states that each year unsafe injections cause an estimated 1.3 million early deaths, a loss of 26 million years of life, and an annual burden of USD 535 million in direct medical costs.

Furthermore, in underdeveloped countries, vaccine storage becomes an issue due to transport delays and lack of proper refrigeration facilities. With uninterrupted electric power supply not available always, it sometimes results in vaccines getting spoiled, becoming ineffective, and potentially life-endangering.

---

[153] http://www.unicef.org/immunization/23245_safety.html

Scientists Disclose Vaccine Deceptions

Fortunately for parents and children, even elite members of the scientific community are beginning to question the ethics and science behind vaccination programs.

On January 12, 2012, the *Annals of Medicine* published a ground-breaking peer-reviewed paper titled, "Human Papilloma virus (HPV) Vaccine Policy And Evidence-Based Medicine: Are They At Odds[154]?"

The paper, written by renowned researchers Lucija Tomljenovic, Ph.D., and Christopher Shaw, Ph.D., with the Neural Dynamics Research Group, University of British Columbia, in Vancouver, reveals the complete lack of scientific evidence demonstrating the safety and efficacy of Gardasil, human papilloma virus (HPV) vaccine (produced by Merck & Co) and Cervarix, a cervical cancer vaccine (produced by GlaxoSmithKline) before they were unleashed on unsuspecting parents of adolescents and directly on teenagers in California.

As it turned out, Merck's clinical trials were heavily flawed because the researchers used an aluminum adjuvant as a placebo, which has well-known, serious side effects. As a comparative for non-serious adverse reactions, they conveniently chose saline, which usually has no adverse effects. To conceal the true rate of serious reactions, these *scientists* pooled the results from the saline placebo group and the aluminum placebo group, thereby claiming there are only few mild side effects. Yet, in real life, there is a huge discrepancy between Merck's stated *mild side effects* and those severe and often deadly adverse reactions experienced by teenagers around the world.

The authors of the report go on to state: "What is more disconcerting than the aggressive marketing strategies employed by the vaccine manufacturers is the practice by which the medical profession has presented partial information to the public, namely, in a way that generates fear, thus promoting vaccine uptake. ...... It thus appears that to this date, medical and regulatory entities worldwide continue to provide inaccurate information regarding cervical cancer risk and the usefulness of HPV vaccines, thereby making informed consent regarding vaccination impossible to achieve."

---

[154]Human papilloma virus (HPV) vaccine policy and evidence-based medicine: Are they at odds? Ann Med. 2011 Dec 22.

In the abstract of the paper, Tomljenovic and Shaw remind medical professionals that "contrary to claims that cervical cancer is the second most common cancer in women worldwide, existing data show that this only applies to developing countries." They further state: "In the Western world, cervical cancer is a rare disease with mortality rates that are several times lower than the rate of reported serious adverse reactions (including deaths) from HPV vaccination. Future vaccination policies should adhere more rigorously to evidence-based medicine and ethical guidelines for informed consent."

They point to the fact that the efficacy of HPV vaccines in preventing cervical cancer has not been demonstrated, while vaccine risks remain to be fully evaluated. "Current worldwide HPV immunization practices with either of the two HPV vaccines appear to be neither justified by long-term health benefits nor economically viable, nor is there any evidence that HPV vaccination (even if proven effective against cervical cancer) would reduce the rate of cervical cancer beyond what Pap screening has already achieved," said Tomljenovic and Shaw.

The researchers explain that cumulatively, the list of serious adverse reactions related to HPV vaccination worldwide includes deaths, convulsions, paraesthesia, paralysis, Guillain-Barré Syndrome (GBS), transverse myelitis, facial palsy, chronic fatigue syndrome, anaphylaxis, autoimmune disorders, deep vein thrombosis, pulmonary embolisms, and cervical cancers. In addition, they offer this sensible, logical piece of advice that no drug company likes to hear: "The almost exclusive reliance on manufacturers' sponsored studies, often of questionable quality, as a basis for vaccine policy-making should be discontinued."

The effect that the vaccine will have on other cancer-causing HPV strains is becoming apparent now. Gardasil confers presumed immunity to only 2 of the 15 HPV strains that are associated with cervical cancer. Results from clinical trials clearly demonstrate that vaccinated women show an increased number of precancerous lesions caused by strains of HPV other than HPV-16 and HPV-18. This is not a new phenomenon and should have been anticipated by the vaccine producer and the FDA. But then, neither of these is interested in preventing disease; that would be akin to committing cancer-medical genocide. The cancer *business* must go on, no matter what.

Under the pretense of preventing cervical cancer which only kills 300 people a year in the US, millions of young girls, and now even boys, are being vaccinated with one of the most dangerous vaccines ever produced, so they can make this rare type of cancer spread like wildfire. Remember, every cancer patient can make the medical industry over a million dollars, not to mention the costs involved in treating all the other debilitating side effects the vaccine causes. Merck has already made billions off young women, and that's just for starters.

Isn't it astonishing that a vaccine purported to *prevent* cervical cancer actually causes it? Isn't it time we start protecting our own and our family's health from those who deliberately wish to see it ruined in order to profit from treating us for the many ailments their so-called *preventative medicine* is causing? It appears that we can only do this by taking care of our own health needs.

This recommendation becomes further reinforced by a recent 72-page report by GBI Research, published on March 14, 2012, that shows that "recalls for vaccines and immunoglobulins were higher than other drug classes." The analysis covered recalls on a year-to-year basis for the years 2007 to 2010. Although it is great to have such an analysis made, this report is cost-prohibitive to those who need to read it the most: the doctors and their patients. Very few people are willing to pay the $3,500 it costs to learn about case studies of recalled biologic products and re-released manufacturing or labeling changes?

Still, for the safety of your life and that of your family, it is very important that you know if a drug, such as a vaccine, has been recalled because it may be contaminated or otherwise unsafe for your child, or useless altogether. Most vaccine recalls result from the discovery that a vaccine potency or strength is too low (after testing blood antibodies following injection). The low potency fails to produce the necessary immune response believed to bestow immunity to a particular infectious agent (pathogen).

For example, in 2009, the vaccine manufacturers Sanofi Pasteur recalled 800,000 pediatric doses of H1N1 vaccine for exactly this reason. Regardless, the CDC told parents and doctors not to get the affected children revaccinated, thereby giving the (false) impression that the recalled vaccine was still potent enough. If the vaccine had been potent enough, why didn't they just leave it on the market? If it was not good enough, why should these kids go without adequate protection? Today's medical practices not only abound with such contradictions, they constitute criminal and corrupt practices that affect millions of children and cost taxpayers enormous sums of money.

One of the most serious vaccine frauds ever committed by a major vaccine producer was reported by Mike Adams, Natural News, in an article titled "Merck vaccine fraud exposed by two Merck virologists; company faked mumps vaccine efficacy results for over a decade, says lawsuit[155]." The article appeared on NauralNews.com on June 27, 2012. "According to two Merck scientists who filed a False Claims Act complaint in 2010[156] - a complaint which has just now been unsealed - vaccine manufacturer Merck knowingly falsified its mumps vaccine test data, spiked blood samples with animal antibodies, sold a vaccine that actually *promoted* mumps and measles outbreaks, and ripped off governments and consumers who bought the vaccine thinking it was 95% effective," writes Mike Adams. More details about the federal antitrust class action against Merck can be found at the web site of Courthouse News Service[157].

What's worse, although the US government was aware of the Merck vaccine fraud that has been going on since the late 1990s, it chose to ignore it. In the meanwhile, millions of children were knowingly exposed to a vaccine that was known to be of little or no use in the prevention of mumps.

The mere assumption that vaccines could work, or work better than no vaccines at all has somehow been turned into the science-backed evidence that doctors often refer to when they try to persuade us that we need all our vaccine shots to be protected against the world's most dreaded infections, including the seasonal flu.

Flu Vaccines are 98.5 % Ineffective

Most people still believe flu vaccines protect against the flu, as they are told by their doctors, the media, and the health protection agencies[158].

Of course, we are not being told that influenza vaccines only prevent influenza in 1.5 out of every 100 adults who are injected with the flu vaccine, according to a large meta-analysis of 5,707 articles and 31 eligible studies, published in the *Lancet* on 26 October, 2011. While the

---

[155]Merck Vaccine Fraud Exposed..., Mike Adams, NaturalNews.com, June 27, 2012
[156]www.naturalnews.com/gallery/documents/Merck-False-Claims-Act.pdf
[157]http://www.courthousenews.com/2012/06/27/47851.htm
[158]The Lancet Infectious Diseases, Efficacy and effectiveness of influenza vaccines: a systematic review and meta-analysis Published Online: 26 Oct., 2011, doi:10.1016/S1473-3099(11)70295-X

effectiveness of the flu vaccine is statistically insignificant (offering almost no protection at all), it often causes flu-like symptoms in those who are injected with it.

Disappointingly, the researchers called for new vaccines with improved clinical efficacy and effectiveness needed to further reduce influenza-related morbidity and mortality. This is hardly surprising, since the currently used flu vaccines are so ineffective in protecting against the flu that they are practically useless.

"Influenza vaccines can provide moderate protection against virologically confirmed influenza, but such protection is greatly reduced or absent in some seasons," conclude the researchers in the study interpretation. Unquestionably, it is highly unpredictable for which season such moderate protection would be or would not be absent. It is anyone's guess, not science. In other words, millions of people may be getting a flu shot this season but with zero guarantee that it will have any protective benefits at all.

What is even worse, "Evidence for protection in adults aged 65 years or older is lacking," admitted the researchers. The older people are the greatest population target for seasonal flu shots, without a shred of evidence that the shots will even offer more than 0.00001 percent protection against the seasonal flu. You may call this form of *preventive* medicine the ultimate practice of quackery. The obvious result of this study is that, overall, flu vaccines do nothing in 98.5 percent of adults.

The main question is whether it is worth injecting 100 people with a toxic sludge of carcinogenic, immune-suppressive chemicals and viruses to protect just 1.5 people against a usually harmless flu? It's certainly worth a lot of money for the multibillion dollar vaccine industry.

For an in-depth analysis of the study's results, see this excellent exposé published by Natural News[159].

Most doctors will also not tell you about the CDC's recent admission, that the flu vaccines' protective effect (if there is any) fades after just a few weeks or months after you receive it, and older people need 3 times the regular dosage for it to work at all (which the *Lancet* study has confirmed). I wouldn't be surprised if the placebo effect is up to 10 times more effective than the actual vaccine. After all, there is good research to show

---

[159]Shock vaccine study reveals influenza vaccines only prevent the flu in 1.5 out of 100 adults (not 60 percent as you've been told), by Mike Adams, Journalist & Editor, NaturalNews.com

happy people are much less likely to catch a cold or the flu than unhappy people.

And what happens when a dangerous vaccine for the innocuous flu involves infants and children? Both the FDA and CDC recently admitted that the number of reports to VAERS of febrile seizures following vaccination with Fluzone. Fluzone (manufactured by Sanofi Pasteur, Inc.) is the main influenza vaccine recommended for use in infants and children 6-23 months of age. Most of these febrile seizures occur in children younger than 2 years of age.

The most often used argument to inject the population against influenza is to save lives, but so far, there is no research to show that it does. To the contrary, there is circumstantial evidence that it doesn't. In years when there is a shortage of vaccine serum, or when the vaccines don't match the dominant strain, the number of seasonal flu deaths remain constant. Obviously, if the flu vaccine was saving the millions of vaccinated people the rest of the time, there would have been a surge in the number of deaths during those times when vaccines were not available (like in the year 2011). Furthermore, the number of people dying during the winter months from respiratory infections such as pneumonia (which is caused by bacteria, not viruses) also remains constant even in the absence of vaccine availability. Many doctors argue that especially patients with an existing respiratory ailment need to be vaccinated against the flu or otherwise it may kill them, but this is just a theory with no scientific basis to it.

In their analysis of 50 studies (including 40 clinical trials) on flu vaccinations, researchers from The Cochrane Collaboration found no reduction in the rate of complications such as hospitalizations and pneumonia, and no evidence whatsoever that flu shots slow the spread of the disease. "The review showed that reliable evidence on influenza vaccines is thin but there is evidence of widespread manipulation of conclusions and spurious notoriety of the studies," wrote the researchers. They also stated that studies not funded by pharmaceutical companies were "significantly less likely to report conclusions favorable to the vaccines."

Perhaps, the most shocking discovery in relation to the 2009 H1N1 influenza outbreak was made by scientists conducting two separate review studies that were both published in the journal *Public Library of Science ONE*. The researchers found that Pandemrix, an H1N1 flu vaccine produced by GlaxoSmithKline (GSK), is responsible for causing an up to

17-fold increase in narcolepsy among children and teenagers less than 17 years of age[160].

Narcolepsy, which affects about one in 2,000 people, is characterized by daytime drowsiness, irregular sleep at night and cataplexy, a sudden loss of muscle tone and strength. Narcoleptics are missing brain cells that produce hypocretin, a hormone that promotes wakefulness. Many narcoleptics can stay awake just for an hour each day. The scientists suspect the vaccine may have contributed to an auto-immune effect linked to narcolepsy.

Families who have a narcoleptic child are often devastated in that the child requires round-the-clock care and supervision. The immense emotional and financial burden is often unbearable for parents who have seen their once healthy child suddenly turn into person who sleeps 23 hours a day, for the rest of his life. I always warn parents they are alone when it comes to protecting their children. All drugs, including vaccines, are potentially dangerous, and it is impossible to foretell how a child will react to them. Some will survive the chemical assault, others won't. In my opinion, it is very irresponsible to play Russian roulette with their lives.

In spite of all the evidence pointing to vaccination as not only being ineffective but actually being a major cause of traumatic and often irreversible illness, the extremely well-organized medical industry has come up with a clever plan to force parents into submitting their children to the full vaccine schedules. Many doctors now openly inform parents that they will not treat their children unless they comply with the vaccination mandates. In the US, when parents of an unvaccinated child cannot find a willing doctor who treats him for an illness, the Child Protective Services can take the children away from them because of *child abuse and neglect*.

While in 2001 and 2006, only 6 percent of physicians admitted that they routinely refused to treat families over vaccine refusal, this number has increased to up to 30 percent, according to some doctor surveys done in 2011. This blunt form of medical arm-twisting is a reminder of the racial discrimination not so long ago when black African-Americans used to be denied adequate medical care because white doctors considered them second-class citizens.

---

[160]Swine flu vaccines cause 17-fold increase in narcolepsy, horrified scientists discover, NaturalNews.com, April 08, 2012

The doctors' main argument behind this medical profiling is that non-vaccinated children pose a serious disease risk to the vaccinated children. Of course, there is no real science or logic to back up their claim. If vaccines were truly effective in providing immunity to infectious disease, why should there be a concern for the non-vaccinated? Which of the two is it: do vaccines protect against disease, or don't they? We cannot have it both ways.

The available scientific evidence now overwhelmingly supports the latter argument. In addition, many of the recent disease outbreaks that were initially blamed by the CDC and the mainstream media on unvaccinated individuals were actually most rampant in vaccinated individuals. For instance, in the 2010 whooping cough outbreak in California, immunized children between ages 8 and 12 were more likely to have the bacterial disease than kids of other ages, suggesting that the childhood vaccine wears off as kids get older. A recent study showed that the vaccine's effectiveness was only 41 percent among 2- to 7-year-olds and a dismal 24 percent among those aged 8-12. What's ironic, the most protected children were those who were never vaccinated against whopping cough.

In a shocking admission by researchers who discovered the waning effectiveness of the whooping cough vaccine, whooping cough occurs mostly in vaccinated children. This story was first broken by Reuters Health on 3 April, 2012. "We have a real belief that the durability (of the vaccine) is not what was imagined," said Dr. David Witt, an infectious disease specialist at Kaiser Permanente Medical Center in San Rafael, California, and senior author of the study[161].

Witt and his team had expected to find the disease to be rampant among unvaccinated kids, assuming they are more vulnerable to the disease than vaccinated kids. "We started dissecting the data. What was very surprising was that the majority of cases were in fully vaccinated children. That's what started catching our attention." Among the tested subjects, 81 percent were fully up to date on the whooping cough vaccine, 11 percent had received at least one shot, but not the entire recommended series, and a mere 8 percent had never been vaccinated. This should tell us a lot about the lack of vaccine-effectiveness and the damage caused to the immune system in the vaccinated population.

---

[161] Whooping cough vaccine fades in pre-teens: study, Reuters, 3 April, 2012

To me, the most astonishing admission in this unfortunate spectacle was this one: "GSK (GlaxoSmithKline, the manufacturer of the vaccine) has never studied the duration of the vaccine's protection after the shot given to four- to six-year-olds," according to a company spokesperson.

Dr. Joel Ward at the Los Angeles Biomedical Research Institute said in response to the finding: "It's still important for parents to get their kids immunized, even though it doesn't provide lasting protection from whooping cough."

Let me summarize this rather awkward situation: Whooping cough occurs mostly in vaccinated children, either because the vaccines have compromised their immune system or have directly caused the disease by infection. To deal with this dilemma, parents are told to continue getting their children vaccinated against it, although it is has now been proven that not vaccinating them keeps them practically safe. Further, parents should give their children a vaccine drug, for which long-term efficacy has not been even tested, but that is known to have many toxic side effects, including giving them whooping cough.

In addition, parents and caregivers are told they should get regular booster shots themselves to prevent passing on the bacterium to children they come into contact with, even though research has clearly demonstrated that this is utterly useless. A Canadian study, published in 2011 in the journal *Clinical Infectious Diseases*[162], found that the number needed to vaccinate (NNV) for parental immunization was at least 1 million to prevent 1 infant death. Given the high number of vaccine injuries in adults and children[163], it is therefore extremely unethical and irresponsible to call for a further expansion of the existing vaccination campaigns to the adult population.

Millions of children have once more become the guinea pigs for an untested, experimental vaccine which makes those who receive it susceptible to the very disease it is purported to protect them against. Like other childhood illnesses, Bordetella pertussis (whooping cough) is a cyclical disease and natural increases tend to occur every 4-5 years. These diseases are not there to harm the population but help to develop a fully evolved immune system in those who require it. This study clearly demonstrates that no matter how high the vaccination rates in a population,

---

[162] The Number Needed to Vaccinate to Prevent Infant Pertussis Hospitalization and Death Through Parent Cocoon Immunization, Clinical Infectious Diseases, 2011: Danuta M. Skowronski, et al.
[163] Vaccine-Memorial, National Vaccine Information Center, www.nivic.org

as it is in the case of whooping cough, this cyclic illness will continue to occur, especially in the most immune-compromised population - mostly comprised of vaccinated individuals.

The bottom line is that vaccines actually *cause* disease outbreaks and *kill* children, as has occurred in the California whooping cough outbreak. In addition, the younger and older vaccinated adults who don't receive booster shots every 3-4 years become passive carriers and active spreaders of the bacterium Bordetella pertussis, which is believed to be behind the infection. Unvaccinated children who naturally go through whooping cough, which is usually very mild and uneventful in children with a healthy immune system and nutritious diet, retain lifelong immunity and cannot pass the bacterium on to others.

What applies to the whooping cough vaccine holds true for all vaccines. Most modern disease outbreaks, unless they are due to a lack of hygiene, sanitation, good nutrition, and clean drinking water, have all been triggered and spread by people who were artificially immunized. Publically available statistical data on infectious disease outbreaks over the past 100 years is replete with supportive evidence to that effect.

Each flu shot or chickenpox vaccine given suppresses the immune system further and makes it increasingly susceptible to environmental toxins and pathogens. Therefore, since mass vaccinations have taken place now for so many decades, most diseases we are facing now are purely man-made.

Nature is not self-destructive but self-preserving. Wild animals in Africa, Asia, or South America don't die from cancer, heart attack, stroke, diabetes, measles, or whooping cough. They certainly don't need mass vaccination to guarantee their survival as a species. They become naturally immunized through regular contact with germs. The human animal is no exception to nature's immunization programs. An infection occurs only when the body needs to clear out toxins or inflame and remove weak or damaged cells.

Also, the flu, which is actually an effective cleansing mechanism that sets in when the body has accumulated too many toxins, is typically far more prevalent among those who receive regular flu shots; this is hardly surprising, given the powerful immune damage caused by such highly toxic vaccine ingredients as formaldehyde, thimerosal, mercury, anti-freeze agents, among many other disclosed and undisclosed immunity-destructive chemicals. For a complete list of ingredients found in different flu vaccines see the vaccination page of the web site healthscents4u.com[164]. To remove these toxins from the body, I strongly recommend organic sulfur crystals (see Chapter 5 for details).

Just recently, a nurse friend of mine working in a large nursing home for the elderly told me that because of a new house rule, all its residents had to receive the new triple dose flu shot. Shortly thereafter, nearly all of the residents developed the flu. The doctor who was fortunate enough to treat these flu shot victims, believes the flu shot didn't work because the flu strain might have changed after the vaccine was developed. Well, that's old news. Vaccine-makers can never produce a vaccine ahead of time that exactly matches the viral strain of the coming season. Besides, research has already shown that flu vaccines have no protective benefits in the elderly. However, this does not deter the nursing home administrators from strictly implementing the house rule next year again. "We are obligated to follow the doctor's advice, no matter what," said my nurse friend.

Unexpected Help from Mother Nature

Of course, vitamin D produced by the body in response to regular sun exposure or to a vitamin D lamp, offers a near 100 percent protection. Although flu viruses are just as prevalent in the summer as they are in the winter, there is no flu season in the summertime when most people have already replenished their body's vitamin D reserves. I have not had the flu for 45 years because I make sure to have enough sun or UV lamp exposure (without using sunscreen and sunglasses, which block the body's ability to produce vitamin D).

Regular exposure to UV light does not only prevent influenza, but other infections, too. It can even help stop the spread of chickenpox, according to new research. A review of 25 studies by University of London researchers on the varicella-zoster virus - one of the eight human herpes viruses which cause chickenpox and zoster - revealed a clear link between UV levels and the prevalence of chickenpox and zoster.

This study, published in *Virology Journal*[165] on April 23, 2011, showed that chickenpox rates are far less common in the tropics where the population is exposed to sunlight year-round. This link is further supported

---

[164] http://www.healthscents4u.com/Pages/FluVaccineIngredients.aspx
[165] Ultra-violet radiation is responsible for the differences in global epidemiology of chickenpox and the evolution of varicella-zoster virus as man migrated out of Africa, *Virology Journal* 2011, **8**:189 doi:10.1186/1743-422X-8-189

by the fact than in temperate regions, chickenpox tends to flare up more often in the cold weather months, when sunlight is scarce.

The researchers noted: "Chickenpox is seasonal in temperate zones, with the highest incidence seen in winter and spring. One explanation for this seasonality could be the significantly higher levels in ultra-violet radiation (UVR) of approximately 10-25-fold seen in summer in temperate zones, which could inactivate the virus [linked with chickenpox] either in vesicular lesions or after their rupture."

Of course, sunlight is able to inactivate or destroy many pathogens directly, given the strong anti-viral, anti-bacterial, antifungal and immune-boosting benefits of Vitamin D. Before the advent of antibiotics about 70 years ago, sunlight therapy was the only effective treatment for numerous life-threatening infections, including tuberculosis[166].

Just go back as far as 60 years and you will find evidence that sunlight is helpful in preventing the spread of infectious diseases. In a 1949 study by the New York State Department of Health, Labany, N.Y., titled, "Effect of Ultra-Violet Irradiation of Classrooms on Spread of Mumps and Chickenpox in Large Rural Central Schools" showed UV lamps installed throughout the classrooms and corridors of schools helped reduce incidence of diseases among school children[167].

The average city-dwelling American spends 22 hours a day indoors, most of that time beneath and around artificial light.

Children, too, are increasingly spending less time outside in nature, and more of their time indoors at home, in school, on the computer, and in front of the television set. Children and college students are, therefore, particularly vulnerable to having a vitamin D deficiency and being the principal population groups to spread infectious diseases. Even if they spend time outside after school or after doing their homework, it may be 3 p.m. or later, at which time the sun is no longer high enough to trigger the production of enough vitamin D in the body.

With the ever-increasing threat of deadly infections caused by antibiotic-resistant organisms and the failure of vaccines to prevent outbreaks of infectious diseases, the reemployment of nature's most powerful healing gifts now makes a lot of sense, once more. Vaccinating the masses endangers millions of lives because vaccines contain antibiotics

---

[166]Bacteriologic Studies in Disinfection of Air in Large Rural Central Schools. I. Ultra-violet Irradiation Am J Public Health Nations Health. 1949 October; 39(10): 1321–1330.
[167] For more details see my book *Heal Yourself with Sunlight*

that directly contribute to the emergence of these superbugs and immune-deficiency. Over 50 percent of all hospital-acquired infections now involve germs resistant to antibiotic treatment.

Antibiotics in pharmaceutical drugs and vaccines, and those routinely given to farm animals, have produced bacteria so resistant to common antibiotics that the phenomenon will bring about the "end of modern medicine as we know it," warns Margaret Chan, the Director-General of WHO[168]. "Things as common as strep throat or a child's scratched knee could once again kill," Chang said. "Antimicrobial resistance is on the rise in Europe and elsewhere in the world. We are losing our first-line antimicrobials."

In other words, every person who opts for the quick-fix versus natural healing approach, who has their kids vaccinated, or who chooses to eat meat of antibiotic-treated farm animals, directly contributes to the downfall of modern medicine. We are at such a crucial stage of this magic bullet misuse where every dose of antibiotics given to someone in whatever form greatly increases the risk of deadly infections where even a simple operation in a hospital will become too risky to perform. According to Chang, every antibiotic ever developed is at risk of becoming useless, making once-routine operations impossible.

Of course, what applies to the irresponsible overuse of antibiotics also applies to the overuse of vaccines for similar reasons. Now, we have vaccine-resistant pathogens putting our children at risk, according an ever-increasing number of studies. By vaccinating the masses against infectious diseases we are now faced with dangerous mutant invaders that never existed before on planet earth and for which vaccines are completely helpless. These mutants consist of microscopic viruses and bacteria that, like antibiotic-resistant bacteria, are outsmarting the vaccines.

This is demonstrated by the fact that in the past few years, there have been a large number of well-publicized outbreaks of infectious diseases, including the 2010 outbreak of whooping cough or pertussis affecting Californians, and the more recent measles outbreaks occurring in both the US and Canada. The incidence of meningitis is also increasing around the globe, including in the US.

---

[168]Resistance to antibiotics could bring "the end of modern medicine as we know it", WHO claim 16 Mar 2012, The Telegraph.

As mentioned before, children who are vaccinated are not immune to these diseases. Many of the outbreaks have occurred in fully immunized populations.

While, to this day, there is still no scientific proof that vaccines offer any protection against infections (according to research published by the CDC medical journal), there is now evidence that common pathogens are not only increasingly becoming resistant to vaccines, but also more deadly. A 2010 study, published in the *Journal of Emerging Infectious Diseases (EID)*[169], for example, shows that the rising number of whooping cough cases may be in part due to the widespread use of acellular pertussis vaccines resulting in mutated pertussis strains. In an earlier 2009 study, epidemiologic data found an association between these new strains and an increased infant mortality rate[170].

What is most astonishing in all this is the admission by the CDC that vaccinated adults and children may actually be putting vulnerable loved ones at risk of infection. The researchers of a 2000 study published by the CDC's medical journal EID[171] state this in the study's conclusion: "We also observed that DPT vaccine does not fully protect children against the level of clinical disease defined by WHO. Our results indicate that children ages 5-6 years and possibly younger, ages 2-3 years, play a role as silent reservoirs in the transmission of pertussis in the community!"

"The effects of whole-cell pertussis vaccine wane after 5 to 10 years, and infection in a vaccinated person causes nonspecific symptoms. Vaccinated adolescents and adults may serve as reservoirs for silent infection and become potential transmitters to unprotected infants. The whole-cell vaccine for pertussis is protective *only* against clinical disease, *not* against infection. Therefore, even young, recently vaccinated children may serve as reservoirs and potential transmitters of infection."

Case in point, the true, non-preventable cause of disease outbreaks are the vaccinated children and adults, according to this research. Vaccinated children and adults are circulating infectious time bombs that can be set off anytime, anywhere, and even alter the infectious bomb material through unpredictable strain mutation.

---

[169]Bordetella pertussis Clones Identified by Multilocus Variable-Number Tandem-Repeat Analysis, Journal of Emerging Infectious Diseases, http://wwwnc.cdc.gov
[170]Bordetella pertussis Strains with Increased Toxin Production Associated with Pertussis Resurgence. Journal of Emerging Infectious Diseases, http://wwwnc.cdc.gov
[171]Pertussis Infection in Fully Vaccinated Children in Day-Care Centers, Israel, Journal of Emerging Infectious Diseases, http://wwwnc.cdc.gov

To spread disease in the name of prevention is an old trick to deceive the population into submission to the health authorities and the pharmaceutical companies, and the masses have willingly submitted to the fear-mongering, at a hefty price, I may add.

The recent emergence of vaccine-resistant measles and pneumococcal strains, responsible for causing serious cases of pneumonia and meningitis infections is only the beginning of this dangerous vaccination policy, and there is a lot more to come, not just for the US population. A research team led by Dr. Claude Muller from the National Health Laboratory in Luxembourg has recently discovered circulating strains of measles in Africa developing a significant level of resistance to the vaccines currently administered in that part of the world.

Lower respiratory tract infections are now the leading cause of death in the world. Vaccines that lead to treatment-resistant respiratory infections may therefore pose the single most dangerous threat to human life on earth, not unlike the threat of antibiotic-resistant organisms, which now kill more people in the US than AIDS.

Since Americans are the most vaccinated population in the world, they are also the most at risk of becoming the victims of this medical insanity. US children following the recommended vaccine schedule are injected with approximately 115 vaccine antigens within the first two years of their life. The majority of doctors still believe that this approach will have no repercussions, the same doctors who have also believed they can prescribe antibiotics for every little infection without incurring serious negative consequences.

Whether it is just medical ignorance or the intention by those who become wealthy by creating an ever-growing number of patients, it is simply astonishing how far ruthless scientists are taking the agenda of performing illegal experiments on humans (just because they can get away with it). A recent study, for example, involved giving 70 infants a total of 5 doses of antibiotics before and after standard vaccinations. Published in the journal Pediatrics, the scientists suggest that giving 8-week-old babies several doses of acetaminophen (Tylenol) before and after the barrage of recommended childhood vaccines received will help them to sleep better, and improve vaccine efficacy. Just because some doctors believe that sleeping after vaccinations is a positive sign that shows vaccines are working, this dangerous protocol could become common practice among pediatric doctors when administering childhood vaccines.

The study led by Linda Franck at the University of California, San Francisco's (UCSF) Department of Family Healthcare Nursing, did, of course, not mention that such large doses of acetaminophen have been shown in numerous studies to cause liver and kidney damage, and even death[172]. There is also well-documented evidence that antibiotics cause serious and permanent damage to an infant's growing immune system and its just-developing gut flora. In fact, one course of antibiotics can ruin a person's digestive health for the rest of his life.

In 2007, a US Food and Drug Administration (FDA) scientific panel actually recommended that acetaminophen no longer be recommended for children under 6 years of age because of its extreme toxicity. Previous studies have shown that that the administration of acetaminophen before and after vaccinations actually obstructs the supposed effectiveness of the vaccines[173].

Parents who don't want to see babies develop oxidative stress, asthma, and lung damage should question their children's pediatricians when they want to give them acetaminophen for any reason. For example, a2008 New Zealand study published in the journal *Lancet* found that babies who are given acetaminophen within the first year of their lives are 46 percent more likely than other babies to develop asthma.

However, to this day the FDA ignores all expert findings and continues recommending acetaminophen for young children.

The new recommendation to fill infants up with antibiotics every time they get vaccinated will dramatically increase the risk of antibiotic resistant organisms in hospitals and pediatric centers; all that just for increasing the number of antibodies to mostly harmless childhood pathogens, something that has not even been proven to offer better protection against them than doing nothing at all.

Mass vaccination campaigns have already led to serious outbreaks of new diseases that otherwise would never have occurred. For example, mandatory use of the chickenpox vaccine by all children can now be held responsible for the massive escalation of shingles in the US population[174].

Instead of blaming pathogens for causing infections, we will have to take a more proactive stance and consider improving all the immune-depleting factors responsible for making us vulnerable to them (the

---

[172]The Little-Known Dangers of Acetaminophen, http://www.lef.org
[173]Post-Vaccine Tylenol May Harm Immune Response, ABC News Oct 16, 2009
[174]Why a Shingles Epidemic is Bolting Straight at the US (mercola.com)

pathogens). Some of the most-immune-depleting factors are the carcinogenic chemicals and antibiotics contained in vaccines.

In addition to regular full body sun exposure and a balanced diet and lifestyle, cleansing of the liver is a highly effective means of strengthening natural immunity and keeping even superbugs and other morphed pathogens at bay.

4. Lifestyle

Disrupting the Biological Clock

The way we organize and live our lives has a tremendous impact on how the body functions. Its efficiency and performance largely depend on predetermined biological rhythms that operate in perfect synchrony with the circadian rhythms of nature. Circadian rhythms are closely linked with the movements of our planet around the sun. They are also influenced by the motions of the moon and the other planets in relation to the position of the earth.

Our body follows more than a thousand such 24-hour rhythms. Each individual rhythm controls the timing of an aspect of our body's functions, including heart rate, blood pressure, body temperature, hormone levels, secretion of digestive juices, and even pain threshold.

All these rhythms are well coordinated with one another and are controlled by the brain's pacemaker device, known as suprachiasmatic nuclei. This area of the brain regulates the firing of nerve cells that seem to set the clocks of our biological rhythms. If one rhythm becomes somewhat disrupted, other rhythms are thrown off balance, too. In fact, numerous disorders can arise from interference with one or more of our biological rhythms because of an unbalanced, irregular lifestyle.

This section deals with some of the more common deviations that particularly affect the functioning of the liver and gallbladder. By attuning your daily routine to the natural schedule of your body, you can greatly assist it in its ceaseless efforts to nourish, cleanse, and heal itself. Moreover, you can also prevent new health conditions from arising in the future.

Natural Sleep/Wake Cycles

The cyclic alternation of night and day regulates our natural sleep/wake cycles as well as various essential biochemical processes. The onset of daylight triggers the release of powerful hormones (glucocorticoids), of which the main ones are cortisol and corticosterone. Their secretion has a marked circadian variation. These hormones regulate some of the more important functions in the body, including metabolism, blood sugar level, and immune responses. Peak levels occur between 4 a.m. and 8 a.m. and gradually decrease as the day continues. The lowest level occurs between midnight and 3 a.m.

By altering your natural daily sleep/wake schedule to a different one, the peak of cortisol's cycle changes as well. For example, if you suddenly start going to sleep as late as after midnight, instead of before 10 p.m., and/or you arise in the morning after 8 or 9 a.m., instead of with or before sunrise at around 6 a.m., you will enforce a hormonal time-shift that can lead to chaotic conditions in the body. This time-shift is not unlike the one you would experience after arriving at a time zone of a different country located far away from your country of origin. The resulting temporary adjustment effort by the body to restore homeostasis is normally referred to as *jet lag*.

Waste materials that tend to accumulate in the rectum and urinary bladder during the night are normally eliminated between 6 and 8 a.m. With a changed sleep/wake cycle, the body has no choice but to hold on to that waste matter and possibly reabsorb a part of it. When you disrupt your natural sleep/wake cycles, the body's biological rhythms desynchronize with the larger circadian rhythms controlled by the regular phases of darkness and light. This can lead to numerous types of disorders, including constipation, acid reflux, chronic liver disease, respiratory ailments, and heart trouble.

An upset cortisol cycle can also bring on acute health problems. In the 1980s, researchers discovered that more strokes and heart attacks occur in the morning than at any other time of day. Blood clots form most rapidly at about 8 a.m. Blood pressure also rises in the morning and stays elevated until late afternoon. At around 6 p.m. it drops off, and it hits its lowest level during the night.

To support the basic hormonal and circulatory rhythms in the body, it is, therefore, best to go to sleep early (before 10 p.m.) and rise no later than the sun does (ideally at around 6 a.m.). (**Note**: These times change according to the seasons. During the winter, we may need a little more sleep; in the summer, we may need a little less)

Of course, the almost globally adopted practice of following an unnatural, altered time schedule, called Daylight Saving Time, proves to the detrimental to our health, according to a 2007-study published online in *Current Biology*. The study finds that our bodies' internal, biological rhythms don't adjust to daylight savings time.

Moreover, a study titled "Shifts To And From Daylight Saving Time And Incidence Of Myocardial Infarction" found that incidences of heart attacks increased significantly for the first three week days after the transition to daylight saving time in the spring. The study, which was published in the *New England Journal of Medicine* on October 30, 2008, also showed that there were fewer incidences of heart attacks after the transition from daylight saving to standard time in the autumn. This research clearly shows how important it is for the human body to remain synchronized with the circadian rhythms of nature.

One of the pineal gland's most powerful hormones is the neurotransmitter melatonin. The secretion of melatonin starts between 9:30 and 10:30 p.m. (depending on age), inducing sleepiness. It reaches peak levels between 1 and 2 a.m. and drops to its lowest levels at midday. The pineal gland controls reproduction, sleep and motor activity, blood pressure, the immune system, the pituitary and thyroid glands, cellular growth, body temperature, and many other vitally important functions. All of these depend on a balanced melatonin cycle. By going to sleep late or working night shifts, you throw this cycle out of balance, and disrupt many other hormonal cycles as well.

Apart from making melatonin, the brain also synthesizes serotonin, which is a very important neurotransmitter/hormone related to our state of physical and emotional well-being. It affects day and night rhythms, sexual behavior, memory, appetite, impulsiveness, fear, and even suicidal tendencies. Unlike melatonin, serotonin increases with the light of day; physical exercise and sugar also stimulate it.

If you get up late in the morning, the resultant lack of exposure to sufficient amounts of daylight reduces your serotonin levels during the day. Moreover, since melatonin is a breakdown product of serotonin, this habit of rising late also lowers the levels of melatonin during the night, a major cause of sleep disturbance and insomnia. Only after we have slept for about half an hour in the early night hours can the pineal gland convert existing serotonin into melatonin. This makes serotonin the real sleep hormone. Without enough serotonin, melatonin will be deficient and render it incapable of inducing rejuvenating, deep sleep.

Any deviation from the circadian rhythms causes abnormal secretions of these two master hormones. This, in turn, leads to disturbed biological rhythms, which can upset the harmonious functioning of the entire organism, including metabolism and endocrine balance. Suddenly, you may feel *out of synch* and become susceptible to a wide range of disorders, from a simple headache to depression to a heart attack or a cancerous tumor.

Why you should not mess with your melatonin cycle

Both these master hormones are not just produced in the brain's pineal gland, but also in your gut. In fact, 85 percent of the body's serotonin is made in the digestive system to regulate digestive functions, and the amount of melatonin made in the digestive system is a whopping 400-fold greater that the amount the brain produces. Melatonin is also found in the pancreas and the liver's biliary system[175].

Sleep deprivation hasn't been, and still isn't, fully recognized as one of the principal causes of illness. Did your doctor ever ask you how many hours you sleep each night, or at what time you usually go to sleep? Yet, there are actually very few chronic diseases that are not caused or worsened by a messed up melatonin cycle.

It is extremely rare for diseases to manifest unless there is a preexisting impairment of the gut immune system. According to a 2005 review study of all existing research on the multiple action of melatonin on the immune system, this powerful hormone is   involved in several immune pathologies including infection, inflammation, and autoimmunity, together with the relation between melatonin, immunity, and cancer[176].

Melatonin is also involved in the production of important growth hormones, also called growth factors. Proper secretion of growth factors, which stimulates growth in children and helps maintain muscle and connective tissue in adults, depends on balanced sleep cycles. Melatonin-

---

[175]Summarizing Melatonin Research: Melatonin for biological rhythms, body health, gut function and inflammation (minochahealth.typepad.com)
[176]A review of the multiple actions of melatonin on the immune system. Endocrine, 2005 Jul;27(2):189-200

induced sleep triggers growth hormone production. Peak secretion occurs at around 11 p.m., provided you go to sleep before 10 p.m. This short period coincides with dreamless sleep, often referred to as *beauty sleep*. It is during this period of the sleep cycle that the body cleanses itself and does its main repair and rejuvenation work.

When you are sleep-deprived, growth hormone production drops dramatically. People who work the night shift have a greater incidence of insomnia, infertility, cardiovascular illness, stroke, stomach problems, diabetes, and obesity. Their immune system becomes suppressed, which puts them at a higher risk of infection, such as hepatitis and pneumonia. In addition, performance falls and accident rates are higher during the night.

Warning about melatonin supplements

Unlike most other complementary health practitioners, I do not recommend taking melatonin as a food supplement or sleeping aid. When you supplement with melatonin, your body will curb production of its own melatonin. Eventually, you will make yourself dependent on melatonin supplements. Besides, the body's own melatonin carries its unique *signature* recognized by the body as the only genuine melatonin.

The body clearly doesn't like externally supplied melatonin, otherwise it wouldn't produce such harmful side effects as daytime sleepiness, dizziness, headaches, abdominal discomfort, mild anxiety, irritability, confusion, and short-lasting feelings of depression. In addition, melatonin supplements can have harmful interactions with blood-thinning medications (anticoagulants) immune-suppressive drugs, diabetes medications, and birth control pills.

Many people with insomnia are now using melatonin, although in most cases, the sleep problem is not really due to a lack of melatonin but results from a serotonin deficiency. While melatonin is secreted in response to darkness, serotonin is secreted in response to daylight.

Lack of sunlight exposure leads to melatonin deficiency, which, in turn, can keep you awake during the night. In the case that a melatonin supplement helps you to fall or stay asleep, you are most likely suffering from a circadian rhythm sleep disorder. This implies that your body is producing melatonin at the wrong time of day, perhaps because you usually go to bed too late and/or sleep during the day.

Simply adding melatonin is just a Band-Aid approach and can contribute to depressive mood disorders. The most effective treatment for circadian rhythm sleep disorder is going to sleep before 10 p.m., sleeping in total darkness (any light source in the bedroom blocks melatonin secretion), avoiding sleeping during daylight hours, using light therapy, and eating only light meals in the evening (no later than 7 p.m.)[177].

Natural Mealtimes

Ayurveda, the *Science of Life*, declared thousands of years ago that in order to maintain physical and emotional well-being, the body must be fed according to a natural time schedule. Like most other functions in the body, the digestive process is controlled by circadian rhythms. Controlled by the regulatory hormone serotonin, the secretions of bile and other digestive juices peak at midday and are at their lowest during the night. Most of the body's serotonin is made in the digestive system in response to the varying intensities of natural daylight. For this reason, it is best to eat the largest meal of the day at around midday when serotonin levels peak, and take relatively light meals at breakfast and dinner times when serotonin levels are low. This enables the body to digest the ingested food efficiently and absorb the nutrients needed for the maintenance of all bodily functions.

To avoid interfering with the secretion of digestive juices at lunchtime, it is ideal to eat breakfast no later than 8 a.m. Likewise, to digest your evening meal properly, it is best to eat it not later than 6:30 or 7 p.m.

Any long-term disruption of this cycle, caused either by irregular eating habits or by placing the main emphasis on the evening meal and/or breakfast, leads to the accumulation of undigested foods in the intestinal tract and congests lymph and blood. This also disturbs the body's natural instincts.

If our instincts were intact and functioning properly, we would naturally want to eat only those foods that are suitable for our body type, and we would eat them only when our digestive system would also be able to digest them. One of the main causes of gallstone formation is the accumulation of improperly digested foods in the bowels. Eating meals irregularly, or having substantial meals at times of the day when the body is not prepared to produce the appropriate quantities of digestive juices, generates more waste than the body is able to eliminate (also see *Disorders of the Digestive System* in Chapter 1).

---

[177] For a complete explanation of the importance of circadian rhythms and related biological rhythms, see my book *Timeless Secrets of Health and Rejuvenation*

5. Miscellaneous Causes

Low Gastric Secretion

One principal cause of gallstones is a deficiency of hydrochloric acid (HCl) in the stomach, which, in turn, can play a major role in causing other reasons for gallstones to develop. To find out whether you are HCl deficient, you may want to perform this simple test:

Buy betaine hydrochloride tablets or capsules at a health food store. Take ½ a tablet or capsule before the last mouthful of a main meal. If you notice a burning sensation you can stop the test right now because your stomach makes enough HCl. If you noticed no burning or indigestion, take 1 tablet or capsule the following day at the end of your next main meal. If there is still no burning or indigestion, take 2 tablets or capsules the next time. Continue in this way by adding 1 tablet or capsule each day until burning or indigestion occurs. When it does, take a teaspoon of sodium bicarbonate to stop the discomfort.

The more HCl you need to take before reaching the point of burning or indigestion, the more severe is the deficiency. Eating half a teaspoon of freshly grated ginger with a pinch of sea salt before meals can increase HCl production. Eating meals in a calm and stress-free manner also increases HCl. Stress and anxiety, on the other hand, suppress gastric secretions.

Eating highly processed foods and drinking beverages with your meals, except a few sips of water, also interferes with gastric secretions. Combining animal proteins with starches is one of the commonest reasons for HCl deficiency[178].

Most people and medical doctors believe that hydrochloric acid is produced and occurs only in the stomach, but this is not true. HCl is also present in the bloodstream and other fluids of the body to serve as the primary agent responsible for the acidity of the white blood cells (immune cells) and the maintenance of a normal pH (acid/alkaline balance). If HCl is deficient in the stomach, it will also diminish in the rest of the body. Besides causing an imbalance of blood chemistry, poor digestion and assimilation, this also renders the immune system ineffective with regard to maintaining natural immunity to pathogens and toxins. Bile duct

---

[178]For details on proper food combining see my book *Timeless Secrets of Health and Rejuvenation*

congestion strongly interferes with proper digestion and absorption of nutrients, including essential minerals and trace minerals. This, in turn, affects the stomach's ability to produce sufficient amounts of HCl. As a result, the body starts to accumulate waste acids such as carbonic acid, diacetic acid, lactic acid, acetic acids, fatty acids, and uric acid to help maintain the acid/base balance. Although this survival measure by the body may have the short-term benefit of keeping the pH somewhat balanced, it also has the dire long-term consequence of interfering with normal blood chemistry.

When the body recognizes the loss of HCl in the blood and fluids, gastric cells try to make up for the loss by secreting more of it in the stomach leading to a condition called hyperchlorhydria. Eventually, though, the overstimulated gastric cells begin to tire, and hydrochloric acid production drops to a level so low that it completely disappears from the blood and lymph. This is known as achlorhydria. Consequently, phagocytic activity (defensive reactiveness against infectious agents) becomes non-existent.

The rise and fall, and eventual disappearance, of hydrochloric acid concentrations in the blood and body fluids predispose a person to large number of different conditions including acute infection, gastric catarrh, dyspepsia, chronic ulcers of the stomach and duodenum, pyloric obstruction, cholecystitis, duodenitis, appendicitis, diabetes, cancer, neurosis, passive congestion, severe anemia, hypertension, arteriosclerosis, chemical poisoning, heart disease, neoplastic growths, metabolic and endocrine disorders, worry, anxiety, and senility.

Pepsin, an enzyme produced in the stomach, is inactive unless a considerable amount of hydrochloric acid is present. Without pepsin, protein cannot be digested but instead becomes decomposed by bacteria. The resulting toxins can impair digestive functions further and lead to overall toxicity in the body. In addition, without enough acid in the stomach, most foods become subject to decomposition, producing toxic, foul-smelling gases, often noticed as bad breath.

If HCl deficiency persists, dyspepsia, abscesses, pyorrhea, nephritis, pneumonia, appendicitis, boils, and other degenerative disorders begin to manifest. Metabolic waste products may remain in the blood and tissues, leading toward systematic tissue destruction. This happens, for example, when carbonic acid rises in the blood, lactic acid in the tissues, uric acid in the joints and blood vessels, and butyric acid in the stomach or intestines.

Normally, hydrochloric acid reacts with the duodenal membrane to produce the hormone secretin, which stimulates the liver to secrete bile. Depleted HCl suppresses the production of bile, which can undermine digestive functions and prevent the liver from removing toxins from the blood and the rest of the body.

Emotional stress, trauma, relationship conflicts, unbalanced diet and lifestyle, sleep deprivation, lack of regular sun exposure[179], poor quality drinking water, dehydration, exposure to environmental toxins, and foremost, the presence of gallstones in the liver and gallbladder which affects the metabolic functions of stomach cells, are causes of HCl depletion in the stomach and elsewhere in the body.

Drinking too many Juices and Smoothies

Similar to our bodies, plants also have immune systems to ensure their own survival and health. They use prickly thorns, poison as in the case of the deadly nightshades, or they envelop themselves in a wax-covering that is impenetrable for microbes and insects such as lice, beetles, etc. If any of these predators somehow manage to enter the plant's interior, inborn defense mechanisms attempt to destroy the invaders, not dissimilar to our own defense responses.

To protect their species from extinction, plants produce antibodies of which 20,000 kinds are known to date, still only a fraction of what they are capable of producing. These antibodies, when ingested by animals or humans (now considered antigens) can make them sick, which stops them from eating the plants, or at least not eat up all of them.

Another potential sensitivity that protects plant species from becoming extinct is a reaction to toxic salicylates - natural preservatives stored in the bark, leaves, roots and seeds of plants and found in many foods. In vegetables, they're mostly concentrated in the peels and rinds or the outer leaves.

The salicylate content in fruit is highest when the fruit is not fully ripened yet, and decreases during the ripening process. Properly sun-ripened fruits (cooked by the sun), versus those ripened after they are harvested, have great beneficial effects on the body. In general, raw foods, dried foods and juices contain higher concentrations of salicylates than cooked food. To avoid the natural poisons contained in many raw foods,

---

[179]Insufficiency of vitamin D, due to inadequate sun exposure, causes the liver to increase cholesterol production, which can lead to the development of gallstones

all major ancient civilizations traditionally used various methods of food preparation for the purpose of detoxifying[180].

The human body can deal with a certain amount of plant toxins without a problem, but there is a limit. Juicing or making green smoothies means that these plant toxins occur freely and unbound, and thus in higher concentrations that would otherwise be there if you ate these as solid foods. Liquefying food may also make you eat more than you would if you ate them in their solid form.

To protect the plants against their own toxins, they also contain neutralizing compounds in the fibrous parts (cellulose) that become released when you masticate them and combine them with salivary enzymes. This makes chewing of food to be so important. Most people who drink juices or smoothies just swallow them like water or tea. They don't realize that more than 80 percent of the ingested carbohydrates in these liquidized foods require enzymes that only the mouth can produce in sufficient amounts during mastication.

If cows were given their foods in liquid form, which would prevent them from producing enough digestive enzymes in their mouth, they would soon suffer from malnutrition, and become sick. Likewise, drinking smoothies or juices, may not offer much, if any, advantage over eating these as solid foods. The following are some other good reasons to avoid *drinking* your food:

1. The body's immune system identifies natural plant toxins and tries to discard them, along with the rest of the juice, as quickly as possible. This greatly reduces nutrient absorption, which is further exacerbated when no fat/oil is added. Most vegetable carbohydrates require fats to digest them.

2. Missing out on salivary enzymes by drinking your food instead of chewing it will leave most carbohydrates undigested or only partially digested. This prompts an increased action by fermenting gut bacteria, including Candida albicans, thereby causing gas and bloating. The toxins these bacteria produce enter the liver and bile ducts, where they can cause bile sludge and obstruction.

3. When the fibrous part of the food is removed through juicing or is cut into tiny fragments during blending, the liquidized foods fail to properly stimulate peristalsis. Indigestible fiber (cellulose) has an

---

[180]For details, see my book *Timeless Secrets of Health and Rejuvenation*

important function in the GI tract, especially in the large intestine. The slowed bowel movement can lead to overall toxicity and liver problems.

4. While juicing or drinking green smoothies may initially lead to strong cleansing reactions (plant toxins stimulate the immune system to clear them from the intestinal tract, which also removes accumulated waste deposits), this can greatly weaken digestive functions in the long-term.

That said, taking 4-6 oz. of freshly pressed carrot juice once every 2-3 days before the lunch meal - properly swished around in the mouth before swallowing - can act as a great tonic, and intestinal cleanser.

I personally start my lunch meal with a good amount of lettuce, cucumber, avocado, cilantro, tomato, grated ginger, olives, and perhaps some pumpkin or sunflower seeds, and olive oil and lemon juice. This stimulates digestive enzymes and prevents the digestive system from becoming *lazy*. To cook foods, I use waterless cookware which keeps vitamins and enzymes intact.

Watching Television for Many Hours

According to a study published in 2011 in the Journal of the American College of Cardiology[181], "Anyone who devotes more than four hours daily on screen-based entertainment such as TV, video games or surfing the web, ups their risk of heart attack and stroke by 113 percent…compared to those who spend less than two hours daily in screen play." This is regardless of their age, gender, exercise routine, and whether or not they smoke.

Further, watching TV for 4 hours a day increases the risk of dying by 46 percent overall and the risk of dying from cardiovascular disease by 80 percent. For each hour of TV viewed, the risk of dying increases by 11 percent.

Over 18 previous studies, reviewed by the *Journal of the American Medical Association* in 2011[182], have already linked TV watching with an increased risk of metabolic disorder that predisposes those affected to cardiovascular risk, obesity, and diabetes. On the other hand, exercising has been shown to reduce it.

---

[181] Too Much Screen Time Means Health Decline ABC News; Jan 11, 2011
[182] Television Viewing Increases Risk of Type 2 Diabetes, Cardiovascular Disease, and Mortality; *JAMA* 305:2448–2455, 2011

Lack of activity also increases the risk of high blood pressure, and, in women, the risk of breast cancer by 33 percent.

Scientific research has also shown that watching television can dramatically increase cholesterol production in the body. Besides being a necessary component of most tissues and hormones in the body, cholesterol also serves as a stress hormone that increases during physical or mental strain. In fact, cholesterol is one of the first hormones transported to the site of an injury to help heal it. Cholesterol forms an essential constituent of all scar tissue formed during wound healing, whether it is a skin-related injury or a lesion in the wall of an artery.

It can be very tiring and stressful for the brain to compute the fast movement of picture frames for long periods of time. Television stress is especially pronounced among children, whose blood cholesterol can rise by 300 percent within a few hours of watching television. Such excessive secretions of cholesterol alter the composition of bile, which causes the formation of gallstones in the liver.

Exposure to television is a great challenge for the brain. It is far beyond the brain's capacity to process the flood of incoming stimuli that emanate from an overwhelming number of rapidly changing picture frames appearing on the television screen every split second. The resulting stress and strain takes its toll. Blood pressure rises to help move more oxygen, glucose, cholesterol, vitamins, and other nutrients to various parts of the body, including the brain. All of these are used up rapidly by the heavy brainwork. Add to this the tension associated with the content of some programs - violence, suspense, the noise of gunshots, screeching cars, people shouting, loud background music - and the adrenal glands respond with shots of adrenaline to prepare the body for a fight-or-flight response. This stress response, in turn, contracts or tightens the large and small blood vessels in the body, causing the cells to suffer a shortage of water, glucose, minerals and other nutrients. This shortage of nutrients, in turn, may create the phenomenon of insatiable hunger that so many people experience in front of the television set.

Several kinds of symptoms may result from this effect. You may feel tired, exhausted, experience stiffness in the neck and shoulders, feel very thirsty, lethargic, depressed, and even too tired to go to sleep. Stress is known to trigger cholesterol production in the body. Since cholesterol is the basic ingredient of stress hormones, stressful situations use up large quantities of cholesterol to manufacture these hormones. To make up for the loss of cholesterol, the liver raises its production of this precious commodity.

If the body did not bother to increase cholesterol levels during such stress encounters, we would have millions of *television deaths* by now. Nevertheless, the stress response comes with a number of accumulative side effects, one of which is the formation of gallstones. Lack of exercise can also lead to stasis in the bile ducts and, thus, cause gallstones.

Emotional Stress

A stressful lifestyle can alter the natural flora (bacteria population) of the bile, thereby causing the formation of gallstones in the liver. One of the leading stress-causing factors in life is not having enough time for oneself. If you do not give yourself sufficient time for the things you must do or want to do, you will feel pressured.

Continuous pressure causes frustration, and frustration eventually turns into anger. Anger is an indication of severe stress. It has an extremely taxing effect on the body that can be measured by the amounts of adrenaline and noradrenaline secreted into the blood by the adrenal glands. Under severe stress or excitement, these hormones increase the rate and force of the heartbeat, raise blood pressure, and constrict the blood vessels in the secretory glands of the digestive system. In addition, they restrict the flow of digestive juices, including stomach acids and bile, delay peristaltic movement and the absorption of food, and inhibit the elimination of urine and feces.

When food is no longer digested adequately, and significant amounts of waste are prevented from leaving the body via the excretory organs, every part of the body becomes affected, including the liver and gallbladder. This congesting effect, resulting from the stress response, gives rise to great discomfort on the cellular level and is felt as emotional upset. Research shows that chronic stress or rather, the inability to cope with stress, is responsible for 85 to 95 percent of all diseases. These are commonly referred to as psychosomatic diseases. Stress-induced obstructions not only require deep physical cleansing, such as liver, colon, and kidney purges, but also require approaches that trigger relaxation[183].

During relaxation, the body, mind, and emotions move into a mode of performance that supports and enhances all the functions of the body.

---

[183]My book, *It's Time to Come Alive*, offers information on profound, effortless methods of relaxation

Contracted blood vessels open again, digestive juices flow, hormones are balanced, and waste is eliminated more easily. Therefore, the best antidote to stress and its harmful effects are methods of relaxation, such as meditation, yoga, Qigong, spending time in nature, playing with children or pets, playing or listening to music, exercising, walking, and the like.

To cope with the fast pace of modern life and to give the nervous system enough time to unwind and release any accumulated tension, it is vital to spend at least 10 to 30 minutes a day by yourself, preferably in silence. Doing something just for yourself has an uplifting effect on you and makes you a happier, more fulfilled person.

If you have had any stressful periods in your life or currently have difficulties calming down or unwinding, you will greatly benefit by doing a series of liver flushes. Having gallstones in the liver is, by itself, a major cause of constant stress in the body. When you eliminate these stones, you will become naturally calm and relaxed. You may also discover that once your liver is clean, you will become much less angry or upset about situations, other people, or yourself, regardless of the circumstances[184].

---

[184]To fully understand emotions and their root causes and to free yourself from their limitations, refer to my book *Lifting the Veil of Duality—Your Guide to Living Without Judgment*

Conventional Treatments for Gallstones

Treatments typically used to deal with gallstones aim at either dissolving gallstones directly within the gallbladder or removing the gallbladder through surgery. However, these treatments have no beneficial impact whatsoever on the large amount of stones congesting the bile ducts of the liver. It is important to realize that every person who has gallstones in the gallbladder has multiple times as many stones in the liver. The surgical removal of the gallbladder or its stones does not substantially increase bile flow, because the stones that are stuck in the liver bile ducts continue to prevent proper bile secretion.

Even in the case of surgical removal of the gallbladder, the situation remains highly problematic for the body. Since the pumping device for bile (the gallbladder) is now gone, the small amount of bile that the liver is able to squirt out through its congested bile ducts comes forth merely in dribbles. Both insufficient bile secretion and the uncontrolled flow of bile into the small intestine continue to cause major complications with the digestion and absorption of food, particularly if it contains fats. Protein foods, which usually contain fats, remain largely undigested.

The result is an ever-increasing amount of toxic waste that accumulates in the intestinal tract and lymphatic system. The intestines practically become a cesspool of rotting matter and bacterial overgrowth. The fat-soluble vitamins A, D, E, and K, as well as important minerals such as calcium and magnesium, remain undigested, too. (**Note**: if your gallbladder has already been removed, to avoid inflammation and hypertension, you may need to regularly apply a good transdermal magnesium oil to your skin (see *Product Information - Magnesium Oil*)

I have heard general practitioners and surgeons making promises like this to their patients: "You will be just fine and all your digestive problems with be gone once your gallbladder has been removed." After all, the medical textbooks claim that the gallbladder is not an essential organ and can be safely removed. However, since only the modified bile in the gallbladder is capable of digesting fats, and the bile passed from the liver directly into the intestines is meant to remove toxins from the liver and blood, not digest food. Simply removing the gallbladder cannot make everything alright.

The restricted ability to digest and assimilate fats stimulates the liver cells to increase production of cholesterol. The side effect arising from this emergency maneuver of the body is the generation of more gallstones in the liver bile ducts. Therefore, removing the gallbladder is not a long-term solution to digestive problems but, rather, a cause of further and more serious complications in the body, such as cancer, obesity, diabetes, kidney disease, and heart disease. Balanced bile secretion and a functional gallbladder, on the other hand, protect the body against most diseases.

Any treatment of the gallbladder, however advanced and sophisticated it may be, can only be considered a drop in the ocean of cure because it does not remove the main problem, which is the hundreds or thousands of gallstones blocking the bile ducts of the liver.

Each year, millions of people fall into the trap of following the most commonly recommended solution to gallstones (in the gallbladder) offered by conventional medicine, that is, to have their gallbladder surgically removed. The recommendation is often coupled with the stern warning, "If you don't get it removed, you may die," which is the oldest method of successfully blackmailing and manipulating people into doing what you want them to do.

A good doctor would never push a patient into choosing a quick-fix solution over achieving a long-lasting cure of their condition. She lays out all the possible options, with all the advantages and disadvantages, and then lets the patients empower themselves and make the decision.

Conventional medicine offers 3 main approaches to treating gallstones, none of which include a long-term solution:

1. Dissolving Gallstones

For patients with mild, infrequent symptoms, or those who do not want surgery, various drugs are available that claim to dissolve gallstones. On the surface, it seems like a good idea to gradually dissolve gallstones through drugs that contain bile salts (oral dissolution therapy). The main drugs used for this purpose are known as CDCA (chenodeoxycholic acid) and UDCA (ursodeoxycholic acid). The preferred single drug now used is UDCA, or it may be combined with CDCA. Given in pill form over a period of 12 to 24 months, these drugs may achieve a decrease in cholesterol levels in the bile and dissolve small gallstones in the gallbladder. But there is no guarantee of this.

In a meta-analysis comprising almost 2,000 patients treated until 1992, complete dissolution was achieved in 18.2 percent with CDCA, in 37.3 percent with UDCA, and in 62.8 percent with combination therapy[185]. Unlike UDCA, CDCA has the disadvantage of often causing severe diarrhea.

After successful dissolution of gallstones with ursodeoxycholic acid, 30-50 percent of patients form new stones within 5 years[186]. Patients with multiple primary stones have an increased recurrence rate. In addition, only cholesterol stones can be dissolved by bile acids, and any significant calcification of the stones will make it very difficult to dissolve them.

Other dissolving agents, such as methyl tert-butyl ether, have no advantage over bile salts. Unsuccessful treatment may lead to surgery.

More recently, solvents have been directly instilled into the gallbladder by means of a small catheter. This approach has been shown to be more effective in dissolving hard gallstones in the gallbladder, but it still fails to resolve the major issue - the accumulation of soft gallstones in the liver. There exists insufficient scientific research to determine what side effects accompany this method of treatment.

In all cases of treatments, side effects can range from mild to severe to death.

2. Shock Waves & Dissolution

Another alternative method to surgery is lithotripsy, a technique by which the gallstones are literally pounded into submission by a series of sound waves. According to a 1993 report by the medical journal Lancet, this therapy has great setbacks because it can result in kidney damage and raise blood pressure - risks that have remained unchanged until today. Both these side effects can lead to an increase in the number of gallstones in the liver (see Disorders *of the Circulatory System and Disorders of the Urinary System* in Chapter 1).

In addition, this procedure, in which gallstones are fragmented through shock waves, leaves toxic gallstone residue behind. This residue can quickly become a breeding place for harmful bacteria and parasites, leading to infections in the body.

---

[185]Efficacy of bile acid therapy for gallstone dissolution - a meta-analysis of randomized trials. May GR, Sutherland LR, Shaffer EA. *Aliment Pharmacol Therapeut.* 1993;7:139-148

[186]Collins C et al. A prospective study of common bile duct calculi in patients undergoing laparoscopic cholecystectomy: Natural history of choledocholithiasis revisited. Annals of Surgery 239:28-33, 2004

Recent studies have confirmed that most patients undergoing this kind of treatment experience internal bleeding, ranging from a small hemorrhage to major blood loss that requires blood transfusion. This treatment also has a high stone-recurrence rate.

There is yet another pulverization method, percutaneous electrohydraulic lithotripsy, which involves energy bursts to break up the stones. This treatment involves inserting a catheter into the gallbladder to accommodate the energy burst delivery device. However, as in the case of using shock waves, the risk of causing serious injury to the gallbladder is high.

There is also a relatively new process of stone dissolution, litholysis, but it may still be in the experimental stage and may not be covered by health insurance. In this approach, a catheter is used (percutaneous cholecystostomy) to deliver a solvent into the gallbladder.

According to Swiss research[187], percutaneous cholecystostomy in association with contact litholysis using methyl tertiary butyl ether is an effective treatment in patients who cannot be operated due to critical conditions.

The success rate in case of cholesterol stones averages 70 to 95 percent depending on the number and size of stones. "Relatively rare complications associated with this procedure usually occur immediately or within days and include hemorrhage, vagal reactions, sepsis, bile peritonitis, pneumothorax, perforation of the intestinal loop, secondary infection or colonization of the gallbladder and catheter dislodgment," according to research conducted in Turkey[188]. "Late complications have been reported as catheter dislodgment and recurrent cholecystitis," said the researchers.

3. Surgery

Nearly 800,000 gallbladder removal surgeries are performed annually in the US at a cost exceeding $6 billion, according to the American Gastroenterological Association. A gallbladder operation costs between $8,000 and $10,000 and takes about 30 to 45 minutes with laproscopy. While cholecystectomy (open gallbladder surgery) is still commonly used for patients with frequent or severe pain, or with a history of acute

---

[187]Contact litholysis of gallstones with methyl tert-butyl ether in risk patients--a case report
Swiss Surg. 2001;7(1):39-42
[188]Percutaneous cholecystostomy, Eur J Radiol. 2002 Sep;43(3):229-36

cholecystitis, laparoscopic cholecystectomy has now become the preferred surgical technique. With traditional surgery, the gallbladder is removed through an open technique requiring a standard skin incision and general anesthesia. During laparoscopic cholecystectomy, also called a keyhole operation, the stone-filled gallbladder is literally pulled through a small incision in the abdomen. Sometimes, open cholecystectomy is required if the keyhole operation fails.

With a keyhole operation, patients seem to recover much faster and often leave the hospital and return to regular activity within days. However, since its introduction, this quick Band-Aid approach to treating gallbladder disease has prompted many more patients to have a gallbladder operation than ever before. The intended benefit of giving this operation is to rid the body of some persistent symptoms of discomfort, but in reality, this may not happen at all.

In a 2011 study, published in the journal *Clinical Gastroenterology and Hepatology*[189], researchers admitted that abdominal pain persists in up to 50 percent of patients after gallbladder removal, and that physicians need a better way to determine who will benefit from surgery. "Given the number of cholecystectomies that are performed, this study underscores the importance of taking a detailed history when selecting patients for surgery," said Johnson L. Thistle, M.D., of Mayo Clinic and lead author of this study.

Many patients suffering from gastroesophageal reflux disease and irritable bowel syndrome may experience similar symptoms as those caused by a gallstone attack and subsequently have their gallbladder removed (completely unnecessarily, I may add). This is particularly concerning since about 80 percent of gallstones never become symptomatic, which means they will never bother the patient for as long as he lives. That said, a person who frequently suffers from gas pains in the transverse colon or stomach and also has some asymptomatic gallstones in the gallbladder, may end up having an unnecessary gallbladder surgery because the treating physician believes the abdominal pain could be due to gallbladder problem.

Apart from having had no proven effect on the overall mortality rate from gallbladder diseases, laparoscopic surgery does have its risks. As many as 10 percent of patients coming out of surgery have stones

---

[189]Factors That Predict Relief From Upper Abdominal Pain After Cholecystectomy. *Clinical Gastroenterology and Hepatology*, 2011; 9 (10): 891 DOI:10.1016/j.cgh.2011.05.014

remaining in the bile ducts, according to the US National Institutes of Health. (**Note**: The bile ducts referred to here are not liver bile ducts).

According to *Mayo Health Oasis*, other hazards include lost gallstones in the peritoneal cavity, abdominal adhesion, and possibly infective endocarditis. Moreover, according to the *New England Journal of Medicine*, the procedure can cause hemorrhage, inflammation of the pancreas (a potentially fatal condition), and perforation of the duodenal wall. There may also be injury and obstruction of bile ducts and the leakage of bile into the abdomen, increasing the patient's chance of suffering a potentially serious infection. About one percent of patients are at risk of dying from this kind of operation.

Bile duct injuries have increased dramatically because of using keyhole surgery. In Ontario, Canada, where 86 percent of all gallbladder operations are performed in this way, the number of bile duct injuries has risen by over 300 percent since this method has become standard practice since the mid-1990s.

In a number of patients, gallstones are caught in the common bile duct (the main bile duct leading to the duodenum). In such cases, the removal of the gallbladder does not alleviate the symptoms of gallstone disease. To help the condition, a flexible tube is placed in the mouth and advanced to the point where the common bile duct enters the duodenum. During the procedure, the opening of the bile duct is enlarged and the stones are moved into the small intestines. Unfortunately, many of the stones may become stuck in the small or large intestine, becoming a source of constant intestinal infection or toxemia.

Conclusion

None of the above procedures addresses the *cause* of gallbladder disease. In fact, they all contribute to further disruption of the digestive and eliminative processes in the body. The short-term relief that a patient may experience after his gallbladder has been removed may lead him to believe that he has been cured. Many others continue to experience the same pain they had when they still had their gallbladder. The continued and often worsened impairment of proper bile secretion by the liver may lead to the development of far more serious health problems than just gallbladder disease.

The following chapter describes a simple procedure that painlessly, safely, and effectively removes not only the few gallstones in the gallbladder, but also, and most importantly, the hundreds and thousands of gallstones in the liver. It is extremely unfortunate that millions of people have had their gallbladder removed unnecessarily or have lost their lives because of liver and gallbladder disease.

Luckily, there is a simple, risk-free, inexpensive approach available to every person who wishes to naturally restore liver and gallbladder health and to prevent diseases from arising in the future.

Those who unfortunately no longer have a gallbladder can also greatly benefit from liver flushes. They tend to have more stones in the liver than those individuals with an inefficient gallbladder. The main reason for gallbladder disease is the occurrence of intrahepatic gallstones. These stones prevent the liver from properly removing toxins and noxious substances that can be responsible for numerous health conditions, including obesity, diabetes, cancer, and heart disease.

If your gallbladder was removed and you have also cleansed your liver through a series of liver flushes, you may still need to take a bile supplement (usually sold in the form of ox bile). Make sure to lower the dosage if you experience diarrhea, or increase it if you are constipated.

To avoid new complications, I strongly recommend abstaining from eating animal proteins such as meat, fish, chicken, eggs, cheese, milk, as well as fried or greasy foods. Besides taking a bile supplement and following a balanced vegetarian diet and lifestyle, you can live a very comfortable and healthy life.

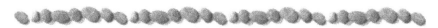

Chapter 4

The Liver and Gallbladder Flush

R idding the liver and gallbladder of gallstones is one of the most important and powerful approaches you can take to improve your health.

The liver and gallbladder flush requires 6 days of preparation, followed by 16 to 20 hours of actual cleansing. To remove gallstones, you will need the following items:

- **Apple juice** - six 32 oz. containers (6 x 1 liter) **or Sour/tart cherry juice** – six 8 oz. portions (6 x 240 ml) **or** choose from other alternatives listed under "Alternatives to Apple Juice or Sour Cherry Juice"
- **Epsom salt*** (or magnesium citrate) - 4 tablespoons (60 g) dissolved in 24 oz. (about 710 ml) of water**
- **Pure extra virgin olive oil**, 4 oz. (120 ml)
- **Fresh grapefruit (pink is best)** - enough to squeeze 6 oz. (about 180 ml) of juice or use the same amount of fresh lemon and orange juice combined***

---

* You can find Epsom salt in most drugstores or natural food stores. Some packaging labels describe it as a natural laxative, oral laxative, or *for internal use*. Do not use Epsom salt labeled *not to be taken internally* or *for baths*, since it contains impurities! If you cannot find Epsom salt, use magnesium citrate instead (same dosage, or if it comes in liquid form, take 3-4 fl. oz. (90-120 ml) at each of the four specified times).

** One tablespoon of Epsom salt equals 3 teaspoons of 5 grams each. The total amount of Epsom salt per tablespoon is 15 grams. Four tablespoons equal 60 grams. If your body weight is below normal, use a total of 40 grams; this amount will still give you frequent watery bowel movements necessary to help expel the released toxins and stones from the liver and gallbladder.

*** If you cannot tolerate grapefruit juice, you may use equal amounts of freshly squeezed lemon and orange juice instead. The effect is the same with either choice. For best results, use organically grown fruits.

Preparation

Drink 1 container of 32 oz. (1 liter) of packaged or freshly prepared apple juice (ideally from organically grown apples) *or* 8 oz. (240 ml) of unsweetened sour/tart cherry juice (see other options below) per day for a period of 6 days.

The malic acid in the apple juice or sour cherry juice softens the gallstones and makes their passage through the bile ducts smooth and easy. Sour cherry juice has about 4 times the concentration of malic acid that apple juice has, and is usually better tolerated by those who cannot deal with the large amount of sugar contained in apple juice.

Both apple juice and sour cherry juice have a strong cleansing effect. Some sensitive people may experience bloating and, occasionally, diarrhea, while on this much apple juice. While some of the diarrhea is actually stagnant bile, released by the liver and gallbladder (indicated by a brownish, yellow color), it may also be due to fermentation of the sugar in apple juice. If this becomes somewhat uncomfortable, you can dilute the apple juice with any amount of water, switch to sour cherry juice, or use any of the other options described later.

I found that apple juice and sour cherry juice are equally beneficial in preparing your liver and gallbladder for an effective flush.

Drink either of these juices slowly and in small portions spread throughout the day, between meals. You want to make sure there is a continuous supply of malic acid almost throughout the day, which is required to help soften the stones. Avoid drinking the juice during, just before, and in the first 1-2 hours after meals, and in the evening past 6 p.m. This is in addition to your normal daily water intake of 6 to 8 glasses.

Note: During Day 6 of the preparation, drink the entire amount of juice during the morning hours only.

What you need to know about apple juice:
- If you choose apple juice as your preparation method, use organic juice; freshly pressed apple juice from organic apples is ideal. Although for the purpose of the flush, any good brand of commercial apple juice, apple concentrate, or apple cider works well, too; commercially produced apple juice may contain high amounts of inorganic arsenic - a naturally occurring mineral that can be toxic in high concentrations.
- It may be useful to rinse your mouth out with baking soda and/or brush your teeth several times per day to prevent the acid from damaging your teeth. The same applies to the alternative options.
- Some people should not drink apple juice in the large quantities required for the liver flush. These include those who suffer from diabetes, hypoglycemia, yeast infection (*Candida*), cancer, and stomach ulcers.

***

What you need to know about sour/tart cherry juice:
- Tart cherries should not be confused with the sweet, black cherry variety.
- Sour cherries contain 4 times the amount of malic acid than found in apples. Hence, you only need a fourth of the quantity, i.e. 8 oz. cherry juice versus 32 oz. apple juice during each of the 6 days of the cleanse preparation.
- Make certain to only buy sour cherry juice in glass bottles! Most health food stores stock organic, preservative-free tart cherry juice.
- Studies suggest sour cherries may help reduce risk factors for type 2 diabetes, which makes tart cherry juice a good option for diabetics who wish to do the liver flushes and cannot use apple juice because of its high sugar content.
- The juice has also shown to help reduce inflammation of joints and inhibit tumor growth, improve blood flow, lower blood pressure, and increase heart and brain health.
- It can be used by those suffering from Candida problems.

Dietary recommendations (for the first 5 days):

During the entire week of preparation and cleansing, avoid foods or beverages that are ice-cold; they chill the liver and, thereby, reduce the effectiveness of the cleanse. All foods or beverages should be warm or at least room temperature. If you are used to eating only raw foods, you may continue doing that. To help the liver prepare for the main part of the cleanse, try to avoid foods from animal sources, including meat, fish, poultry, eggs, dairy products (except butter), fried food items, and refined sugar or foods that contain it. Otherwise, eat normal meals, but avoid overeating. It is best to consume fresh salads, cooked vegetables, grains, legumes, nuts, seeds, natural fats and oils, herbs, spices, and fruits during the preparation time. Please note the important dietary instructions for Day 6 of the preparation phase below.

The best times for cleansing:

The main and final part of the liver flush is best done over a weekend, or when you are not under any pressure and have enough time to rest. Although the liver flush is effective at any time of the month, it should preferably coincide with a day between full moon and new moon, or new moon and full moon. If possible, avoid doing the actual flush on full moon day when the body tends to hold on to extra fluids in the brain and tissues and is, therefore, more reluctant to release toxins[190]. The days around new moon are the most conducive for cleansing and healing.

Please read this if you take any medication!

While some people on prescription medication have done liver flushes successfully, others have reported that they did not release any stones, or felt very sick for a day or two.

In 99 percent of all cases, pharmaceutical medications are merely symptom-suppressive and non-cause-oriented, and therefore, useless, unnecessary, and increasing harmful, especially if taken long-term. For instance, blood pressure medication is now known to cause congestive heart failure, hypertension, and kidney disease; arthritis medication

---

[190]For a detailed explanation about lunar influences on the body, see my book *Timeless Secrets of Health and Rejuvenation*

damages the liver and kidneys and causes more pain and more arthritis; statins increase the risk of heart disease, stroke, and liver damage; anti-cancer drugs cause more cancers and spread them in the body, etc. (for more details, see Chapter 3)

There are numerous simple, proven, and completely natural methods of restoring balance in the body that are far more effective and also void of any harmful side effects. For instance, vitamin D alone, which the body produces in response to regular sun exposure, can balance blood pressure, normalize blood sugar and cholesterol, prevent and reverse cancer, stop infections such as tuberculosis, heal skin diseases, and help with almost every other illness.

In many cases, hypertension is *just* due to chronic dehydration and can be corrected in a matter of days. This book contains plenty of information you can use to make the necessary changes to your diet and lifestyle and escape the vicious cycle of taking toxic drugs that only further the occurrence of illness and debility and which, in turn, requires new drugs that cause further symptoms of disease.

If you have already become drug-dependent, I recommend you work under the supervision of a naturopathic doctor to gradually wean yourself off the medication while you also follow the guidelines for diet and lifestyle outlined in this book, or in greater detail, in my book *Timeless Secrets of Health and Rejuvenation*.

While liver flushes help the body to detoxify and heal itself, medications like antidepressants, anti-inflammatory drugs, or antibiotics do the exact opposite. It is risky for the body to undergo two incompatible and opposing processes at the same time. In fact, taking medication while doing a liver flush, may alter its concentration in the blood to undesirable levels; hence, the warning. Once off pharmaceutical drugs, you can then safely do liver flushes.

Cautionary note about cancer drugs

Those who have undergone chemotherapy and wish to do liver flushes need to wait 6-8 months after the last round of treatment. Chemo drugs produce an excessive amount of intrahepatic gallstones because of their high toxicity, but it takes a while before all the chemical toxins are absorbed by bile and formed into stones. Doing a liver flush too soon after receiving these drugs would release much of the unbound poison into the intestinal tract and literally burn holes through it.

A Note on thyroid medication

Those who have had their thyroid removed (or have an underactive thyroid) and are taking thyroid medication will need to continue taking the medicine when doing the liver flushes. It is one of the few exceptions to the rule. I have not seen any diminished effectiveness of the liver flush when taking thyroid hormone.

Food supplements

If you take natural food supplements, such as minerals and non-synthetic vitamins, you may continue taking them, but it is best to avoid taking any supplements or medicines during the actual liver flush, unless they are absolutely essential. Besides, they are wasted as they are flushed out with the bile and Epsom salt.

Age Considerations

Children as young as 9 or 10 years old can do liver flushes, but they should only take half the amounts of cleanse ingredients (see separate instructions below). I have also had people in their 90s who also had excellent results with liver flushing.

Cleanse your colon BEFORE and AFTER you do a liver flush

Having regular bowel movements is not necessarily an indication that your bowel is unobstructed. Colon cleansing, done either a few days before or, ideally, on Day 6 of preparation, helps to avoid or minimize any discomfort or nausea that may arise during the actual liver flush. It prevents back-washing of the oil mixture or waste products from the intestinal tract into the stomach and it also assists the body in swiftly eliminating the released gallstones. Most cases of nausea during liver flushes are due to not properly cleansing the colon beforehand. Colonic irrigation (colon hydrotherapy) is the most thorough method to prepare the colon for the liver flush. Colema-board irrigation is an almost equally effective method, followed by water enemas (see details in the section *Keep Your Colon Clean* in Chapter 5).

This is what you need to do on Day 6 of the preparation:

Drink all the 32 oz. (1 liter) of apple juice or all the 8 oz. of sour cherry juice, or any of the other chosen options, in the morning. You may start drinking the juice soon after awakening. If you feel hungry in the morning, eat a light breakfast, such as fruit or a hot cereal like oatmeal. Avoid regular sugar or other sweeteners, spices, milk, butter, oils, yogurt, cheese, ham, eggs, nuts, pastries, cold packaged cereals, and other processed foods. Freshly-pressed fruit juices or vegetables juices are fine.

For your lunch meal you may eat plain cooked or steamed vegetables with rice (preferably white basmati rice), buckwheat, quinoa or similar grains, and flavor it with a little unrefined sea or rock salt. If you prefer to eat fruit or raw vegetables, that's fine, too.

Please *do not eat any protein foods, nuts, avocado, butter, or oil,* or you might feel ill during the actual flush. The main thing is to save as much bile as possible for the liver flush, which is required to remove as many stones as possible from the liver and gallbladder. Eating fat or oil-containing foods would use up that bile and render the liver flush ineffective.

Also, do not eat or drink anything except water after 1:30 p.m., otherwise you may have difficulty passing stones! Follow the exact schedule below.

Please do not attempt the liver cleanse until you have carefully read the rest of this chapter!

The Actual Flush

Evening

6:00 p.m.: Add 4 tablespoons (a total of 60 grams) of Epsom salt (magnesium sulfate) to a total of 24 US-fluid oz. (710 ml) of filtered water in a glass jar. This makes four 6-oz. (180 ml) servings. Drink your first portion of 6 oz. (180 ml) now.

You may take a few sips of water afterward to neutralize the bitter taste in your mouth, or add a little lemon juice to improve the taste. If you still cannot stand the taste, you may add a small amount of apple juice. Some people drink it with a large plastic straw to bypass the taste buds on the tongue. Closing the nostrils while drinking it works well for most people. It is also helpful to brush your teeth afterward or rinse out the mouth with baking soda. One of the main actions of Epsom salt during the liver flush is to relax and dilate (widen) the bile ducts, as well as the sphincter of Oddi[191], thereby making it easy for the stones to pass.

Epsom salt also causes the gallbladder to contract to a third of its original size, according to published research[192]. This effect greatly assists in the removal of stones from the gallbladder. Moreover, Epsom salt clears out waste that may obstruct the release of the stones.

If you are allergic to Epsom salt (which is rare), or if it makes you feel nauseated or you are just not able to get it down, you may instead use the second best choice, magnesium citrate (see details below).

Set out the citrus fruit you will be using later, so that it can warm to room temperature.

8:00 p.m.: Drink your second serving of Epsom salt.

9:30 p.m.: If the Epsom salt has not prompted at least one bowel movement until now, it is usually because you have already done a thorough colon cleanse (colonic irrigation, Colema, or water enema) within the past 6-8 hours. However, this may also be because you have not cleansed your colon beforehand; in this case, take a water enema at this time (see instructions on how to perform a water enema in chapter 5). This will trigger a series of bowel movements and also make it easier for the liver and gallbladder to release stones.

Note: Congestion in the colon can prevent the proper opening of the gallbladder and reduce the flush's effectiveness.

9:45 p.m.: Thoroughly wash the grapefruits (or lemons and oranges). Squeeze them by hand and extract the juice. You will need about 6 oz. (180 ml) juice. Pour the juice and 4 oz. (120 ml) olive oil into a glass jar that has a lid. Close the jar tightly and shake hard, about 20 times or until

---

[191]Sphincter of Oddi is a muscular valve that controls the flow of digestive juices (bile and pancreatic juice) through the ampulla of Vater into the intestinal duodenum.
[192]Correlation Between Gallbladder Size and Release of Cholecystokinin After Oral Magnesium Sulfate in Man Kazutomo Inoue, Isidoro Wiener, Charles J. Fagan, Larry C. Watson, and James C. Thompson; Ann Surg. 1983 April; 197(4): 412–415

the solution is watery. For best results, drink this mixture at 10:00 p.m., but if you feel you still need to visit the bathroom a few more times, you may delay this step for up to 10-15 minutes.

10:00 p.m.: Stand next to your bed (do not sit down) or near there and drink the mixture, if possible, without interruption. Closing the nostrils while drinking it and holding your breath seems to work best. Some people, though, prefer to drink it through a large plastic straw. If necessary, use a little honey between sips, which helps the mixture go down more smoothly. Most people, though, have no problem drinking in one go. It's best not to take more than 5 minutes for this. You may wish to quickly brush your teeth to get rid of the taste of the concoction.

PLEASE LIE DOWN IMMEDIATELY!

This is essential for helping to release the gallstones! Turn off the lights and lie flat on your back with one or two pillows propping your head up. Your head should be higher than your abdomen. If this is uncomfortable, lie on your right side with your knees pulled toward your head, but also keep your head elevated. **Lie perfectly still for at least 20 minutes, and try not to speak!** You want to use all the available energy to release stones and not divert it elsewhere. Close your eyes and put your attention on your liver.

(**Note**: To relax the bile ducts further, you may place a piece of cloth soaked in castor oil or warm apple cider vinegar over the liver area. This is not necessary, but some people find it to be beneficial)

You may feel the stones traveling along the bile ducts like marbles. There won't be any spasms or pain because the magnesium in the Epsom salt keeps the bile duct valves wide open, dilated, and relaxed, and the oily bile that is discharged along with the stones keeps the bile ducts well lubricated. (The situation is very different in the case of a gallstone attack where magnesium is not present and bile concentration is relatively low)

After the first crucial 20 minutes, you may remove the extra pillows and go into your normal sleeping position; however, avoid sleeping on your stomach.

It is best to remain in bed, but if at any time during the night you feel the urge to have a bowel movement, do so. Check if there are already small gallstones (pea-green or tan-colored ones) floating in the toilet.

In the rare case you feel sick at any time during the liver cleanse, please follow the instructions provided under "Feeling Sick During The Flush" in this chapter.

The Following Morning

6:00–6:30 a.m.: Upon awakening, drink a glass of warm water. Shortly after, drink your third portion of Epsom salt. Rest, read, or meditate. If you are very sleepy, you may go back to bed. However, it is best if the body stays in an upright position. Most people feel fine, but low in energy until later in the morning.

8:00–8:30 a.m.: Drink your fourth and last portion of Epsom salt.

10:00–10:30 a.m.: You may drink freshly pressed fruit juice at this time. One half-hour later, you may eat one or two pieces of fresh fruit. One hour later, you may eat regular (but light) food, preferably vegetarian. Make certain you don't overeat, and stop eating when you still feel a little hungry.

By the evening or the next morning you should be back to normal and feel the first signs of improvement. Continue to eat light meals during the following 2-3 days. Remember, your liver and gallbladder have undergone major *surgery*, albeit without the harmful side effects or the expense.

Drinking Enough Water During the Cleanse

During the entire process of liver cleansing, including the 6-day preparation, make certain to drink enough water, especially when thirsty. However, avoid drinking water right after taking Epsom salt (allow 10-15 min) and for the first 2 hours after drinking the oil mixture.

To produce enough bile and to remove stones from the liver and gallbladder during the liver flush, the body has to be well hydrated. Dehydration can, in fact, render the liver flush ineffective.

Contraindications

(When the liver flush is not recommended):

Bowel obstruction: If there is an obstruction in the small bowel, the liver flush should not be attempted. A small-bowel obstruction (SBO) is caused by a variety of pathologic processes. These include postoperative adhesions, followed by malignancy, Crohn's disease, and hernias. Surgeries most closely associated with SBO are appendectomy, colorectal surgery, and gynecologic and upper gastrointestinal (GI) procedures.

Weakness: Individuals who are very weak and emaciated (underweight) should not attempt liver flushes. If this applies to you, regaining your strength and stamina through the other recommendations made in this book, should be your first priority. Once your body has regained a more healthy weight and feels stronger, you may attempt your first liver flush.

Bowel Diseases: If a part of the large bowel has been removed, it is still possible to do the liver cleanses. However, they should be avoided if there is any inflammatory disease, such as ulcerative colitis, Crohn's disease, diverticulitis, diverticulosis, numerous polyps, and large hemorrhoids. Please refer to my book, *Timeless Secrets of Health and Rejuvenation,* to address the dietary and lifestyle causes for these disorders. Once healed up, you can safely do liver flushes.

Acute Infection, Prescription drugs: Do not cleanse your liver when you suffer an acute infection; take prescriptions drugs (except mild thyroid medication); have fissures or large hemorrhoids; experience strong abdominal pain, nausea or vomiting; are dehydrated; or have frequent diarrhea or bloody stools.

Constipation and Hemorrhoids: Hemorrhoids, which are congested, varicose veins in the lower intestinal tract, usually result from chronic constipation.

If you are constipated and still attempt to do the liver flush, the oil mixture may back up or remain in the stomach unduly long. Eventually, the esophageal valve opens and you may feel nauseous, feel faint and throw up. If you still pass stones, the stone material and/or liver toxins may cause any existing hemorrhoid(s) to rupture and bleed. Although passing some blood may appear to be scary, it actually helps remove the toxins these varicose veins harbor. This can greatly improve intestinal health.

However, it is still best if you can do everything you can to avoid constipation, so that hemorrhoids won't develop. Then you can also do the proper colon cleanse before the liver flushes, and thereby avoid the undesirable nausea and potential vomiting of the oil mixture.

To improve constipation, go to sleep before 10 p.m., drink enough water, and eat the main meal of the day at around noon. When choosing foods, eat more water-containing foods and less dry foods, more fat and oil, sea salt, and sour food items. Also spend more time relaxing, listen to music, go for walks (which massages the bowels), and spend enough time in the sun to obtain vitamin D which is required for maintaining optimal digestive functions.

Pregnancy and Nursing: Although many pregnant women and nursing mothers have successfully done liver cleanses, for legal reasons I cannot make a recommendation to that effect. If you are pregnant and still wish to do a liver flush, make certain you are not constipated, and thoroughly cleanse the colon before and after each liver flush (also see Chapter 5).

Menstrual Cycle: Although the liver flush may still be effective when done during menstruation, it is more convenient and comfortable for women to flush their liver before or after the monthly cycle. Besides, menstrual bleeding is another form of cleansing the body, and it is best for the body not to cleanse on two fronts at the same time. Menstrual cleansing takes much energy, and doing the liver flush at the same time could reduce its effectiveness and also interfere with removing menstrual waste products.

Chemotherapy: I strongly advice against doing liver flushes until 6-8 months after the last chemotherapy treatment. It can take this long for the highly toxic chemo chemicals to become thoroughly absorbed and encapsulated in biliary stones, which in this case is desirable. Otherwise, doing liver flushes too soon after chemotherapy may leak chemo poisons via bile into the intestines, causing multiple perforations and inflammation in the intestinal walls. In other words, cleansing the body after chemotherapy can be life-endangering; in this case, it is best to be in a state of congestion for the suggested duration and first focus on the other health-enhancing approaches suggested in this book.

Stent in biliary duct: The problem with having a plastic or metal stent inserted into the bile duct is that it cannot dilate like normal bile ducts do during liver flushes (in response to taking Epsom salt). So when stones are being released, they may not be able to pass through the stent. This can cause a blockage, especially if the stones are larger than the diameter of the stent. Most people with stents have to have them replaced on a regular basis. If I were in this situation, I would have the stent removed and do liver flushes, or at least use Epsom salt and some of the other suggestion made in this book to prevent the bile ducts from constricting again. I know of some people who have had their stent removed, and they were able to do liver flushes successfully

Diabetes: I know of many diabetics who have done liver flushes successfully, but if you have diabetes you may need to modify the procedure outlined in this chapter. Keeping your blood sugar balanced at all times is a legitimate concern. Fasting may, of course, upset blood sugar levels, but all the same, *not* eating food on Day 6 of the preparation is important to avoid feeling sick and to allow for maximal release of stones during the liver flush.

Yet, strangely and much to my own surprise, I have found that most diabetics were able to follow the normal regimen without any problems at all. Perhaps, this was due to the colon cleansing before the actual liver flush, the effect of Epsom salt, the drinking of the oil mixture, or a combination of the above. In some few cases, though, having 1-2 teaspoons of raw honey or eating a few soaked, dried figs in the mid-late afternoon and again in the early morning helped them get through the cleanse without any major issues. You may need to find out what works best for you, but I strongly recommend you do not eat any protein foods, for they can make you feel so sick that the liver flush will be of no benefit at all.

To understand the underlying causes of type 2 diabetes, you may wish to read the diabetes chapter of my book, Timeless Secrets of Health and Rejuvenation. In my work with type 2 diabetes over the past three decades, I have found that animal protein consumption is its leading cause, followed by the consumption of refined sugars and artificial sweeteners, and vitamin D deficiency due to lack of regular sun exposure.

Simply by adopting a balanced vegan diet and getting regular sun exposure and exercise, I have seen diabetes vanish within as little as 6-8 weeks. So if you are not able to do a liver flush right away, I recommend you first implement the necessary dietary and lifestyle changes and start doing the liver flushes once your blood sugar has naturally stabilized itself.

(**Note**: Unless there is an existing small-bowel obstruction (SBO), stones will not accumulate or get caught in the small intestine. The high water, oil and bile content in the small intestines acts like a super-efficient toilet flush. The situation is different in the large intestine which absorbs water, compacts feces and stores it in the rectum until it is being removed via the anus in defecation. However, if the colon is not cleansed before doing a liver flush, especially if there is constipation, stones may not pass from the small intestine and remain there until the colon opens up again.

This must be avoided, or otherwise it may lead to toxemia. Hence the importance of cleaning out the whole colon before and after each liver cleanse (see details under *Follow the Liver Flush Protocol for a Safe Flush*)

The Results You Can Expect

During the morning and, perhaps, afternoon hours following the liver flush, you will have a series of watery bowel movements. Expect up to 15-

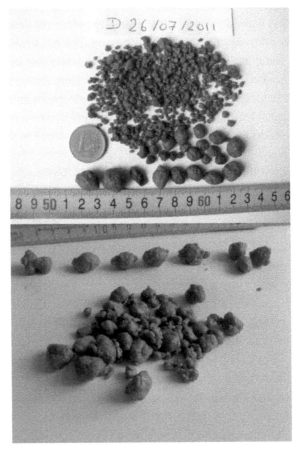

20 evacuations. These initially consist of gallstones mixed with some food residue, and then just stones with colored water. Most of the gallstones are pea-green or tan-colored and float in the toilet because they contain fatty bile components (see **Figure 13a**). As shown in the photographs, some

green stones may be bright-colored and shiny like gemstones. Only bile from the liver can cause this green color.

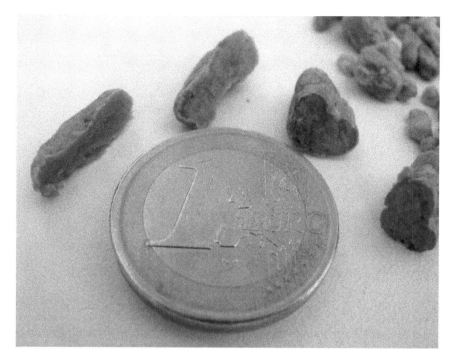

Figure 13a: Green-colored gallstones (cut)
Image source: http://www.agirsante.fr

Gallstones can come in many sizes, colors, and shapes. The light-colored stones are the newest. Dark-green stones are the oldest. Some are pea-sized or smaller, and others are as big as 1 inch in diameter or larger. There may be dozens and, sometimes, even hundreds of stones (of different sizes and colors) coming out at once (see **Figure 13b**). Most of them are green, beige, yellow, white, brown, red and black. The different colors are due the varied percentages of the bile pigments found inside of every stone, such as bilirubin (yellow/red/brown) and biliverdin (green/blue/black).

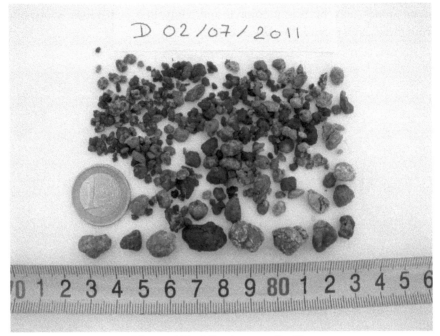

Figure 13b: Mixed types of gallstones
Image source: http://www.agirsante.fr

Also, watch for tan-colored and white stones. Some of the larger tan or white stones may sink to the bottom with the stool. These are calcified gallstones that have been released from the gallbladder, although some may also come from the liver as I have discovered recently. They contain heavier, solid mineral substances, consolidated cholesterol crystals, and only small amounts of bile fats, if any (see **Figure 13c**). All the green and yellowish stones are gel-like or as soft as putty, which is due to the action of the malic acid in apple juice or cherry juice and the low concentration of calcium.

You may also find a layer of white or tan-colored chaff, or *foam*, floating in the toilet. The foam consists of millions of tiny white, sharp-edged cholesterol crystals, which can easily rupture small bile ducts. They are equally important to release.

Don't be alarmed if you see any red stones (see **Figure 13d**). They have a very high concentration of the blood pigment bilirubin. If you release any, it's good to get rid of them, too.

Black stones are increasingly common and usually form in the gallbladder in people with hemolytic anemia or cirrhosis.

Some stones that look like chick peas, and can be hollow inside. Don't be surprised to see other *strange* objects coming out during liver flushes, including dead parasites and worms.

I receive dozens of pictures each month from readers who have released all sorts of *things* that obviously don't belong in the body. If you also pass something that has not been described here, just be happy that it has come out. Remember, it's better out than in.

This popular health website, www.curezone.com, has a large gallery of pictures of gallstones and parasites released by people from all over the world during liver flushes[193].

Addressing Common Concerns

Is Parasite Cleansing Before Liver Flushing a Good Idea?

Some health consultants say that one must do a parasite cleanse before every liver cleanse for it to work and to be safe. Unless a parasitic infection is extreme I don't recommend killing parasites, such as liver flukes. It is far more effective to clean out the liver bile ducts than targeting these organisms directly. Once the bile ducts are clean, the resulting normal bile flow causes them to pass naturally.

Having worked with the liver/gallbladder flush for nearly two decades and having introduced it to millions of people around the world, I receive a lot of feedback, but there is no indication that this is the case. Initially, I put many people on parasite cleansing prior to liver flushes or added parasite-killing extracts to the procedure. However, in all the people I tested, I could not detect that doing a parasite cleaning made any difference or offered any advantage over not doing one.

The 6 days of preparation, as well as the colon washes before and after liver flushes turned out to be good enough. I found that about 10 percent of people doing liver flushes pass dead parasites during one or several of their liver flushes (see photos of parasites released[194]). Killing them directly can actually cause parasites to develop resistance to treatment. While initially,

---

[193] Curezone Liver Flush Gallery, http://curezone.com/ig/f.asp?f=12&p=2
[194] Parasites passed during liver flushes: http://curezone.com/ig/f.asp?f=12&p=3

the parasite cleanse may produce good results, this approach can very well backfire. Parasites become smarter the more you try to kill them.

On the other hand, by changing the intestinal terrain from contaminated and congested to clean and open, the parasites lose their ability to thrive and proliferate. Although I am aware that there are exceptions to the rule, overall, my experiences and research in this regard led me to being very cautious about recommending killing parasites.

There seems to be new evidence that contrary to previously held beliefs, parasites can actually help a person afflicted with chronic illness to reduce severity. For example, a team of British and Vietnamese scientists found that parasitic worms in the intestine protects against asthma and allergy in prone individuals[195].

When circumstances are dire, and severe congestion exists, parasites are actually very useful and helpful, and may even prevent cancer. I have found that nothing in nature is ever wasted or wrong. We just don't always understand nature's wisdom in conducting its affairs and our misinterpretations may subsequently lead to actions that are not in our best interest. Setting the preparations for the body to help itself through cleansing is a much wiser strategy than merely targeting symptoms and interfering with the body's sometimes unusual cooperation with microorganisms.

How Often Should One Cleanse?

Try to make a rough estimate of how many stones you have eliminated. To permanently cure bursitis, back pain, allergies, or other health problems, and to prevent diseases from arising, you need to remove *all* the stones. This may require a minimum of 8 to 12 flushes, which can be performed at 3- or 4-week intervals. (It is best to not flush more frequently than that) Some people with a history of drug use (any kind), alcohol abuse, cigarette smoking, vaccinations, unhealthy diet and lifestyle, emotional trauma or conflict, or severe illness, may need a lot more than 12 flushes. An old friend of mine (age 55) who died following aggressive treatment for liver cancer, had over 70,000 stones in his liver, according to the autopsy report. He never had the chance to clean out his liver, but it would have taken him at least 30 or more flushes.

---

[195] Asthma And Allergy Protection From Parasitic Worms in the Intestine | MedIndia

The 3-week break between flushes may include the 6-day preparation for the next liver flush, but most ideally, it should start after the 3 weeks have passed. If you cannot flush this often, you may take a little more time between flushes, but no more than 6-7 weeks.

The important thing to remember is that once you have started cleansing the liver, you should keep cleansing it until no more stones come out during two consecutive flushes. Leaving the liver half clean for a long period of time (3 or more months) may cause greater discomfort than not cleansing it at all, for reasons explained below.

The liver, as a whole, will begin to function more efficiently soon after the first flush, and you may notice sudden improvements, sometimes within 12 hours. I have received thousands of reports of greatly reduced pains, increase in energy, sudden improvement of eyesight, more calmness and clarity of mind, and an overall sense of euphoria.

However, within a few days, stones from the rear of the liver will have traveled *forward* toward the two main exiting bile ducts (hepatic ducts) in the liver, which may cause some or all of the previous symptoms of discomfort to return. In fact, you might feel disappointed because the recovery seems so short-lived. Any existing, old symptoms may become even stronger because now the liver recognizes that the opening up of the clogged bile ducts provides it with the opportunity to dump even more stones and toxins into the exiting bile ducts than before. All this indicates that the stones left behind have moved to the parts of the liver where they can be removed during the next round of cleansing. Regardless whether or not the improvements remain noticeable, the liver's self-repair and cleansing responses will have increased significantly, adding a great deal of effectiveness to this extremely important organ of the body.

As long as there are even a small number of stones traveling from some of the thousands of small bile ducts to any of the hundreds of larger bile ducts, these stones may combine to form larger stones and cause previously experienced symptoms, such as backache, headache, earache, digestive trouble, bloating, irritability, anger, and so forth, to remain or return. However, in the majority of cases, these symptoms will be increasingly less severe than they were before.

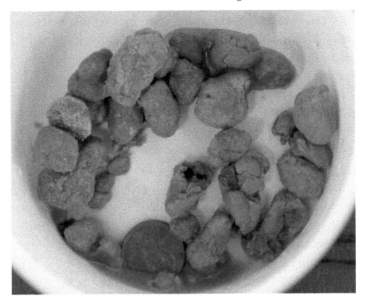

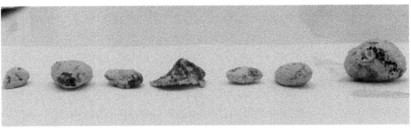

Figures 13c: Mostly semi-calcified gallstones

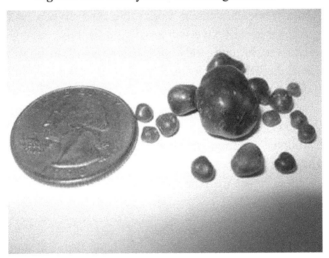

Figure13d: Red bilirubin stones

I am well aware of the advice given by some health practitioners to not cleanse the liver more often than once or twice a year. However, from my extensive experience with the liver flushes and the feedback that I have received from hundreds of thousands of people who have done them, I find this advice to bear considerable health risks.

Keeping the bile ducts clogged or semi-clogged is a major risk factor for disease, and I cannot support the idea that keeping the bile ducts clogged up serves the body any better than unclogging them. It is tremendously more stressful for the liver and the rest of the body to have to hold on to toxic bile and accumulated stones which causes it to keep producing new stones, than to go through the mild draining of energy during the 12-24 hours period of liver cleansing. In 95 percent of the people doing liver flushes, the liver and the body are more energized and revitalized by the afternoon of Day 7 than they felt the day before, and the rest of the people feel they are back to normal or better by Day 8.

If 2 consecutive new cleanses no longer produce any or no more than about 15 small stones, which is unlikely to happen before you have done at least 8 flushes(in severe cases it may take many more), your liver can be considered *stone-free*.

Nevertheless, once your liver is clean it is recommended that you repeat the liver flush every 6 to 8 months. Each flush will give a further boost to the liver and take care of any toxins or new stones that may have accumulated in the meantime. If you follow a fairly healthy diet and lifestyle as I do, though, you may not produce any new stones ever again. I completed my own series of 12 liver flushes about 15 years ago (with 3,500 stones released) and have not passed any more stones since.

How Do Large Gallstones Safely Pass Through the Narrow Bile Ducts?

I often hear the argument that it is impossible for large gallstones to pass through the narrow bile ducts and into the intestinal tract. Most medical doctors and surgeons will tell you that such stones would get stuck either in the common bile duct or the ampulla of Vater, requiring immediate surgery. "You absolutely cannot get a stone through a duct that is half the diameter of the released stone," one doctor told me during a phone conversation. One surgeon told me, "The ampulla of Vater is way too small for a large stone to pass through it. If it gets stuck there, it will give you life-threatening pancreatitis and jaundice."

Of course, most patients have no medical expertise whatsoever and have no reason to doubt what their doctor is telling them, especially if it sounds as logical as the above statements. There are literally hundreds of medical myths that have survived to this day because nobody has tried dispelling them. Fortunately some brave scientists are starting to do their own investigations into commonly used medical practices and speak out against them.

One of the most stunning examples of medical myths is the use of stents used to presumably save the lives of heart attack patients and those at risk of having one. One 2012 study published in the American Medical Association's journal *Archives of Internal Medicine*[196] took the medical industry by total surprise. Being the Holy Grail of interventional cardiology, implanting stents to stretch open plaque-clogged arteries in people with non-acute coronary artery disease is not only completely useless, but actually causes definite harm, according to the study conclusion. This new meta-analysis of all randomized clinical trials compared initial coronary stent implantation with medical therapy to determine the effect on death, nonfatal myocardial infarction (MI), unplanned revascularization, and persistent angina.

This surgical procedure is performed between 300,000 and 500,000 times a year in the US at the cost of billions of dollars, without any benefit, except to fill the coffers of the medical industry. That it often causes serious harm to patients doesn't seem to bother anyone. The procedure continues to be used as aggressively as before the study results became known.

In fact, stent and bypass operations have never been shown to be beneficial. In the first 1998-edition of my book *Timeless Secrets of Health and Rejuvenation,* I wrote: "The emerging understanding of the causes of heart attack raises the question of the value or usefulness of opening blocked arteries. For one thing, the increasingly popular aggressive treatments of opening arteries with bypass surgery, angioplasty[197] and stents[198] do little or nothing to prevent the recurrence of an occlusion.

---

[196]Initial Coronary Stent Implantation With Medical Therapy vs Medical Therapy Alone for Stable Coronary Artery Disease: Meta-analysis of Randomized Controlled Trials. Arch Intern Med. 2012 Feb 27;172(4):312-9
[197]Opening of arteries by pushing plaque back with a tiny balloon and then, often, holding it open with a stent
[198] Stents consist of wire cages that hold plaque against an artery wall; they can alleviate crushing chest pain. They *appear* to rescue someone in the midst of a heart attack by holding the closed artery open, something that has turned out to be wrong assumption.

Although bypass surgery was believed to extend the lives of some patients with severe illness (at least until very recently), it does nothing to prevent heart attacks. As we shall see, heart attacks don't occur because of an arterial blockage, as most people assume....Overall, none of the currently used surgical procedures have been shown to lower the high mortality rate resulting from heart disease."

In the book, I provide an in-depth understanding of what causes heart attacks, how the body creates its own arterial bypasses when coronary arteries become clogged, and why stent or bypass surgery is so utterly useless as found in the above meta-analysis of all randomized clinical trials in this field.

While it is relatively easy to persuade a heart disease patient to have a stent inserted into his clogged coronary artery, it takes even less persuasion to convince a gallbladder disease patient to undergo gallbladder surgery. After all, most doctors tell their patients that they can live just as well or better without their gallbladder; yet, there is no scientific proof to that effect, and only very little scientific evidence to support the need for having this invasive procedure.

A 1985 study titled, "Large Gallstones May Pass Spontaneously"[199] found that these medical assumptions are not backed by science at all and may just be medical myths. In this study, published in the prestigious *Journal of the Royal Society of Medicine,* researchers at the Frenchay Hospital in Bristol, England, proved that gallstones greater than 19 x 15 mm (0.74 x 0.60 inches) in diameter can pass spontaneously from the common bile duct into the duodenum. Their recommendation, "The possibility of spontaneous passage should be borne in mind in the management of patients with common duct stones," is rarely followed.

While the researchers acknowledge that it is widely believed that all stones in the bile ducts should be removed as soon as possible, they argue that "an expectant policy may be justified if there is a possibility that the stone may pass spontaneously." This possibility clearly exists and is, of course, greatly amplified by the application of the liver and gallbladder flush.

The members of the research team point out that they have seen cases in which quite large stones (nearly 2 cm diameter) passed spontaneously from the common bile duct (CBD).

---

[199]Large gallstones may pass spontaneously. *Journal of the Royal Society of Medicine* (Volume 78 April 1985 305)

The medical consensus is that most people have a common bile duct diameter of around 5 mm, +/- 1 mm. According to currently practiced medical doctrine (myth), a stone that is 4 times larger than the diameter of the duct could never make it through without surgical intervention.

Whereas it is known that small stones frequently pass spontaneously, it is less widely appreciated that this may occur without any associated symptoms or complications such as pancreatitis[200].

In yet another report published in the journal Endoscopy[201], three German scientists described a large biliary stone that passed spontaneously into the lumen of the gut.

The researchers from Frenchay Hospital also mention the Bergdahl & Holmlund study (1976) which described 38 patients with retained stones in the CBD after cholecystectomy, who were observed for one month after diagnosis. According to the study's results, in 24 cases the stones passed spontaneously. Two of these stones were 10 mm or more in diameter, and 13 measured 5-9 mm. In 18 cases there were no symptoms related to the passage of the stone.

"We have successfully managed retained stones by waiting four weeks and then, if necessary, flushing the T-tube with normal saline," states the study. Two cases demonstrate that stones up to 19 x 15 mm may pass spontaneously, even in the absence of the gallbladder.

This conclusive statement sums up the invaluable implications derived from this research: "Such an expectant policy of management would avoid unnecessary bile duct instrumentation in those patients - which might be as many as two-thirds in whom the stones will pass spontaneously." (Bergdahl & Holmlund, *Journal of the Royal Society of Medicine*, Volume 78, April 1985, 307 1976)

Given that fact that millions of people from around the world have already used the protocol in this book to safely rid their liver and gallbladder of hundreds of gallstones, from the size of a pinhead to the size of a golf ball, shows that not only two-thirds of all gallbladder surgeries are unnecessary, but almost all of them are.

As mentioned before, according to research published in the *Annals of Surgery,* oral magnesium sulfate (Epsom salt) greatly dilates and relaxes the bile ducts and the sphincter of Oddi, thereby allowing stones to pass easily and without getting caught.

---

[200] Gallstone Size and Risk for Pancreatitis, *Arch Intern Med.* 1998;158(5):543-544. doi:

[201] Large gallstone passes spontaneously into lumen of gut. Endoscopy. 1980 Jul;12(4):191-3

Unless the gallbladder is completely dysfunctional, has atrophied or burst, or is packed full with calcified stones that no amount of bile can move in or out, there is no good reason to have this organ removed.

If large stones have been proven scientifically to pass painlessly and spontaneously without doing a liver flush, it is clear that any doctor who is telling you that this cannot happen when you actually perform a series of them is either ignorant about it or has a financial interest in getting you to have surgery and making money off you. With 800,000 gallbladder surgeries performed annually at the cost of $11,000 each, this 8 billion-dollar business would be difficult to give up by those who make a living from it.

Follow the liver flush protocol for a safe flush

The liver and gallbladder flush is one of the most invaluable and effective methods to regain your health. There are no risks involved if you follow all the directions to the letter. Please take the next cautionary note very seriously. There are many people who have used a liver flush protocol that they received from friends or through the internet, and they suffered unnecessary complications. They did not have complete knowledge of the procedure and the way it works, believing that just expelling the stones from the liver and gallbladder was sufficient and safe enough.

It is very likely that, on their way out, some gallstones will be caught in the colon. They can quickly be removed through colonic irrigation, (see **Figure 14**), Colema, or enemas. Doing a Colema-board enema, is the closest you can get to a professional colonic. The colon-cleansing method MyPerfectColon is one of the most affordable devices available. (To acquire a Colema-board or a MyPerfectColon device, see *Product Information* at the end of the book)

The colon needs to be cleansed on the 2nd or 3rd day after each liver flush. If gallstones, which may be loaded with toxins, remain in the colon longer than that, they can cause irritation, infection, headaches, abdominal discomfort, bloating, loss of appetite, thyroid problems, itchy skin, skin eruptions, and so on. These trapped stones can eventually become a source of toxemia in the body.

If colonics are not available where you live, or you don't have a Colema-board or similar colon cleansing equipment, you can do 2 or 3 back-to-back, one after the other, consecutive water enemas (at least 1 liter each). You can do the first enema and then release. Then do another one, and release. Repeat if necessary. However, if you are already experienced in doing water enemas, one may be sufficient. You will know if one enema is enough when the water reaches the entire right side of your colon, causing it to balloon out somewhat, and if you feel empty and clean after having had a number of evacuations(for more on how to do an effective water enema, see the section *Keep Your Colon Clean* in Chapter 5).

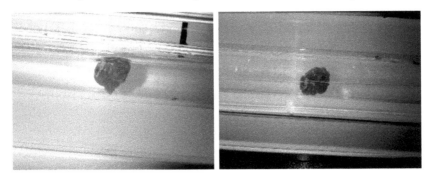

Figure 14: Stones passing through colonic tube
Image courtesy of Leis Keith (Certified colon hydrotherapist)

The importance of colon and kidney cleansing

Although the liver cleanse on its own can produce truly amazing results, it should ideally be done *following* a colon cleanse and a kidney cleanse if there is a preexisting kidney condition, such as kidney stones, or frequent urinary tract infections.

Cleansing the colon before a liver flush ensures that the expelled gallstones are more easily removed from the large intestine. Cleansing the kidneys before the first liver flush makes certain that toxins coming out of the liver during the liver flush do not put any burden on these delicate, vital organs of elimination. However, if you have never had kidney trouble, kidney stones, or a number of persistent bladder infections, you may go ahead with the 'colon cleanse - liver flush - colon cleanse' sequence.

Nevertheless, make certain that you cleanse the kidneys at a later stage. You should do a kidney cleanse (for 3 weeks) after about every third or fourth liver flush until your liver has been completely cleaned out (see also *Keep Your Kidneys Clean* in Chapter 5). Alternatively, you may drink a cup of kidney cleanse tea for 3 to 4 days after each liver flush. Follow the same directions given for the preparation of the main kidney cleanse.

Note: If you have a history of kidney trouble, such as kidney stones, you are better off doing the full kidney cleanse of 3 weeks.

You may combine the kidney cleanse with the liver cleanse, but be sure to avoid drinking the kidney tea on the 2 main days of the actual liver flush. You may stop the kidney cleanse on Day 5 of the liver cleanse preparation and resume on Day 8, and add the 2 missed days to the normal 21-day duration of the kidney cleanse.

People whose colon is severely congested, or who have a history of persistent constipation, should consider doing at least 2 or 3 colon cleanses, like one per week, before attempting their first liver flush.

Moreover, to reemphasize, it is very important that you cleanse your colon within 3 days of completing each liver flush. Removing gallstones from the liver and gallbladder may leave some of the stones and other toxic residues in the colon that can ruin your health if left behind. It is better not to cleanse your liver if you cannot also clean out your colon afterwards! I have seen such serious complications in people who followed other liver cleanse protocols without following this all-important recommendation, that I consider it highly irresponsible to omit this warning.

Alternatives to Apple Juice/Sour Cherry Juice

If you cannot tolerate apple juice or sour cherry juice for some reason, you may substitute one of the following substances or alternate, i.e., use one option during one day, and another option the next day, and so on). I have listed various options because not everyone can find all of them in their country or region.

1. **Pure malic acid** does exceptionally well at dissolving some of the stagnant bile and making the stones softer. Avoid malic acid capsules, especially if they contain other ingredients. It is important for the malic acid to be properly dissolved and diluted before ingesting it. Take about 1 teaspoon of malic acid (5-6 g) dissolved in 24 to 32 oz. (0.75 to 1 liter) or more of room-temperature water during each of the 6 days of preparation. Sip this solution in small amounts throughout the day. Food-grade malic acid powder (which is not mixed with magnesium or other ingredients) is inexpensive and can be purchased over the internet or from some natural health food stores. All wineries

use it for winemaking. (see Product Information at the end of the book) Diabetics and those with Candida issues do particularly well using this option.

2. **Cranberry juice** also contains malic acid and can be used instead of apple juice or sour cherry juice. Combine 16 oz. (0.5 liter) of unsweetened cranberry juice mixed with 8 to 16 oz. (0.25 to 0.50 liter) of water, sipped throughout the day for 6 days. Instead of water, it can be combined with the same amount of apple juice. There is added benefit if some cranberry juice is used each day for 2 or 3 weeks before liver cleansing.

3. **Organic apple cider vinegar** is another good alternative because it is devoid of sugar and is rich in malic acid. Combine 3 oz. (90 ml) in 24 to 32 oz. (0.75 to 1 liter) of water and sip throughout the day, for 6 days. However, if Candida overgrowth is an issue, be aware that vinegar may cause a flare-up of the condition.

4. **Gold Coin Grass & Bupleurum tincture** is also effective in softening gallstones and, therefore, can be used as a preparatory step for the liver flush, although it may take a little longer than with using apple or cherry juice, or malic acid solution. The proper dosage for the tincture is 1 tablespoonful (0.5 oz. or 15 ml) once daily on an empty stomach, about 30 minutes before breakfast. Keep this regimen for 8 to 9 days before the day of the liver flush. These 2 herbs are usually made into a tincture and sold as Gold Coin Grass (GCG), 8.5 oz. (see Product Information at the end of the book)

    Note: GCG tincture is particularly helpful for those having difficulties with releasing stones during the first few liver flushes and/or who no longer have a gallbladder. In both these cases, it can be used in addition to any of the other options.

5. **Orthophosphoric acid** (75 percent). Take 30 drops a day for 3 to 4 days, and gradually increase the dosage to 50 drops daily for an additional 10 days. Perform your liver flush on Day 14. Each dose of 30 drops contains 390 mg of orthophosphoric acid. It is best to dilute the drops in a total of 16 oz. (0.5 liter) of water and sip it throughout the day.

Use Only Authentic Extra Virgin Olive Oil

Please be aware that some brands of olive oil are actually not 100 percent pure olive oil, which can cause intolerance to it. Make certain to only use extra virgin and 100 percent pure olive oil for the liver flush. Usually, olive oil that bears the label *Extra Virgin Olive Oil* means it is a safe choice but, nevertheless, read the label carefully. It should imply that the oil has not been combined with other oils.

Unfortunately, in some countries, olive oil bottles are sold as *100 % Extra Virgin Olive Oil,* which may be true, but in addition to some pure extra virgin olive oil, it may also contain up to 80 percent soy oil or different, cheap, inferior oils. It is an old labeling trick that allows these manufactures to sell their brands very inexpensively under the label *extra virgin olive oil*.

Real olive oil has a greenish color and it is relatively expensive. Avoid olive oil that comes in plastic bottles or cans. Be on the safe side by buying a more expensive brand imported from Italy, Greece or Spain.

Organic olive oil has the best taste. If you are still not sure about its authenticity, test it by using the kinesiology muscle test[202]. Olive oil combined with inferior oils will make your arm muscle become very weak.

Is fasting a good idea while preparing for the liver flush?

Although some individuals who had abstained from eating food in preparation of doing liver flushes successfully released stones, I generally don't recommend it, except after 2 p.m. on Day 6 and the morning of Day 7. In order to take out as many stones as possible, it is best to keep bile secretions going and well stimulated during the preparation phase so that there is enough bile available for the actual liver flush. When you fast, the bile secretion slows significantly and bile may even dry out in the gallbladder, which can actually prevent stones from coming out altogether. However, fasting from 2 p.m. onward helps to save and accumulate any

---

[202] There are many books and videotapes available that can teach you how to apply this simple testing method. Kinesiology muscle testing can tell you immediately whether a food product is suitable for you or not. There is also an exact description of the testing procedure in my book *Timeless Secrets of Health and Rejuvenation*.

unused bile for the flush at 10 p.m. I found this regimen to be the most effective in almost 2 decades that I have worked with it.

Having Difficulties with the Flush?

Problem sleeping during the flush night

While most people sleep right through the night of the liver flush, some people just cannot. If you are usually a light sleeper you may take 4 to 8 ornithine capsules with the olive oil/lemon juice solution. This will help you have an uninterrupted sleep. There are no side effects.

Intolerance to Epsom Salt

As mentioned before, you may try taking a few sips of water after ingesting the Epsom salt to neutralize the bitter taste in your mouth, or add a little lemon juice to improve the taste. Adding a small amount of apple juice and drinking it with a large plastic straw may make it more tolerable for you. Closing the nostrils while drinking it and chasing it down with a small amount of water works best for most people. It is also helpful to brush your teeth afterward or rinse out the mouth with baking soda.

If you have an allergy to Epsom salt (magnesium sulfate), or just cannot tolerate it (throwing it up) even after taking the aforementioned measures for easier ingestion, you may use magnesium citrate (MC) instead. Test MC for allergy by taking, let's say, ¼ teaspoon in a cup of water on an empty stomach, and if there is no reaction (as with Epsom salt), then you should be fine using it for the liver flushes. It is extremely rare for a person to be allergic to magnesium, since most natural foods contain it. With sulfate, though, there is has a higher chance for reactiveness. The citrate in MC is only problematic for people who are allergic to citrus or citrate.

As far as I know, no research has ever been conducted to show that MC can dilate and relax bile ducts as well as Epsom salt does it. However, those who have used it as part of their liver flushes have found it to be just as effective. I attribute this benefit to the nerve and muscle relaxing effect of magnesium. Magnesium citrate is available at most drugstores.

Add 4 tablespoons of magnesium citrate to a total of 24 oz. (three 8-oz. glasses or 710 ml) of filtered water in a jar. If you can find it in liquid form, typically available in 8-oz. (250 ml) bottles, get 3 bottles and divide them into four 6-oz. (180 ml) portions. Drink 6 oz. at each of the four specified times, followed by a glass of water. It has a lemon flavor and is not bitter like Epsom salt.

I do not recommend taking Epsom salt or MC in capsule form. The salts require proper dissolving in sufficient amounts of water to avoid irritation and to achieve proper and prolonged relaxation of the bile ducts, as well as the necessary laxative effect.

Reservations About Ingesting Epsom Salt

Some people have read on the internet that Epsom salt is dangerous. However, it is easy for someone to blame Epsom salt for a health problem they have so that they don't have to make some inconvenient changes to their diet or lifestyle.

For example, if a person suffers from chronic heart condition, one should not blame natural salt for causing it, but must look at the *proven* underlying causes, such as heart medication, statins, severe stress at home or at work, chronic lymph congestion, eating flesh foods, alcohol and cigarette consumption, sleep deprivation, and an unhealthy lifestyle. If this person, let's say, also suffers from constipation and takes Epsom salt for relief, it is farfetched to say that his heart condition is due to the Epsom salt. You can just as well say that in spite of taking Epsom salt a person may have suffered a heart attack (for a number of reasons). Still, some people prefer to blame something natural than a failed treatment for a particular health condition.

I have worked with Epsom salt for over 40 years and never seen any harm done by it when used as part of the liver flushes and on an empty stomach. Like everything else, one must not use Epsom salt carelessly. While water is essential for us to survive, drinking too much of it can cause water intoxication and death. Likewise, we cannot live without oxygen, but if oxygen levels in the air are higher than normal, we can die from that, too. A person can use nearly anything that's normally natural and healthy and yet use it to commit suicide.

Regardless, there is nothing inherently harmful in Epsom salt. It is a naturally occurring mineral found in spring water containing magnesium, sulfur, and oxygen, with the formula $MgSO_4$. Magnesium is an essential mineral used in hundreds of biological processes. Sulfur is equally essential. All cells require sulfur for normal function. In fact, sulfate is among the most important macronutrients in cells and enzymes. Organically bonded sulfur is a component of all proteins. Without it, we would not have skin, hair, or nails on our body, and suffer from chronic inflammation, brain and heart defects (also see *Eat Ionic, Essential Minerals and Get Regular Sun Exposure,* Chapter 5).

The two main elements dissociate in solution, which means they break apart and separate in liquid, easily seen when you place the salt in water. Neither of these two minerals, magnesium and sulfate, have been shown to cause health problems, quite to the contrary.

Epsom Salt is used medically as:

- A replacement therapy for magnesium deficiency[203]
- A first-line antiarrhythmic agent for *torsades de pointes* in cardiac arrest
- A bronchodilator after beta-agonist and anticholinergic agents have been tried, e.g. in severe exacerbations of asthma
- A nebulizer to reduce the symptoms of acute asthma
- An IV treatment for the management of severe asthma attacks
- A preferred treatment to control seizures in pregnant women due to certain complications of pregnancy (such as toxemia)
- An effective method to delay labor in the case of premature labor, and to delay preterm birth
- An effective IV treatment to prevent cerebral palsy in preterm babies
- A first aid treatment for barium chloride poisoning
- An effective method to control high blood pressure, severe brain function problems (encephalopathy), and seizures in children who have sudden, severe inflammation of the kidneys (acute nephritis)
- A treatment for seizures by decreasing certain nerve impulses to muscles

The only known science-backed contraindications for its internal use are as follows:

- you are allergic to any ingredient in magnesium sulfate
- you have a severe irregular heartbeat (e.g. heart block)
- you are pregnant and expect to deliver the baby within 2 hours

---

[203]The most effective way of providing the body with magnesium (without causing any discomfort or irritation) is to apply magnesium oil to the skin, by spraying it under the armpits or on the back of the hands (see *Product Information - Magnesium Oil*). The magnesium will travel to where it is needed

- you are pregnant, planning to become pregnant, or are breast-feeding
- you are taking prescription or nonprescription drugs
- you have severe kidney problems or too much magnesium in the body

Epsom salt has been medically used to save millions of lives. It could not have so many different benefits if it were, in fact, to have toxic effects. Millions of people have used Epsom salt as part of the liver flush program and regained their health. Almost every one of them has done the flush at home, safely and effectively. They would not have had these good results if Epsom salt had done them harm.

If you are still concerned about Epsom Salt, you may use magnesium citrate (same dosage), as an alternative. I don't know of any other substance that can be used for safe and successful liver flushing.

Intolerance to Olive Oil

If you are allergic to olive oil or cannot tolerate it, you may use clear macadamia oil, expeller-pressed or cold-pressed grape seed oil, sunflower oil, or other expeller-pressed oils instead. Don't use canola, soy oil, or similar processed oils (for more information on healthy/harmful oils and fats, please refer to my book *Timeless Secrets of Health and Rejuvenation*). Please be aware that extra virgin olive oil is still the most effective oil for the process of liver cleansing. Oftentimes, intolerance is due to using an inferior olive oil that contains other refined oils such as soy oil.

If you already have gallbladder problems or your gallbladder has been removed, and you avoid eating foods with fats and oils in them, you may feel concerned about ingesting all that oil during the liver flush. In fact, you do need to be careful about not eating oils or fats when your body is unable to digest them because of accumulated stones in the liver bile ducts and the gallbladder. However, the oil mixture taken during the liver flush cannot be compared with eating fats/oils during mealtimes. The way the flush is designed, the oils will trigger a strong bile release that helps move stones out of the liver and gallbladder. Since bile is very oily, and the bile ducts remain relaxed due to the action of Epsom salt, the passage of stones is easy and non-eventful. Doing liver flushes is about the best approach to improve your body's ability to digest and utilize fats.

Intolerance to Citrus Juice

Usually, those who are allergic to grapefruit or oranges are often able to tolerate lemon juice, and substituting lemon juice would be the best solution for them. Those having problems with lemon juice, which is quite rare, often have no problem with using lime juice.

Otherwise, mix the olive oil with ⅔ cup (6 oz.) of sour/tart cherry juice, and if this is not available, use apple juice. However, neither of these alternative options is ideal. Citrus has the most stimulating effect on bile secretion among all the fruits, which we want to increase during a liver flush.

Most people with food allergies find they tend to lessen or disappear after a series of liver flushes.

If you don't have a gallbladder, you can still do liver flushes

If your gallbladder has already been removed, you can certainly still do liver flushes. In fact, people without a gallbladder tend to have many more stones in their liver than those who still have a gallbladder. Intrahepatic stones hinder the liver in removing toxins and waste products from the blood, which can lead to an overload of toxins in the body's connective and fat tissues. This can lead to lymphatic congestion and weight gain - a protective measure taken by the body to temporarily keep toxins from doing harm - and many other conditions, including diabetes, heart disease, and cancer.

When you do your first liver flush, you may not pass many stones right away because your liver's bile ducts tend to be more blocked than average. It may take 1-2 liver flushes to start softening and releasing these more compacted obstructions. Still, many people without a gallbladder start releasing quite a few stones right from the beginning.

If stones don't come out as readily or you don't pass more than about 50 stones, before you flush again, you may extend the preparation period by at least 6 days, making it 12-14 days long. This will make it a lot easier for the liver to release the stones. In this case, you may alternate between the different options, such as apple juice, sour cherry juice, malic acid, Gold Coin Grass, etc.

(**Note**: Although I rarely suggest taking supplements, as a general recommendation, you may wish to consider taking a bile supplement. Most bile supplements contain ox bile. This is the reason for it: without a gallbladder you can never again have the right amount and viscosity of bile required for the proper digestion of food. If you develop symptoms of diarrhea, lower the dosage or discontinue it and resume at a lower dosage once the diarrhea has subsided. Consult with your health practitioner about which product may be the most suitable for you. Doctors are supposed to recommend a bile supplement to their patients after surgical removal of their gallbladder, but they rarely do.

Why calcified gallstones may not be released

...and what you need to know to dissolve them and stop them from forming again

I passed several fully calcified gallstones over 2 cm large during my own series of liver flushes in 1995, and my wife passed one that was at least twice as large (see **Figure 6d**) during her ninth flush. Some people have passed dozens of fully calcified stones from their gallbladder during their very first liver flush.

If all the steps are followed properly, including taking the Epsom salt, which according to research[204] relaxes all the bile ducts, and doing the colon washes before and after liver flushing, these stones can pass quite easily. However, I found that while small calcified stones can even be released during the first liver flush, larger calcified stones in the gallbladder may not come out as easily and readily. Being heavier than bile, they usually sit in the lowest part of the gallbladder and won't move toward the gallbladder duct (cystic duct) unless the gallbladder is pretty emptied out of other non-calcified stones.

Calcified stones are most certainly the more reluctant types of stones to come out, and in some cases, they may never come out. That said, some people pass them right away, like this well-known radio host, Paul Nison, who recorded an interview with me, which can be found on www.youtube.com/enerchiTV. In the video titled "Andreas Speaks About The Liver Flush With Host Paul Nison[205]", Nison is holding up a glass jar

---

[204] The effect of magnesium sulphate upon the sphincter of oddi of man; George S. Bergh and John A. Layne, American Journal of Digestive Diseases; Volume 9, Number 5, 162-165, DOI: 10.1007/BF02997291

[205] Andreas speaks about the Liver flush with host Paul Nison, www.youtube.com/enerchiTV

with fully calcified stones that he had released during his very first liver flush.

If the former situation is the case (no calcified stones were released even after 12 or more liver cleanses) and there are only a few of these gallstones in the gallbladder, it should not be a big concern as long as the liver bile ducts are kept open and clean. As already mentioned, 80 percent of all people who have gallbladder stones will never experience any adverse effects or even have an increased risk of suffering a gallstone attack.

There is something known as *bile ejection rate* which can be low in some persons whose gallbladder walls are weakened over a number of years. This means it is very difficult for these calcified stones to move out of the gallbladder. The only stones these individuals may be able to pass are the ones that impacted the bile ducts in the liver. Of course, unblocking the liver bile ducts is very important because when they are clogged, the liver cannot properly rid the blood and body of toxins. Nevertheless, I have seen a gradual improvement of the gallbladder's bile ejection rate after a series of liver and gallbladder flushes.

In addition to cleansing of the liver and gallbladder, eating foods that can gradually reduce calcium deposits as those found in kidney stones, gallstones, plaque in blood vessels, the prostate and breast glands, etc., is also helpful. They include beetroot juice, lemon juice, asparagus, ginger root, cayenne pepper, the kidney cleanse tea, and yes, even a cup of organic coffee a day (as shown by research).

Excessive calcium in the body is a leading cause of aging and chronic, degenerative disease. The following natural nutritional approach directly strips the body of unused, metallic calcium and assists it with general detoxification and healthy growth of hair, skin, nails, and bone tissue:

Take MSM Organic Sulfur Crystals daily. Start at a comfortable dose and work your way up to 1 teaspoon (5 g) two times a day. This product, which is one of the most common substances in the body, can be taking ongoing and it has no harmful effects. However, initial cleansing reactions may occur. You may increase it up to a tablespoon (15 g) twice a day, for more powerful effects. Besides breaking down calcium deposits, MSM Organic Sulfur effectively removes toxic metals, chemicals, and poisons from the body and it is also excellent for building healthy hair, skin, nails, and bone (for more detailed information, see the section *Give Us Our Daily Sulfur*, Chapter 5).

(**Note**: While drinking coffee has been shown to trigger gallbladder contractions and thus discourage stone formation, it is best to rely on cleansing the gallbladder and using fats/oils in foods to serve as the main trigger, or at least to not exceed drinking more than 1 cup of coffee a day. Taken in excess, caffeine can cause headaches, anxiety, insomnia, cardiac arrhythmia [palpitations], high blood pressure, gastrointestinal and urinary disorders, prostate trouble and PMS. Caffeinated beverages tend to be harmful only when you are tired or suffer from chronic energy depletion. It should not be used as a stimulant, for it depletes the energy-deficient body of even more energy. This can be extremely stressful for the body. On the other hand, drinking a cup of coffee when you feel vital and energetic has no negative consequence, but can even be beneficial)

High-density lipoprotein (HDL), or good cholesterol, naturally prevents calcifications; eating foods that raise HDL is therefore very beneficial. Coconut oil, olive oil, and other natural oils raise HDL levels, whereas fried foods (abundant in trans fats) as well as low-cost and hydrogenated vegetable oils decrease it and directly cause plaque buildup.

Animal proteins and refined/processed sugar leach calcium from the bones and teeth, which can then turn into mineral deposits in joints, kidney stones and calcified gallstones.

Fluoride added to municipal water in the US and other countries is a major culprit in the formation of calcium deposits in the body. Fluoride is magnetically attracted to the pineal gland where it forms calcium phosphate crystals even more than in the gallbladder and kidneys. A calcified pineal gland can cause a defective sense of orientation, among other health problems.

Calcium supplements are by far the biggest cause of calcification and should not be taken by anyone. Use foods rich in organic, ionic calcium instead, such as sesame seeds (or tahini paste), almonds, walnuts, Brazil nuts, chia seeds, curly kale and other leafy green vegetables, broccoli, green beans, chick peas, most beans, fresh figs, and apricots.

Almost all processed food contains some form of added metallic calcium, such as calcium phosphate, or calcium carbonate. Many food supplements contain these as fillers as well. Since calcification represents one of the most serious causes of mental and physical debility, we ought to avoid processed foods and calcium-enriched supplements as much as possible.

Drinking the juice of 1-2 lemons/limes each day for at least 3-4 months helps reduce the size of calcified stones. Chamomile tea is good stone-dissolver/breaker, too, although it is slow-acting. The herb Chanca piedra (stone breaker), ideally taken as a liquid extract (20 drops in a glass of water 3 times daily) has traditionally been used to gradually dissolve calcifications in the gallbladder and kidneys. However, it is important to know that what works for some doesn't necessarily work for everyone. Different things work for different folks and one may need to try out various approaches to determine which one of them is the most effective.

Headache, Nausea, or Feeling Sick During or After Liver Flushing

If you experience a headache or nausea in the days after a liver flush, it is usually because you have not followed the cleanse instructions properly, especially those related to cleansing of the entire colon before and after each liver flush.

However, on some rare occasions, gallstones may continue to pass out of the liver after completing a liver flush. Some toxins released by these stones can enter the circulatory system and cause discomfort. In such a case, it may be helpful to drink about 4-6 oz. apple juice or 2-3 oz. sour cherry juice for as many days as the discomfort lasts. It is best to drink the juice at least ½ hour before breakfast. In addition, a repeat colon cleanse may be necessary to clear out any late-coming stones.

The tissue-cleansing method (ionized water), as described in Chapter 5, also helps to remove the circulating toxins. If you place a small piece of fresh ginger into the thermos flask, drinking this water will quickly stop the nausea. Taking a tablet of hydrochloric acid or a couple of tablespoons of aloe vera juice is another good option. Drinking 2 to 3 cups of chamomile tea per day helps to calm the digestive tract and the nervous system. Chamomile is also a good stone-breaker for calcified stones.

Some people feel nauseated during the night and/or in the early morning hours. This may be due to a strong, sudden outpouring of gallstones and toxins from the liver and gallbladder, pushing some of the oil mixture back into the stomach, especially if the colon wasn't cleaned out beforehand. However, the nausea is more likely to occur if the stomach is chronically deficient in hydrochloric acid, thereby leaving the sphincter of the esophagus open and allowing stomach contents to regurgitate.

Usually, the nausea passes as the morning progresses. However, if the nausea is very uncomfortable and you feel faint or feel like throwing up, take one tablet of Betaine hydrochloric acid or one ounce (30 ml) of aloe vera juice. This will quickly close the sphincter of the esophagus and thereby stop the nausea. Two teaspoons of apple cider vinegar taken with an ounce of water may also work.

During one of my 12 liver flushes, I spent a miserable night and despite throwing up most of the oil mixture, this flush was just as successful as all the others I had done. By the time I vomited, the oil had already done its job, that is, it had prompted the release of gallstones. If this happens to you, remember that this is only one night of discomfort. Recovery from conventional gallbladder surgery may take many weeks or months. Surgery may also lead to major pain and suffering in the years to come.

When to use lower dosages of olive oil and Epsom salt:

In rare cases, especially if you are of small or petit build, or weigh no more than a healthy teenager, the normal amount of olive oil may be too much for you and you may feel sick as a result or taking it. Try to reduce the amount of olive oil, citrus juice and Epsom salt to two thirds or half of the regular amounts. You may find that the reduced amount of each cleanse ingredient will still be sufficient to achieve the desired results, while also allowing you to feel comfortable during the flush.

The Liver Flush Did Not Deliver the Expected Results

In some cases, albeit very rarely, the liver flush does not produce the results you expect. The following are the main reasons, and their remedies, for such difficulties:

1. It is likely that severe congestion in your liver's bile ducts, due to extremely dense structures of stones, has prevented the malic acid in apple juice, cherry juice or other alternative source from softening them sufficiently during the first cleansing attempt. In some individuals, it may take as many as 2 or 3 liver flushes before the stones start coming out.

Chanca piedra, also known as stone-breaker, can help prepare your liver and gallbladder for a more efficient release of stones, especially if you have calcified stones in the gallbladder. Take 20 drops of Chanca piedra extract (see *Product Information* at the end of the book) in a glass of water, 3 times daily for at least 2 to 3 weeks before your next flush.

Another method is to drink 3 tablespoons of undiluted, unsweetened lemon juice, 15 to 30 minutes before breakfast daily for one week before doing the actual liver flush. This stimulates the gallbladder and makes it ready for a more successful liver flush. This can also be done long-term to reduce calcifications in the body.

Enteric peppermint oil, taken in capsule form, is also very useful in dissolving calcified gallstones or reducing their size. It may not be easy to find it in pure form, though, and not every person can tolerate it. It is often mixed with other ingredients, which can reduce its effectiveness.

Drinking 2 to 3 cups of chamomile tea per day also helps to dissolve calcified stones.

Another useful method to help support the liver and gallbladder during the flush, and to encourage the release of more stones, is to soak a piece of flannel with heated apple cider vinegar and apply it to the liver/gallbladder area during the 20- to 30-minute period of lying still. Some people have found increased benefits from doing this using warm castor oil instead.

The herbs Chinese gentian and bupleurum help to break up some of the congestion and can, thereby, prepare your liver for a more successful flush. These herbs are prepared as a tincture. They are more commonly known as Chinese bitters (see *Product Information* at the end of the book). The proper dosage for this tincture is ½ to 1 teaspoonful (2.5 - 5 ml) once daily on an empty stomach, about 30 minutes before breakfast. This regimen should be followed for 3 weeks before drinking the apple juice, sour cherry juice, or one of the other options. Any unpleasant cleansing reactions usually disappear after 3 to 6 days; they can be minimized by following the tissue-cleansing method of using hot, ionized water and by keeping the intestines clean with capsules of Colosan, a Colema, or an enema (see Chapter 5).

2. You may not have followed the directions properly. Leaving out any one item from the procedure, or altering the dosages or timing of the steps laid out may prevent you from obtaining the full results.

3. In some people, the liver flush does not work at all unless the colon has been cleansed first. The backup of waste and gases cuts down adequate bile secretion and prevents the oil mixture from moving easily through the upper GI tract. In people who are severely constipated, the gallbladder may barely open up during the liver flush. Ideally, do the colon cleanse on the day of the actual liver flush.

4. If the gallbladder's bile ejection rate is very low, there is simply not enough bile coming out of the gallbladder to remove any of its accumulated stones. There may also not be enough space for bile to enter the gallbladder from the liver, which is necessary to remove gallstones. Although this may be a difficult situation, with patience and perseverance, bile ejection rate can be greatly improved; at least, this is what I have seen in a number of individuals who have reported back to me.

Interruption During the Liver Flush Preparation

If you start preparing for the liver flush, but for some reason (such as getting a cold) you cannot follow through with doing the actual flush on Day 6, do not be concerned; it is not going to do you any harm. The malic acid that's doing the softening of stones helps to break some of them down into smaller stones and also helps remove toxins from the liver. This will make it easier for your liver when you begin a new flush preparation. If you just need to postpone the flush for 1-2 days, continue drinking the apple juice/cherry juice/malic acid solution (or the other alternative option) during those additional days.

SOS: Gallstone attack (how to deal with it)

I am frequently asked the question if there is an alternative way of stopping a gallbladder attack, other than emergency gallbladder surgery. Many gallstones attacks involve calcified gallstones that may pass from the gallbladder distally into other parts of the biliary tract such as the cystic duct, common bile duct, pancreatic duct, or the ampulla of Vater.

Presence of gallstones may lead to acute cholecystitis, an inflammatory condition characterized by retention of bile in the gallbladder and often secondary infection by intestinal microorganisms. In other parts of the biliary tract, gallstones can cause obstruction of the bile ducts, which can lead to serious conditions such as ascending cholangitis or pancreatitis. Either of these two conditions is considered to be life-threatening, and is therefore considered to be a medical emergency.

First of all, if you have a gallstone attack, it doesn't mean that you are a candidate for surgery. I wouldn't want you to have this extremely important organ removed unless it has been severely inflamed, is perforated, or is lifeless. In almost every case I know of, where unsuspecting patients let a surgeon remove their gallbladder, they continued having gallstone attacks, digestive problems, gained a lot of weight, and increased their risk of cancer.

In the vast majority of the cases, a trapped gallstone passes on its own. I personally had over 40 painful gallstones before I did my own series of liver flushes, and even though some lasted for up to 3 weeks, the stones always passed on their own. I never suffered another attack after my first liver flush, and if you are prone to suffering gallstone attacks, this may hold true for you as well.

However as long as you have any remaining stones in the liver and gallbladder, there is still a chance for you to have an attack after eating a greasy meal, eggs, meat, fish or other proteins. To prevent the possibility of an attack, it's important to make the necessary changes to your diet and lifestyle, as outlined in my book *Timeless Secrets of Health and Rejuvenation*.

If I had known back then what I know today I wouldn't have had to suffer the pain when I actually had an attack. The following recommendations have helped thousands of people to stop a gallstone attack almost right away. Once it has stopped, I would suggest you wait for about a week and then start the preparation for a liver and gallbladder flush. Make certain that you follow the instructions in this chapter to the letter, especially those concerning colon cleansing before and after each flush.

I have found that if you have a gallstone attack after eating a heavy/fatty/protein meal, drinking a glass of Epsom salt (one tablespoon dissolved in 8 oz. of water (about 240ml) on an empty stomach and placing a hand towel that has been soaked in warm apple cider vinegar over the abdomen, and also vigorously massaging and squeezing the second, third, and fourth toes of the feet, will help stop the attack quickly.

As already mentioned, scientific research has shown that Epsom salt sufficiently relaxes and dilates the bile ducts and the ampulla of Vater for any trapped stones to pass into the small intestines and out of the body. It is therefore not surprising to see why all these people who followed the above recommendations were able to stop a gallstone attack, prevent or stop acute pancreatitis and avoid gallbladder surgery.

In addition to the above, I also recommend that those having a gallstone attack should drink one 6-oz. cup (180 ml) of red beet juice during each of the 3-4 meals following the attack. This alone has helped a number of people pass a stuck stone.

Some individuals have done a liver flush to end an ongoing attack and it worked very well, even before they drank the oil mixture. However, I always warn not to attempt a liver flush without cleaning out their colon beforehand, and of course, within 3 days afterwards.

To prevent new attacks or relieve pain from an existing attack, eat 2-3 tablespoons of grated, raw red beets (washed if organic, peeled if not), before breakfast and lunch meals, or add to your salad. It can be combined with the juice of ¼ lemon, ¼ teaspoon of turmeric and 1-2 tablespoons of olive oil. This can be repeated every day until there is no more pain or discomfort.

While going through a gallstone attack, and for at least 3 days afterwards, make certain you strictly avoid eating eggs, meat, seafood, poultry, milk, cheese, grapefruit, oranges, corn, beans and nuts, alcohol, sugar, pastry, hydrogenated oils and partially hydrogenated oils. Cooked vegetables, salads, light grains like Basmati rice, some coconut or olive oil, ghee or butter in small quantities is fine, and fruits (except grapefruit and orange) are fine. Make sure you don't overeat.

Hundreds of millions of people have gallstone attacks each year. There are many triggers, some of which I have already listed in this book. For me, it used to be lifting heavy objects or particular stretching exercises that put pressure on the gallbladder and squeezed out one or several stones. Other people have an attack after drinking a glass of orange juice (citrus stimulates the gallbladder). Mostly, though, it is caused by a high protein meal (meat, fish, chicken, pork, ham, etc.), fried food, stir-fried food, a lot of butter, cream, ice cream, chocolate, eating a lot of nuts, cow's milk, cheese, chips, crisps, etc. Eggs are the leading trigger among all foods. Overeating, regardless of what kind of food, has also been found to trigger gallstone attacks.

If a stone or bile sludge has caused pancreatitis and the inflammation has stopped after following the above recommendations, it would be good to do a series of liver cleanses to prevent recurrence. This is just as important if your gallbladder has already been removed. Remember, surgical removal of the gallbladder does not address the real problem, which is bile duct congestion in the liver.

Can Or Should Children Do Liver Flushes?

It is becoming increasingly obvious that gallstones can form in children just as easily as they do in older people. In fact, age is not a risk factor at all for gallstones. Regardless of whether it is a child or an adult who gets vaccinated, receives antibiotics or other medical drugs, regularly drinks diet sodas or fluoridated water, eats hamburgers, consumes low-fat foods, sugar, or other junk foods, both of them will form gallstones in direct response to such dietary choices.

Many children are literally being poisoned by what they eat or drink (see Chapter 3 on medicine and food colorings), including the popular *healthy* breakfast cereals[206]. Therefore, it is not surprising to find that many children today have already accumulated hundreds, and sometimes thousands, of gallstones in their liver. The more they have gathered, the more likely they are to suffer from some serious illness or another in the future.

I personally developed gallstones before age 6 and began to experience debilitating illnesses from age 8, just from eating foods rich in animal protein.

Children age 10 or older can do liver flushes; however, they should use only *half* the dosage of all the ingredients, that is, apple juice/sour cherry juice, Epsom salt, olive oil and the juice added to it. Children aged 16 or older can use the adult dosage, unless their body frame is still very small.

In addition, it is best for children to begin the entire process on Day 6 of the preparation about 1 hour to 1 ½ hours earlier than laid out at the beginning if this chapter, including their lunch meal (ideally taken at noon time). This means they take their first dose of Epsom salt between 4:30 and 5:00 p.m., and the oil mixture between 8:30 and 9:00 p.m. The instructions for Day 7 remain the same for them as for adults.

Some mothers have administered the liver flush to their children at a much lower age than 10. One Chinese woman had her children aged 4 and 6 who suffered from various conditions do a number of liver flushes (after they requested it) and they passed a lot stones. Most parents, though, wouldn't even consider having their children go through liver flushes at

---

[206]To learn more about the astounding scientific research conducted on breakfast cereals, see my book *Timeless Secrets of Health and Rejuvenation*.

that age. Although there is nothing in the cleanse that could harm children after the age of 4, I would only have them do liver flushes if they insisted on doing them. Liver flushes require their full involvement and a willingness to follow all the necessary instructions.

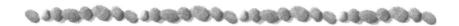

Chapter 5

Simple Guidelines on Keeping the Liver Free of Gallstones

O nce you have eliminated all your gallstones[207] through a series of liver flushes, there are a number of healthful practices you can easily apply that will help your liver to remain permanently clear of stones.

1. Flush your liver twice a year

I strongly recommend that you cleanse your liver once or twice a year. A good time for liver flushes is at around the time of seasonal change, although it is best to avoid flushing on full moon day. When the seasons change, the body also undergoes major physiological changes and is more inclined to release accumulated toxins and waste matter (as seen in an increased incidence of head colds or the flu). Since the immune system is naturally weaker during the days of seasonal adjustment, cleansing the liver supports it greatly in its effort to keep the rest of the body healthy.

2. Keep Your Colon Clean

A weak, irritated, and congested large intestine becomes a breeding place for bacteria that are simply doing their job - decomposing potentially hazardous waste material. As a side effect of their life-saving activities, though, the microbes produce toxic substances. Some of these toxins enter the blood, which sends them straight to the liver. Constant exposure of the liver cells to these toxins impairs their performance and reduces bile secretion. This leads to a further disruption of digestive functions.

---

[207] If you have passed only 10-20 small, soft stones for two consecutive flushes, you may go on the maintenance schedule and just do liver flushes once or twice a year

When you eat highly processed foods that have been stripped of most nutrients and natural fiber, the body has no choice but to leave much of it undigested. Processed foods tend to make for dry, hard, or sticky stools that pass only with difficulty through the intestinal tract.

Normally, the muscles wrapped around the colon can easily squeeze and push fibrous, bulky feces along, but they struggle greatly dealing with gooey, sticky feces that is devoid of fiber. When fecal matter sits too long in the colon, it becomes harder and drier. If that were the only thing that happened, we would only need to worry about constipation (from which millions of Americans suffer) and taking laxatives. But there is more to it.

After the sticky feces are plastered onto the walls of the colon, they will undergo biochemical changes and do the following things. They will:

- Ferment or putrefy, thereby becoming a breeding ground for parasites and pathogens as well as a storehouse for toxic chemicals. These can contaminate the blood and lymph and, thereby, increasingly poison the body.
- Form a barrier that prevents the colon from interacting with the fecal mass and absorbing water and certain nutrients from it.
- Restrict peristaltic movement by the colon walls, making it difficult for the colon to rhythmically contract in order to force the fecal excrement along its way.

How well could you do your job if you were covered with thick sludge? The following are some of the typical symptoms that can result from impaired colon performance:

Lower back pain, neck and shoulder pain, pain in the lower and upper arms, skin problems, brain fog (difficulty concentrating), fatigue or sluggishness, increased risk for colds and flu, constipation or diarrhea, flatulence/gas or bloating, Crohn's disease, ulcerative colitis, polyps, colitis/irritable bowel syndrome (IBS), diverticulitis/diverticulosis, leaky gut syndrome, and pain in the lower part of the stomach.

The large intestine absorbs minerals and water. When the membrane of the large intestine is impacted with mucoid plaque, it cannot assimilate and absorb minerals (as well as some vitamins). A congested colon can lead to nutrient-deficiency diseases and dehydration. Most health problems are, in fact, deficiency disorders. They arise when certain parts of the body suffer malnourishment, particularly of minerals (see also *Eat Ionic, Essential Minerals* in this chapter).

The following are the 3 colon-cleansing methods that I recommend in combination with liver flushes:

1. Keeping the colon clean through colonic irrigation, for example, is an effective preventive method to safeguard the liver against toxins generated in the large intestine. Colonic irrigation, also known as colon hydrotherapy, is one of the most effective colon therapies. A 30- to 50-minute session can eliminate large amounts of trapped waste that may have taken you many years to accumulate. During a colonic session, the therapist uses a total of 3 to 6 quarts of distilled or purified water to gently cleanse your colon. Through gentle abdominal massage, old deposits of *mucoid fecal matter* are loosened, detached from the colon wall, and subsequently removed with the water.

Colonics tend to have a tremendously relieving effect. You will usually experience a feeling of lightness, cleanness, and increased clarity of mind following a colonic. However, during the procedure itself, you may feel slight discomfort from time to time, whenever larger quantities of toxic waste detach themselves from the intestinal walls and move toward the rectum. In some rare cases, old fecal matter and toxins continue to be discharged for a day or two afterwards, which can give rise to a headache, lack of energy, or other symptoms of prolonged cleansing.

During the procedure, rubber tubing carries water into the colon and waste out of the colon. The released waste material can be seen floating through a tube, showing the type and quantity of waste eliminated.

Once the colon has been thoroughly cleansed through 2, 3, or more colonics, thereafter diet, exercise, or other health-promoting regimens are likely to be much more effective.

It is estimated that 80 percent of all immune tissue resides in the intestines. Therefore, cleansing the colon from immune-suppressive toxic waste and removing gallstones from the liver can make all the difference in the treatment of cancer, heart disease, AIDS, or other serious illnesses.

Colonic irrigation is a safe and hygienic system for cleansing the colon. Those who have never experienced a colonic and are afraid of having one, or who have a vested interest in dissuading others from having one, are the people most likely to raise safety concerns about colonics.

I have worked with hundreds of colon hydrotherapists around the world during the past 25 years and I can only support this often life-saving method of intestinal cleansing. There are hospitals in Israel and Russia that don't even accept patients unless they can prove they just had a colonic. This policy rules out a large number of other disease origins and thereby makes their job a lot easier.

2. If you do not have access to a colon therapist, you may greatly benefit from using a Colema board (see *Product Information* at the end of the book) as the second-best choice. The Colema board allows you to clean your colon in the comfort of your own home. The Colema is a do-it-yourself enema treatment that is easy to learn and perform.

Or else, you can do 2-3 back-to-back water enemas to achieve a similar benefit.

3. A water enema is the oldest known procedure of introducing purified water into the rectum and colon via the anus, dating back thousands of years. The increasing volume of the liquid causes rapid expansion of the lower intestinal tract, often resulting in uncomfortable bloating, probable cramping, powerful peristalsis, a feeling of extreme urgency and complete evacuation of the lower intestinal tract. A person skilled in doing enemas can easily make the water reach the far end of the colon and clean it out. An enema has the advantage over any laxative in its speed and certainty of action, which makes it a very valuable and effective tool of intestinal cleansing.

In fact, an enema has an immediate effect on nearly all parts of the body. It alleviates constipation, distension, chronic fever, the common cold, headaches, sexual disorders, kidney stones, pain in the heart area, vomiting, low backache, stiffness and pain in the neck and shoulders, nervous disorders, hyperacidity, and tiredness. Moreover, disorders such as arthritis, rheumatism, sciatica, and gout may greatly benefit from regular enemas.

Use filtered room temperature or lukewarm water for this type of intestinal wash. For greater effectiveness, add one teaspoon of natural sea salt per liter/quart of water used (for a detailed description of other types of enemas that involve certain herbal teas, coffee, or oil, see my book *Timeless Secrets of Health and Rejuvenation*).

To perform a water enema you will need an enema bag (see Figure 15). Much of the enema equipment that is used in homes for colon cleansing is made out of latex (rubber). If you are allergic to latex, make sure to choose different equipment made of plastic, vinyl, or silicone.

Enemabag.com offers some good alternatives to latex bags. Most chemists or pharmacies stock enema bags, usually for pregnant women who are often constipated. Enemasupply.com has a large selection of different enema bags (also see *Product Information*).

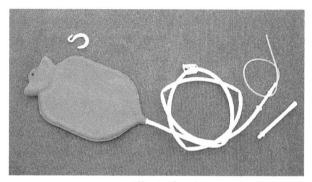

Illustration 15:
A 2-quart latex enema bag kit as sold on healthandyoga.com

Here's How to do a Water Enema:

1. Spread out an old towel or blanket on the bathroom floor near the toilet, and keep a small head pillow next to it.
2. Wash the enema tip thoroughly with soapy water. Rinse it well and attach it to the end of the plastic/rubber hose.
3. Completely fill up the enema bag with chlorine-free water.
4. Attach the one end of the hose to the top of the bag and insert the tip in the other end of the hose.
5. Clamp off the hose but ensure the clamp is positioned low enough so you can reach it when lying down.
6. Hang up the enema bag on a door knob or towel rack in the bathroom, at a minimum of 2 feet (0.60 m) above the floor.
7. Lie down on the towel on your back with your knees up or on your right side with your left knee bent. If this is uncomfortable for some reason, lie on your left side, with your right knee bent. Find your most comfortable position. You may place your head on a pillow.
8. Generously lubricate the tip, as well as the opening to your anus and the area around it, with aloe vera gel, coconut oil, olive oil, or butter.
9. Gently insert the tip into the anus, pushing it in about 3-4 inches (7.5-10 cm). Do not use force!

10. Release the clamp on the hose and allow the liquid to flow into the rectum. If you use a one-liter bag, this may take less than 2-3 minutes. If the inflow rate is too fast for you (indicated by sudden cramping), you can slow down this process by clamping the hose halfway or more.

11. If you are using a larger enema bag (2 liters or more), you may need to stop the flow when you feel full. If the urge to eliminate goes away, you can allow more water to flow in; the further into the colon you are able to let the water reach, the better.

12. Clamp off the hose completely when you see the bag is empty, and remove the tip/hose from your anus.

13. Rest comfortably and gently massage your abdomen.

14. Hold the water inside for as long as you possibly can. Lying on the right side often helps to bring the water into the ascending part of the colon more easily.

15. Do not give in to milder urges right away. However when you have a strong urge to empty your bowels, which may happen quite quickly, be prepared to get off the floor and on to the toilet.

16. You may have several bowel movements, more watery at first, and more solid later on. The entire enema (including the evacuations) rarely takes longer than 10-15 minutes.

17. Wash the tip and bag with hot soapy water, rinse them well and allow them to dry.

Repeat this entire process if you feel you have not removed all the fecal matter from your colon. This is especially important for the colon cleanse which you will need to do following a liver and gallbladder flush. You want to ensure that no stones remain in the colon!

Enemas are best done in the morning soon after a bowel movement. After an evacuation, the flow of the water into the colon is less obstructed and can therefore make its way into the ascending colon more easily. If this is inconvenient, though, later in the afternoon (but before 5:30 p.m.) is a good time, too. If chronically constipated, it may be necessary to prepare the colon for the enema by taking a mild intestinal cleanser or laxative like Colosan or Epsom salt the night before (see details on *Other Intestinal Cleansers* below).

Are Self-administered enemas safe?

If done as instructed, enemas are completely safe. There are no citations for enemas to be harmful. If done often, like once a day, there may be a chance for rectal muscles to lose their natural disposition. However, usually, the more the rectal muscles are used, the stronger they become (as is the case with all other muscle exercises). The *bottom* line is that doing enemas never weakens the intestine and rectum.

An enema quickly improves the blood circulation to the large intestine and also to the rest of the gastrointestinal tract. By removing waste from the colon, it directly helps increase the secretion of the digestive juices/enzymes and digestion.

A note on coffee enemas: If you are doing the liver cleanses, there is no need for you to do coffee enemas. Coffee enemas do not cleanse the colon per se; they are designed to release toxins from the liver. Those individuals who are not able to do liver cleanses for some reason, can benefit from doing coffee enemas instead. However, please be aware that coffee enemas cannot release gallstones. For details on how to perform a coffee enema, see my book *Timeless Secrets of Health and Rejuvenation*.

Other Intestinal Cleansers:

1. Colosan is a blend of various oxides of magnesium designed to gently release oxygen into the digestive tract for cleansing it. Colosan is a powder that you either mix with water and chase down with citrus juice or take in capsule form, which is more convenient. Colosan releases large amounts of oxygen in the intestinal tract, thereby eliminating waste deposits, toxins, old fecal material, as well as parasites and hardened mucus (see *Product Information*). Oxypowder and OxyCleanse are similar products that work just as well. Follow suggested directions provided on the bottle.

2. Another method of cleansing, which uses Epsom salt, cleanses not only the colon but also the small intestine. This may become necessary if you have major difficulties absorbing food, have repeated kidney/bladder congestion, experience severe constipation, or are simply unable to do a colonic. For 3 weeks, add a teaspoon (5 g) of oral Epsom salt (magnesium sulfate) to a glass of warm water and drink this first thing in the morning. This oral enema flushes your entire digestive tract and colon, from top to bottom, usually within an hour, prompting you to eliminate several times. It clears out even some of the plaque and debris from the intestinal walls, along with the parasites that have been living there.

Expect the stools to be watery for as long as there is intestinal waste to be disposed of. Stools adopt a more normal shape and consistency once the entire intestinal tract is clean. This treatment can be done 2 to 3 times per year. Expect some cramps or gas formation, at times, while on this cleanse (a result of releasing toxins). Your tongue may become white-coated and be thicker than normal. This indicates increased intestinal cleansing. Epsom salt is not tolerated by everyone and since it is a laxative, it should not be used ongoing. It is also not effective enough to serve as a replacement for colonics, Colemas, or enemas for the purpose of liver flushing.

3. Castor oil is a traditionally used, excellent remedy to clear waste material from the intestines. It is less irritating than Epsom salt and has no side effects other than normal cleansing reactions. Take 1 to 3 teaspoons (5-15 g) of castor oil in about ⅓ cup (2.5 oz. or 75 ml) of warm water on an empty stomach in the morning or before going to sleep at night (depending on which works better for you). It is a very beneficial treatment for stubborn cases of constipation. It can also be given to children (in smaller dosages).

Avoid using castor oil on Day 6 of the liver flush preparation and during the actual liver flush. Only use Epsom salt or magnesium citrate for that purpose.

4. Aloe vera juice is another effective way to cleanse the GI tract. However, it also is not a replacement for the colonics, Colemas, or enemas before and after a liver flush. Aloe vera has both nourishing and cleansing effects. One tablespoon of aloe vera juice, diluted with a little water, taken before meals, or at least once in the morning before breakfast, helps to break down old deposits of waste and bring basic nutrients to cells and tissues. Those who feel their liver is still releasing many toxins several days after a liver flush may greatly benefit from drinking aloe vera juice.

Aloe vera has been found to be effective in almost every illness, including cancer, heart disease, and AIDS. It is helpful for all kinds of allergies, skin diseases, blood disorders, arthritis, infections, Candida, cysts, diabetes, eye problems, digestive problems, ulcers, liver diseases, hemorrhoids, high blood pressure, kidney stones, and strokes, to name a few.

Aloe vera contains over 200 nutrients, including the vitamins B1, B2, B3, B6, C, E, and folic acid; iron, calcium, magnesium, zinc, manganese, copper, barium, sulphate; 18 amino acids; important enzymes; glycosides; and polysaccharides, among others. Make certain you purchase only pure, undiluted, and organic aloe vera, available in health food stores. One of the best brands is produced by the company Lily of the Desert (in Denton, Texas). It is made of 99.7 percent organic aloe vera juice, with no water added.

A Word of Caution for diabetics: With regular drinking of aloe vera juice, diabetics may improve the ability of their pancreas to produce more of its own insulin. Therefore, diabetics should consult their physician to monitor their need for extra insulin, for too much insulin is dangerous. Many diabetics report a reduction in the amount of insulin required. Make certain you purchase only undiluted aloe vera juice.

If you experience diarrhea after taking aloe vera juice, try reducing the dosage. Not everyone benefits from aloe vera.

3. Keep Your Kidneys Clean

If the presence of gallstones in the liver, or any other situation, has led to the development of sand, grease, or stones in the kidneys or urinary bladder, you may also need to cleanse your kidneys. The kidneys are extremely delicate, blood-filtering organs that congest easily because of dehydration, poor diet, weak digestion, stress, and an irregular lifestyle.

The main causes of congestion in the kidneys are kidney stones. Most kidney grease/crystals/stones, however, are too small to be detected through modern diagnostic technology, including ultrasounds or x-rays. They are often called *silent* stones and do not seem to bother people much. When they grow larger, though, they can cause considerable distress and damage to the kidneys and thereby seriously harm the rest of the body.

An estimated one million Americans develop kidney stones each year. Once you have had even just one kidney stone attack, your chance of recurrence is about 70 to 80 percent, unless, of course, you know how to prevent it.

Kidney stones are formed when there are problems with the way your body absorbs and eliminates calcium and other substances. The most commonly occurring stones are calcium oxalate stones, struvite stones, uric acid stones, amino acid stones (such as cystine stones), and phosphate stones. However, most kidney stones contain crystals of multiple types. By determining the predominant type you may be able to identify the underlying cause. For example, uric acid stones are often caused by high fructose corn syrup (HFCS) or products that contain it, such as sodas.

Kidney stones can range in size from a grain of sand to larger than a golf ball. If the stones move inside the kidney or pass through the ureters, their rugged, razor-sharp edges can cause serious injuries to the urinary tract, and excruciating pain.

While most kidney stones will actually pass on their own, in some cases, they are simply too large to pass. In any case, it is very beneficial to do a kidney cleanse to dissolve all the smaller stones and to *polish* the rugged edges of larger stones so that they can pass without pain or major discomfort.

The currently used medical procedures and surgical techniques for treating kidney stones come with such high risks of causing kidney damage that physicians tend to avoid recommending them, unless they believe there's no other choice.

Besides chronic liver bile duct congestion, the following are the most common underlying causes of kidney stones, according to an article by *Harvard Health Publications* published in September 2011[208], titled "Six Ways to Keep Your Kidney Stones At Bay." I have added my own comments to the points given.

1. Dehydration

The number one cause of kidney stones is not drinking enough water. Dehydration increases the concentrations of substances in urine that can form stones. Drinking a lot of other beverages such as alcohol, coffee, black tea and soft drinks instead of water can easily lead chronic dehydration, and therefore, kidney stones.

One easy way of verifying whether you are at risk of developing these stones is to check the color of your urine. If it is dark-yellow and you are not taking multivitamins or B vitamins (which darken urine), you are at

---

[208]Six Ways to Keep Your Kidney Stones At Bay, Harvard Health Publications, September 2011

risk of making kidneys stones. So make certain your urine has a very light-yellow color, which happens when you drink at least 6 to 8 glasses of water a day. You may need to drink more if you live in a warmer climate or increase your physical activity, such as during exercise.

2. Magnesium deficiency

Magnesium regulates more than 300 biochemical reactions in the body, including absorption and assimilation of calcium, and deficiency of this mineral has been linked to kidney stones. Even if you consume normal amounts of calcium without adequate magnesium, the excess calcium can contribute to the development of kidney stones, gallbladder stones, and cancers. Magnesium helps prevent kidney stones by preventing calcium from combining with oxalate.

To maintain balanced magnesium/calcium levels it is best to rely on eating leafy green vegetables like kale, spinach and Swiss chard, as well as avocados, almonds, pumpkin seeds, chia seeds, sunflower seeds, and sesame seeds. Eating the typical American diet is a sure way to develop a magnesium deficiency. However, all minerals require the presence of bile to digest and absorb them. Besides eating a balanced diet, you will need to ensure that your liver and gallbladder are unobstructed.

If you assume that supplementing with magnesium is going to eliminate an existing deficiency of this important mineral, you may be mistaken. For magnesium to be useful and active in the body, you will need twice the amount of calcium. However, if you take a calcium supplement to meet this requirement, this may backfire and you are most likely going to create more calcifications in the body, including in the kidneys.

Not relying on real food and a clean liver as the principal pillars of balanced mineral presence in the body, can have consequences that hide behind a vast number of disease symptoms, including kidney stones, gallstones, cancer, heart disease, diabetes, rheumatoid arthritis, osteoporosis, arrhythmia, asthma, attention deficit disorder, autism, Alzheimer's disease, multiple sclerosis, menstrual tension, menopausal symptoms, abnormal widening of blood vessels (vasodilation), convulsions, tremor, depression, psychotic behavior, and many more.

There are over 300 published papers/studies[209] to attest to the important role of magnesium in preventing common diseases.

That said, there is one highly effective application that bypasses the digestive system and delivers the right amounts of magnesium to the area needed for healing an existing condition related to magnesium deficiency, that is, the use of transdermal magnesium oil. I believe that about 70 percent of patients who complain of muscle pain, cramps, and fatigue suffer from chronic magnesium deficiency.

This simple test will show whether a condition like fibromyalgia, migraines or constipation results from a lack of magnesium or not. For one week, apply some magnesium oil to the skin, for example, under the armpits, the back of the hands, or the leg calves. If there is improvement, continue until the condition has cleared up. (See *Product Information - Magnesium Oil*)

3. Regular Sugar Consumption

You cannot expect to have stone-free kidneys if you consume a diet high in sugar. Sugar has been proven to upset the balance of minerals in your body by interfering with calcium and magnesium absorption. Sugar also greatly increases blood uric acid levels, leading to blood vessel damage and uric acid stones. The consumption of unhealthy sugars contained in foods and beverages is a major contributing factor to developing kidney stones and calcified gallstones in children as young as age 5 or 6.

A South African study[210] found that drinking soda beverages increases the incidence of calcium oxalate stones. Sugar can also cause enlargement of the kidneys and other pathological changes leading to kidney damage.

4. Lack of Exercise

Not moving the body on a regular basis can increase your chances of developing kidney stones. A sedentary lifestyle causes your bones to release more calcium into the blood, and also raise blood pressure. Both factors contribute to stone formation. The situation worsens if you are bedridden.

---

[209]Magnesium Research Archives, 2003-Present. John Libbey Eurotext, Magnesium Research 2003 - 2011, www.jle.com
[210]South African study, Effect of cola consumption on urinary biochemical and physicochemical risk factors associated with calcium oxalate urolithiasis. Urol Res. 1999;27(1):77-81

5. Calcium Supplements, Calcium-Low Foods, Animal Protein

To this day, most doctors advise their kidney stone patients to avoid calcium-rich foods because calcium is a major component of most kidney stones. However, scientific research contradicts this widely given medical recommendation (which turns out to be a medical myth), and avoiding calcium-rich foods may actually do you more harm than good. A Harvard School of Public Health study[211] conducted on over 45,000 men found that the men whose diet was rich in calcium had a one-third lower risk of kidney stones than those with lower calcium diets. By the way, the study also found that intake of animal protein was directly associated with the risk of stone formation.

As it turns out, food calcium combines with food oxalates in the intestines, thereby preventing both from being absorbed into the blood and subsequently transferred to the kidneys. Calcium-poor foods, on the other hand, may allow excessive amounts of unbound oxalates to enter the kidneys where they combine with calcium and form calcium-oxalate crystals and stones.

In other, words, what your doctor may be telling you, can, in fact, cause you to ruin your kidneys. It's always good to do your own research before blindly following a doctor's advice.

As previously mentioned, taking calcium supplements increases your risk of kidney stones, gallstones, osteoporosis, cancers, and many other health conditions. To reemphasize, many doctors still recommend to their osteoporosis patients to take calcium supplements, although research has clearly shown that this increases their risk of kidney stones by 20 percent[212]. In contrast, "a high dietary calcium intake decreases the risk of symptomatic kidney stones," write the researchers in the study conclusion. All this makes sense since there is a major difference between the toxic, metallic calcium found in most food supplements and the ionic calcium found in natural, unprocessed foods.

However, make sure to avoid eating milk or cheese. These products contain crude calcium which is bound by the milk protein casein and designed to build the massive, bulky bones of cows, not the relatively slender bones of the human body. The high phosphorus content in dairy

---

[211] A prospective study of dietary calcium and other nutrients and the risk of symptomatic kidney stones. N Engl J Med. 1993 Mar 25;328(12):833-8
[212] Comparison of dietary calcium with supplemental calcium and other nutrients as factors affecting the risk for kidney stones in women. Ann Intern Med. 1997 Apr 1;126(7):497-504

foods (except butter) further prevents the proper utilization of milk calcium by the human body.

6. Avoid Non-Fermented Soy

Soybeans and soy-based foods may promote kidney stones in those prone to them. Soy is rich in oxalates, which can bind with calcium in your kidneys to form kidney stones.

In addition, non-fermented soy - the type found in soy milk, soy burgers, soy ice cream and tofu - is a high-risk food because of its high concentration of nutrient-inhibitors and estrogen-mimicking chemicals. This has been confirmed by a large body of research. This article by Dr. Joseph Mercola, titled "Doctor Warns: Eat This And You'll Look Five Years Older," offers a good summary of the current scientific information available on the adverse effects of soy food[213].

I find it strange that scientists who study the benefits or ill-effects of soy still don't differentiate between fermented and non-fermented soy, but somehow presume it's all the same. Properly fermented soy has completely different bio-chemical effects in the body than non-fermented soy.

Fermented soy, even in small amounts, like most other fermented foods, helps restore a disturbed intestinal flora. Since a balanced gut flora constitutes an essential part of our immune system, the beneficial bacteria found in fermented food can offer excellent protection against any type of cancer.

The Japanese tradition requires that soy undergoes several years of fermentation, like a good wine, before it is consumed. And of course, people who choose a vegetarian diet have the natural advantage of having lower cancer rates anyway, even if they add some non-fermented soy to their diet. However, there is still a risk because of the estrogenic and anti-nutrient compounds in non-fermented soy products. I have personally seen women completely reverse tumors in their breasts and abdomen, sometimes within a matter of 10 days, after I recommended they go off soy milk, tofu or soy-based power drinks. On the other hand, I have never seen anyone develop a cancerous tumor who added fermented soy like tempeh or natto to their diet.

---

[213]Doctor Warns: Eat this and You'll Look Five Years Older, *Dr. Joseph Mercola, December 08 2011,*www.mercola.com

I would also like to add the use of pharmaceutical drugs to the list issued by *Harvard Health Publications*. Numerous medical drugs, such as Lasix (furosemide), Topomax (topiramate), and Xenical, or combination of several prescription drugs, can also affect proper urine filtration and lead to stone formation.

To prevent kidney problems and kidney-related diseases, it is best to eliminate kidney stones before they can cause a serious crisis such as kidney failure. You can easily detect the presence of sand or stones in the kidneys by pulling the skin under your eyes sideways toward the cheekbones. Any irregular bumps, protrusions, red or white pimples, or discoloration (dark-brown or black) of the skin indicates the presence of kidney sand or kidney stones.

The following herbs, when taken daily for a period of 20 to 30 days, can help to dissolve and eliminate all types of kidney stones, including uric

Ingredients:	
Marjoram -1oz (28 g)	Uva ursi - 2 oz (56 g)
Cat's claw - 1oz (28 g)	Hydrangea root - 2oz (56 g)
Comfrey root -1oz (28 g)	Gravel root - 2oz (56 g)
Fennel seeds - 2oz (56 g)	Marshmallow root - 2oz (56 g)
Chicory herb or root - 2oz (56g)	Golden rod herb - 2oz (56 g)

acid, oxalic acid, phosphate, and amino acid stones. If you have a history of kidney stones, you may need to repeat this cleanse a few times, at intervals of six weeks.

Directions for making the Kidney Cleanse Tea:

1. Take 1 oz. (28 g) each of the first three herbs and 2 oz. (56 g) each of the rest of the herbs, and thoroughly mix them together. Keep them in an airtight container. You may put them in the refrigerator to maintain potency.
2. Before bedtime, soak about 2 heaping tablespoons of the mixture (10 grams) in 16 oz. (240 ml) of water, cover it, and leave it covered overnight. The following morning, bring the concoction to a boil; then strain it. The second best preparation method is to boil the mixture in the morning, and let it simmer for 5 to 10 minutes before straining.

3. Drink a few sips at a time throughout the day. Do not drink it all at once but divide it into 7-8 portions or more. It's best to sip the tea, and not drink it down like water. Taking a few sips from each portion at a time is ideal. The reason why it should not be consumed at one time is to achieve slow and continuous dissolution of crystals and stones throughout the day, otherwise the benefit may only be minimal.
(**Note**: This tea does not need to be taken warm or hot, but do not refrigerate it. Also, *do not* add sugar or sweeteners! Leave at least one hour after eating before taking your next sips)

Do this for 3 weeks. If you experience stiffness or ache in the area of the lower back, this is because a lot of mineral crystals from kidney stones are passing through the ureter ducts of the urinary system. The crystals' sharp edges may irritate the ureter lining somewhat. This is a good sign and there is no need for concern. Usually, the stiffness lessens and disappears after a few days. Most people pass fewer crystals and don't experience any discomfort, and the kidney cleanse may seem uneventful.

Any strong smell and darkening of the urine at the beginning of, or during the kidney cleanse indicates a major release of toxins from the kidneys. Normally, though, the release is gradual and does not significantly change the color or texture of the urine.

Important additional instructions:

1. Support the kidneys during the cleanse by drinking enough filtered water or spring water, a minimum of 6 and a maximum of 8 glasses per day, unless the color of the urine is dark-yellow (in which case you will need to drink more than that amount).
2. During the entire duration of cleanse, try to avoid consuming animal products, including meat, dairy foods (except butter), fish, eggs, tea, coffee, alcohol, carbonated beverages, chocolate, and any other foods or beverages that contain caffeine, preservatives, artificial sweeteners, coloring agents, and the like.
3. If you are doing liver flushes, make certain that you do a kidney cleanse after every 3 or 4 liver flushes. If you feel your body is toxic or you have had a history of kidney problems, make certain to do a kidney cleanse before attempting your first liver flush.
4. You may also combine the kidney cleanse with the liver flush preparation, except don't take the kidney cleanse tea on Day 6 and Day

7 of the liver flush. Interrupting the kidney cleanse for these two days will not significantly interfere with its effectiveness; simply make up for the lost days by adding 2-3 extra days at the end.

5. If you happen to have a large kidney stone, in addition to kidney cleaning you may also benefit from drinking the juice of one to two lemons or limes (as concentrated as possible) per day for about 10-14 days. After that, drink the juice of half a lemon or lime per day indefinitely. You can then add some of the lemon or lime juice to your drinking water. This helps prevent new stones from being formed.

6. In the rare case that you experience abdominal bloating while on the kidney cleanse, you may reduce the dosage to one heaping tablespoon a day. The herbs in the tea don't just help to dissolve kidney stones and crystals, but they also act as powerful intestinal cleansers. They may open up and dislodge old pockets of accumulated mucoid fecal matter and toxins, which when being released can cause bloating.

Cleaning out the whole colon through a colonic, Colema, or enema once or twice while on the kidney cleanse can greatly accelerate the cleansing process and make it a lot more comfortable.

Can pregnant women do the kidney cleanse?

I have received numerous reports from pregnant and nursing mothers who have done both the liver and kidney cleanses successfully and without causing any adverse reactions for the mother and the baby. However, for reasons of legality, I am not in the position to make recommendations to that effect.

Strong cleansing or purgative herbs are usually not recommended for pregnant women, but this is an area of medicine that is not entirely clear. Obstetricians warn pregnant women against taking herbal remedies but they readily prescribe them drugs like antibiotics and toxin-packed vaccines, which is far more risky than taking a few herbs that have never been shown to cause harm. For example, antibiotics and vaccines damage the mother's liver and cause birth defects in the baby, and the H1N1 vaccine that was given to pregnant women throughout the United States during the 2009 swine flu epidemic has been linked to a 700 percent increase in miscarriages compared with previous years[214]. Still, it is

---

[214] H1N1 vaccine linked to 700 percent increase in miscarriages, NaturalNews.com (December 08, 2010)

perhaps best to be on the safe side and avoid all medicinal substances, including natural ones, while pregnant and even while nursing.

What about the claimed "toxic effects" of Comfrey Root?

I am very well aware of some doctors referring to comfrey as having toxic effects on the liver. I am also aware of the strong pressure exerted by the pharmaceutical industry on the medical establishment and the US *protective* agencies like the FDA, CDC, FTC, etc. to warn the public against using natural remedies or ban them altogether - the stated goal of Codex Alimentarius.

Ratified by the WHO and already implemented by the European Union, Codex is a UN-backed, global cartel designed to hand over the control of all natural remedies from those who sell or use them to the pharmaceutical companies. Whereas the US Dietary Supplement Health and Education Act(DSHEA) scientifically classifies nutritional supplements as *food* and prevents dosage restrictions, Codex unscientifically classifies them as toxins and sets ultra-low doses, thereby rendering natural remedies effectively ineffective. This way, natural remedies will never be able to show greater benefits than medical drugs. The FDA already made a recommendation to limit the use of comfrey with the intention to eventually ban it altogether. It is obvious that this agency is going after the most beneficial herbal remedies first.

It is very easy for a protective agency to infer that a powerful healing herb must be toxic for the human body because it has been found to be toxic when fed to test animals. However, to give rats excessively large amounts of powdered comfrey to eat and then determine that this can harm or destroy their liver has hardly anything to do with science. You can also kill a rat by having it breathe twice the amount of oxygen normally found in the air. Does this mean that oxygen is a dangerous molecule?

First, brewing a tea from comfrey is very different than grinding and eating the herb. Second, the small amount of comfrey used as part of the kidney cleanse is no more harmful or harmless than the 21 percent oxygen normally found in air.

Many people have died from water intoxication (drinking too much water), but this doesn't mean water is dangerous if taken in normal amounts. In fact, we cannot live without it. Likewise, if garlic juice is injected into the blood, it kills the person within minutes. It can weaken the intestinal wall and cause hernias. If eaten only occasionally and in moderation, it can be beneficial. If eaten in excess, it destroys brain cells.

There is hardly any natural food or substance that doesn't have potentially toxic effects. For comfrey to be harmful for the body, you have to consume a lot of it, and for a very long time (years). It's like water, oxygen, alcohol, sugar, caffeine, food, etc; any of these can be useful if taken in moderation, but harmful if taken in excess.

Most medical research is designed to prove a certain outcome, which makes it very biased from the start. For example, study subjects are told they are participating in a drug trial to show efficacy of new drug in the treatment of the particular disease they are suffering from. Since the excitement, hope, and positive expectation among the study's subjects act as a powerful placebo[215], the objectivity of the research is already undermined before the study begins. The way the research is conducted, there is simply no way to determine whether any improvement of the disease condition is due to the drug or the placebo which the subject generates in his body when he takes the drug. So much for objective science!

In a similar way, researchers cannot differentiate between the beneficial effects of a herb and its potentially harmful effects. Alkaloids are bitter (like most green herbs and grasses). Bitter foods act as a medicine; they cleanse the blood and the tissues (hence the term *bitter medicine*). When the body cleanses itself, otherwise normal blood values and enzyme populations show up as *unbalanced* in tests. A regular doctor trained in symptomatology would call this a disease, and start treating the symptoms (suppress them). In reality, though, there is no disease, just the body trying to heal itself and rid itself of toxins.

Pain, for example, is not a disease, but the body's way to inform the brain about an existing area of congestion and to send specialized cells, water, and healing hormones (steroids) to the affected area. In order to remove the congestion, inflammation may be necessary. Inflammation is not a disease either, but a healing response by the body (yet doctors treat is as if it were a disease). When the congestion is finally broken up, the pressure and pain subside and the body returns the blood values and organ functions back to normal.

Most medical research is based on the idea that when something in the body is not showing up as *normal*, there must be something wrong with it. In truth, it is the body's correct and natural way to return to a state of

---

[215]Positive Expectation – A Medical Miracle? - my article on www.ener-chi.com

homeostasis. Comfrey clears out and breaks down toxins and waste, putting these into circulation for elimination, and thereby saving organs and systems from their demise. That's why it has been such a popular healing herb for thousands of years. When researchers study subjects, they often get a lot of congested, unhealthy people.

Pharmaceutical drugs suppress symptoms (healing efforts) which prevents the body from cleansing and healing itself. Herbs, on the other hand, allow symptoms of congestion to emerge or even increase, and thereby, assist the body to actually heal itself. Medical doctors are no longer trained in the science of herbs and, therefore, lack any scientific understanding about the beneficial effects of medicinal herbs on the human body, and how these make it easier for the body to heal. The following benefits may explain more clearly why comfrey is considered a threat to the medical industry:

Comfrey has been extensively used in folk medicine to soothe and heal gastritis, gastric and duodenal ulcers; act as a blood purifier; heal cuts and wounds, burns, sprains, strains, and tendinitis; inhibit wound infection and prevent scarring; heal respiratory ailments of the lungs and bronchial passages; to be a soothing expectorant for dry coughs, pleurisy and bronchitis; heal ulcers of the liver and gallbladder; reduce the swelling and inflammation around a broken bone; help with gout, arthritis, bleeding piles, varicose veins, phlebitis; heal skin problems such as psoriasis, eczema, acne, and boils; reduce soreness and inflammation of eyes when used as an eyewash; support digestive and urinary systems; reduce irritation-causing diarrhea, dysentery and ulcerative colitis; relax urinary spasms; soothe cystitis and clear urinary irritation and infection.

4. Drink Ionized Water Frequently

The sipping of hot, ionized water has a profound cleansing effect on all the tissues of the body. It helps reduce overall toxicity, improves circulatory functions, and balances bile. When you boil water for 15 to 20 minutes, it becomes thinner (its molecule clusters are reduced from the normal number of about 10,000 to one or two clusters), and it is charged and saturated with negative oxygen ions (hydroxide, $OH-$). When you take frequent sips of this water throughout the day, it begins to systematically cleanse the tissues of the body and help rid them of certain positively charged ions (those associated with harmful acids and toxins).

Most toxins and waste materials carry a positive charge and, thus, naturally tend to attach themselves to the body, which in the most part is negatively charged. As the negative oxygen ions enter the body with the ingested water, they are attracted to the positively charged toxic material. This neutralizes waste and toxins, turning them into fluid matter that the body can remove easily.

For the first couple of days or even weeks of cleansing your body tissues in this way, your tongue may take on a white or yellow coating, an indication that the body is clearing out a lot of toxic waste and yeast germs. If you have excessive body weight, this cleansing method can help you shed many pounds of body waste in a short period of time, without the side effects that normally accompany sudden weight loss.

Directions: Boil water for 15 to 20 minutes and pour it into a thermos. Stainless steel thermoses are fine. The thermos keeps the water hot and ionized throughout the day. (**Note**: once the water has turned warm, it has lost its charge and offers none of the described benefits) Take 1 or 2 sips every half hour all day long, and drink it as hot as you would sip hot tea. You may use this method anytime you do not feel well, have the need for decongesting, wish to keep the blood thin, or simply want to feel more energetic and clearheaded. Some people sip ionized water for a certain duration, such as 3 to 4 weeks; others do it ongoing.

The oxygen ions are generated through the bubbling effect of boiling water, similar to water falling on the ground in a waterfall or breaking against the seashore. In the thermos, the water will stay ionized for up to 12 hours, or for as long as it remains hot. The total amount of water you need to boil to give you enough hot, ionized water for one day would be about 20-24 oz. This specially prepared water should not substitute for normal drinking water. It doesn't hydrate the cells like normal water does; the body uses it mostly to cleanse the tissues of toxins.

The ionized water prepared in the above way is far more concentrated with negative oxygen ions than regular machine-generated ionized water. If you wish to, you may also drink water produced by a water ionizer, but this does not have the same, powerful cleansing effects as the boiled, ionized water.

5. Eat Ionic, Essential Minerals

Your body is like *living soil*. If it has sufficient minerals and trace elements to work with, it is able to nurture you and produce everything you need to live and grow. These essential materials, however, can easily become depleted when you do not get enough of them from the food you eat. Centuries of constant use of the same agricultural fields have led to foods that are highly nutrient-deficient. The situation worsened with the onset of chemical fertilizers, which force crops to grow more rapidly without regard for nutrient availability. When minerals and trace elements run low in the body, important functions can no longer be sustained, or they become subdued. Disease is generally accompanied by a lack of one or more of these important substances.

Because of the unnatural situation of mineral depletion in our soil today and, therefore, in our bodies, it may be useful to supplement with minerals. The crucial question is whether the minerals sold in nutrition stores or pharmacies are capable of replenishing the mineral supply to the cells of the body. The answer is: "Highly unlikely!"

Minerals are commonly made available in 3 basic forms: capsules, tablets, and colloidal mineral water. Before the depletion of soils, plant foods were our ideal mineral provider. When a plant grows in a healthy soil environment, it absorbs existing colloidal minerals and changes them into ionic, easy-to-digest form.

The ionic minerals are an angstrom in size, whereas the colloidal minerals, also known as inorganic, metallic minerals, are about 10,000 times larger (micron-size). Ionic, water-soluble plant minerals are absorbed readily by body cells. In contrast, colloidal particles packed into complex compounds, and delivered in pill form, stand less than one percent chance of absorption. The minerals found in colloidal mineral waters are not absorbed any better. They are not water-soluble, but simply suspended between water molecules.

Common colloidal particles, such as the compounds calcium carbonate and zinc picolinate, tend to get caught in the bloodstream and are subsequently deposited in various parts of the body. In the form of deposits, they can cause major mechanical, structural, and functional damage. Many health problems today, including osteoporosis, heart disease, cancer, arthritis, brain disorders, kidney stones, gallstones, and so on, are the direct result of ingesting such metallic minerals, including calcium.

Fortunately, there are some naturally occurring foods that are still extremely rich in minerals - marine phytoplankton being one of the best. Marine phytoplankton, which is the smallest possible micro-algae in ocean water, feeds the world's largest and longest living animals and fish, including blue whales, bowhead whales, baleen whales, gray whales, and humpbacks.

Phytoplankton has the unique ability to transform sunlight, raw inorganic minerals, and carbon dioxide into food for an extraordinary number of living creatures. It is also the single-most rich source of essential fatty acids on Earth, according to a large number of research studies[216]. Phytoplankton is a far more efficient provider of omega-3 fats, for example, than seafood, fish oil, or krill oil.

Marine phytoplankton contains more than 90 ionic and trace minerals, and is loaded with high-energy super anti-oxidants, vitamins, and proteins in microscopic form. In fact, marine phytoplankton is considered to be one of the most complete foods on Earth. It is a tiny little plant (about the size of a red blood cell) which allows for fast absorption on the cellular level, especially when it is taken as a liquid extract (see *Product Information*) versus a powdered form. Phytoplankton is considered a whole food.

Other good foods rich in ionic minerals are olives (olive trees tend to grow in soil that is extremely rich in metallic minerals, especially calcium). Chia seeds, pumpkins seeds and sesame seeds, as well as beans and legumes, also are packed with ionic minerals, and so are nuts from large, mature trees that have been around for many years.

Organically grown green leafy vegetables, cabbage, carrots, cauliflower, broccoli, artichokes, spinach, and pumpkin contain large amounts of calcium, potassium, and magnesium. Among the vegetables, spinach, leeks, broccoli, and zucchini are especially high in calcium. Tomatoes, potatoes, sweet potatoes, and avocados contain high amounts of potassium.

Unprocessed, or minimally processed, organically grown grains are good sources of molybdenum, manganese, magnesium, copper, phosphorous, and chromium. Organically grown fruits offer a whole range of important minerals.

---

[216]Transfer of essential fatty acids by marine plankton, a Thesis presented to The Faculty of the School of Marine Science, by Adriana J. Veloza

A well-balanced diet consisting of a large variety of the above foods is still going to be sufficient to provide the body with most minerals. Processed foods, on the other hand, are mostly depleted of these minerals, which makes them a major cause of illness. If you are not able to eat a balanced diet for reasons not under your control, I would definitely recommend marine phytoplankton.

Himalayan crystal salt and natural sea salts or rock salts contain a large number of different trace minerals, and thus may help enrich your diet as well.

One of the most efficient ways of making these minerals available to the body is to place up to a dozen chunks of Himalayan salt crystals (do an online search for Himalayan Crystal Salt Sole) in a jar of water (10-12 oz.), and take a minimum of 2 tablespoons a day of the *brine* which is the salt water that forms after a few days. You can add it to your foods, or some of it, to your drinking water. After a few weeks, you may add some more crystals to the jar to keep the water saturated with the salt. Of course, you will also need to add more water from time to time. This salt water has about 84 minerals and trace minerals in it.

6. *"Give Us Our Daily Sulfur!"*

Sulfur is an essential mineral which the body uses to make many of its amino acids and proteins, according to a study done at the Institute of Human Nutrition, School of Medicine, University of Southampton in the UK, in 2006[217]. The researchers of the study titled "The Effects of Sulfur Amino Acid Intake on Immune Function in Humans" revealed sulfur's important role in keeping our immune system healthy and efficient. The study shows that sulfur in the form of methylsulfonylmethane (MSM) may provide natural and effective support in alleviating inflammation throughout the body.

The best study on sulfur is perhaps the ongoing "Live Blood Cellular Matrix Study" (12 years at the time of writing this), which is not a scientific study by any means, but it consists of collecting anecdotal evidence from those who have benefited from using sulfur for a large

---

[217]The Effects of Sulfur Amino Acid Intake on Immune Function in Humans, The American Society for Nutrition J. Nutr. 136:1660S-1665S, June 2006

number of different conditions[218]. In my opinion, when scientific research is truly controlled, as it is being done in this study, valuable real-life information can be gained that otherwise may remain concealed in the so-called *properly conducted* scientific studies.

In essence, sulfur makes it possible for proteins and other nutrients and gases to pass across the membranes into the cells. Without it, cell membranes become leathery and less permeable, thereby forcing cells to become anaerobic and accumulate acid metabolic wastes. This can cause them to either turn cancerous, or to degenerate and die. Since sulfur cannot be stored in the body, not being amply supplied with it each day through food and drinking water causes us to die each day a little more through cell degeneration (disease and aging).

Sulfur is naturally found in hard water. The populations in some Mediterranean countries where the water is partially hard tend to have a low incidence in heart disease and dementia. Iceland, which is particularly blessed with sulfur-rich water (sulfur springs), is ranked as the healthiest country in the world, according to a Forbes report, followed by Finland and Sweden.

Water softening, as well as fluoridation and chlorination of water strip the water of all its sulfur. This is one of the reasons sulfur deficiency is more pronounced in larger cities or communities supplied with treated, municipal water.

Before the era of chemical fertilizers, our food was grown through the applications of sulfur-rich manures to the soil. The extensive use of chemical fertilizers and pesticides, on the other hand, has stripped our foods of almost all sulfur. Whatever sulfur is left in these foods, is removed through food processing, heating, and preservation methods. After chemical fertilizers were mandated in the US in 1954, the incidence of cancer and other major degenerative illnesses increased by an astounding 4,000 percent.

Finland was one of the first countries in the world to recognize the fundamental dangers of modern farming methods and food production. In 1985, alarmed by the same obscene increase in degenerative disease at similar levels to those found in the US, Finland altogether banned the use of chemical fertilizers. This resulted in their disease rates to drop to a tenth of their 1985 rates. Today, Finland does not only boast one of the

---

[218] Live Blood Cellular Matrix Study 1999 – 2012, http://www.encognitive.com/node/1123

healthiest populations in the world, it is also the leading supplier of organically grown foods in Europe.

In the body, sulfur is responsible for allowing cells to use oxygen effectively and for undergoing repair, if damaged. In fact, without enough sulfur in the body, healing cannot take place. Unless you eat mostly organically grown foods and drink natural, untreated water, you may not be able to keep the body at its optimal level of health and vitality.

Aging has very little to do with one's age. Aging is rather a nutrient-deficiency syndrome that increasingly prevents the nourishment of the body's organs and systems and forces the cells to hold on to their own waste products.

Sulfur is that one single mineral that regulates cellular nourishment and waste removal. To do this successfully, the body requires about 750 mg of sulfur each day. The sulfur can draw toxins out of the cells, even fat cells and brain cells. It increases circulation, enzyme activity, strengthens the immune system, reduces recovery time after injury, reduces muscle pain and soreness, promotes healthy growth of hair and nails, helps with cancer, osteoporosis, depression, Parkinson's disease, Alzheimer's disease, and diabetes. I cannot think of any inflammatory illness where sulfur-deficiency does not also play a key role. Almost all diseases are due to inflammation.

Toxins in our environment, food additives, pesticides and herbicides sprayed on foods and into the air, chemtrail toxins (such as aluminum oxides and barium), vaccines, radiation toxins created by cell phones and wireless devices, etc., all deplete sulfur in the body. Remember, it takes a lot of sulfur to remove just the internally generated waste products each day. There is not much sulfur left to deal with the unnaturally supplied toxins, which can then easily overtax the liver, kidneys, heart, and brain.

Cleaning out the liver and gallbladder, colon, and kidneys; combined with eating mostly organically grown foods and drinking natural untreated water, are among the basic steps to restore the body's health and slow the aging process.

Vegetarian foods that are particularly rich in sulfur include broccoli, cauliflower, kale, Brussels sprouts, watercress, and radish. If you suffer from an illness, though, and require extra sulfur to support the healing and repair of damaged cells in your body, you may consider eating extra sulfur as part of your daily diet.

If you are taking any medication, make sure to leave at least 30 minutes between taking the medication and taking sulfur. The chemicals would quickly deplete the sulfur and thus render it ineffective.

Note: The sulfur typically sold in the form of MSM (methylsulfonylmethane) supplements is usually ineffective. Most MSM products sold commercially contain less than 35 percent sulfur, and some MSM products contain no sulfur at all! This is largely due to the crushing of the methylsulfonylmethane crystals into powder and adding anti-cake agents. Additives of packaging may also block or neutralize the bio-availability of the sulfur contained in the MSM. I recommend that you only use organic sulfur in its crystal, lignin (wood pulp-based) form (see *Product Information*).

I strongly advice against using synthetically produced methylsulfonylmethane.

Possible cleansing reactions:

Because sulfur is an effective cleanser, it may initially lead to mild cleansing reactions such as intestinal gas. Do not become discouraged if it doesn't make you feel good right away. It can easily take 3-4 weeks before the body's cell membranes become unclogged and proper cell oxygenation kicks in. The less toxic the body is, the faster the results will become apparent. In any case, the sulfur is equally effective for everyone because it is an essential food, not a medicine (although natural food acts like medicine). Without sulfur, we could not live even for one minute.

If taking the sulfur at the recommend dosage makes you feel uncomfortable at first, use a smaller dosage and slowly work up to a teaspoon (5 g) twice a day. Those with a severe degenerative disease may take as much as 1 tablespoon (15 g) twice daily but should also start at no more than 1 teaspoon twice a day.

It can take up to 3-4 months for damaged or weak cells to reach the end of their natural cycle and for new, healthy, properly oxygenated cells to replace them. In addition, a lifetime of absorbing toxins buried under layers of fat and insulating mucopolysaccharides (mucus) cannot be undone overnight. So be patient. It is far better to know something as pure and cleansing as sulfur is causing a little temporary discomfort than not to notice the body slowly suffocating in a pool of toxins.

A simple taste test: When eaten straight, organic sulfur has a bitter taste to it, which is much more noticeable when the body is quite toxic.

The less toxins there are in the body, the less bitter the sulfur tastes. So if it tastes very bitter to you, you can be certain you are quite deficient in it.

To make it easier on your taste buds, you can put the sulfur in your mouth and immediately swig a little lime or lemon juice and its flakes will melt in your mouth as you swallow. Then drink an 8-oz. (240 ml) glass of non-chlorinated, non-fluoridated water (these chemicals will nullify the benefits of the ingested sulfur). Alternately, dissolve it in a glass of warm water with some lime or lemon juice added, and perhaps a little raw honey.

Organic sulfur has no known toxicity. Even if you took too much of it, it would simply be excreted by the body.

When choosing a product, there is a simple test that you can perform to determine its effectiveness. Dissolve some of the crystals in a little bit of hot water and let it stand until it evaporates. Once evaporated, the crystals will be larger than they were when you started the process. If not, the product is worthless. Most commercial MSM products, especially those in powder form fail this test (see *Product Information* for good product sources that have passed the test).

7. Drink Enough Water

To produce the right amount of bile each day (1–1½ quarts), which the body requires for proper digestion of food, the liver needs plenty of water. In addition, the body uses up a lot of water to maintain normal blood volume, hydrate the cells and connective tissues, cleanse out toxins, and carry out literally thousands of other functions. Since the body cannot store water the way it stores fat, it is dependent on regular, sufficient water intake.

To maintain proper bile production and bile consistency, as well as balanced blood values, you need to drink about 6 to 8 glasses of water each day. The most important time to drink water is right after getting up.

First, drink one glass of warm water to make it easier for the kidneys to dilute and excrete urine formed during the night. This is of great importance because urine is highly concentrated in the morning; if it is not diluted properly, urinary waste products may settle in both the kidneys and the urinary bladder.

Second, drink another glass of warm water to which you can add the juice of a wedge up to ½ of a fresh lemon or lime and a teaspoon of raw honey. This helps to cleanse the GI tract. Lemon has strong cleansing properties, and raw honey kills harmful germs and heals intestinal cuts and wounds. It also breaks down excessive mucus in the stomach and intestinal tract.

Besides when feeling thirsty, other important times for drinking a glass of water (not chilled) are about ½ hour before and 2-2½ hours after meals. These are the times when a well hydrated body would naturally signal thirst. Having enough water available at those times ensures that the blood, bile, and lymph remain sufficiently fluid to conduct their respective activities in the body. Since hunger and thirst signals use the same hormonal alert system in the body, if you happen to feel *hungry* even though your stomach is not empty yet, it is more likely that you are actually running out of water. Therefore, it is best to drink a glass of room temperature or warm water first and then see whether your hunger has subsided or not.

If you suffer from high blood pressure and use prescription drugs for this condition, make sure you have your blood pressure monitored regularly when you begin drinking more water. With an increase in your water consumption, your blood pressure may return to normal within a relatively short period of time. This would make the intake of medication redundant and even harmful.

By drinking enough water, you may also start to lose weight if you are overweight, or gain weight if you are underweight.

However, I strongly recommend you avoid bottled water, unless it comes in glass bottles. Toxic plastic chemicals such as Bisphenol A (BPA) seep from the bottle into the water and accumulate in your body when you drink it.

BPAs can cause abnormal weight gain, insulin resistance, prostate and breast cancer, excessive mammary gland development, neurological problems, deranged dopamine activity resulting in hyperactivity, attention deficits, a heightened sensitivity to medical drugs, and possibly a significantly increased risk of heart disease, according to new data from a long-running British health survey, the NHANES study[219].

As mentioned before, BPAs are also prevalent in canned goods, food packaging, dental sealants, and paper money.

---

[219] Association of urinary bisphenol a concentration with heart disease: evidence from NHANES 2003/06.PLoS One. 2010 Jan 13;5(1):e8673

It is equally important to choose a water treatment system that gives you fresh, healthy water. The most commonly used methods to remove chlorine and numerous other contaminants from your drinking water (and possibly shower water) are filtration and reverse osmosis. Although some of these systems can be high priced, they are still an affordable option if you consider the cost of suffering through a bout of cancer. To help replenish some of the minerals lost when using these two types of systems, add a few grains of uncooked basmati rice to the water jug or bottle (avoid plastic containers) and leave the rice in the jar for up to a month at a time. Adding a pinch of or unrefined sea salt to a glass of water also helps to give you some of the lost minerals back.

Distilled water, which is the closest to natural rainwater, is excellent for hydrating the body cells, but when produced by a commercial water distiller, it is lifeless. Adding 3 to 4 grains of uncooked basmati rice to 1 gallon of distilled water gives it minerals and vitamins (or else use the sea salt option), and exposing the water to direct sunlight or placing a clear quartz crystal in the water for an hour helps to restore some of its lost vitality. Of course, the old-fashioned method of boiling your drinking water for several minutes causes any chlorine to evaporate.

Another inexpensive way to get rid of most chlorine in water is to use vitamin C. One gram of vitamin C will neutralize 1ppm (part per million) of chlorine in 100 gallons of water. This is particularly useful if you want to lie in the bathtub without suffering the irritating effects of chlorine on your skin and in your lungs.

Prill beads are another, far less expensive, form of water treatment. Although they cannot replace a water filter, they still cleanse your drinking water and make it *thinner*. This has a positive effect on the blood, lymph, and basic cellular processes. Prill beads are available on the internet (see *Product Information* at the end of the book). I can attest to the good taste of the water, its *thinness*, and its excellent hydrating and cleansing effects.

Quite affordable, yet still very effective, and excellent for people who not only are interested in proper hydration but also want to cleanse the body from toxins, are water ionizers. These are widely available on the internet (see *Product Information*). I personally use a LIFE water ionizer.

I am a great friend of *structured water*, which restores the lost vitality of treated municipal water, reversed osmosis water, and even distilled water. An online search of this term will provide you plenty of options to choose from. Aqua-Lyros is probably the best structured water device I have come across. It is available in Europe and shipped worldwide.

I have also had very good experiences with the low-cost Adya Ceramic Water Filtration System (see *Product Information* for details about the above recommendations).

8. Cut Down on Alcohol

Alcohol is liquefied, refined, fermented sugar and is highly acid-forming. It makes no valuable contribution to cell metabolism, like the sugar glucose does, but this does not prevent it from having a strong mineral-depleting effect in the body. The organ most affected by alcohol is the liver. If a generally healthy person drinks 2 glasses of wine within an hour, the liver is not able to detoxify all the alcohol. Much of it is converted into fatty deposits and, eventually, gallstones in the liver and gallbladder. If the liver and gallbladder have already accumulated a certain number of gallstones, alcohol consumption will make these stones grow faster and cause them to become more plentiful.

Like coffee or tea, alcohol has a strongly dehydrating effect. It reduces the water content of the body's cells, blood, lymph, and bile, thus impairing blood circulation and the elimination of waste products. The effects of a dehydrated central nervous system are delirium, blurred vision, loss of memory, disorientation, slow reaction time, and poor mind-body coordination, all of which we generally refer to as a *hangover*. Under the influence of alcohol and the dehydration it can cause, the nervous and immune systems go into depression. This leads to a slowing of the digestive, metabolic, and hormonal processes in the body. All of this promotes the development of even more gallstones in the liver and gallbladder.

It is best for those who have had a history of gallstones to avoid alcohol altogether, at least until they are sure all their stones have been cleared out. Many of my clients who stopped drinking any kind of alcohol, including beer and wine, often spontaneously recovered from such problems as panic attacks, arrhythmia, respiratory problems, various heart conditions, sleeping disorders, gallbladder attacks, pancreatic infections, prostate enlargement, colitis, and other inflammatory diseases. If you suffer from any disease at all, it is best to stay away from all dehydrating beverages, such as alcohol, coffee, tea, and soda (especially diet drinks). This allows the body to direct all its energy and resources toward healing the affected part(s) of the body.

Once you have recovered, it is fine to consume coffee, tea, or alcohol in moderation, as long as you also drink enough water. Among the wines, red wines are preferable. It takes at least one hour for a healthy liver to remove the alcohol contained in one glass of wine from the blood. Having excessive amounts of alcohol in the blood is very toxic to the brain, liver, and kidneys.

However, women tend to metabolize alcohol more slowly than men, and are therefore markedly less able to tolerate alcohol than men, according to numerous research studies.

Women with estrogen dominance (those whose liver cannot remove excess amounts of estrogens from the blood) are particularly vulnerable to the potentially harmful effects of alcohol. Even small amounts increase their risk of developing fibroids, endometriosis, heavy bleeding, and breast cancer. Alcohol may also inhibit ovulation and sexual functions, and in menopausal women, it can worsen hot flashes, mood swings, night sweats, insomnia, and dryness of skin.

9. Avoid Overeating

One of the greatest causes of gallstones is overindulging in food. Eating more than the stomach can process without suffering indigestion or fullness causes the liver to secrete excessive amounts of cholesterol into liver bile. This, in turn, leads to the development of gallstones in the bile ducts. Therefore, one of the most effective methods to prevent gallstones is *under eating*.

Eating in moderation and observing an occasional day of fasting on just liquids (e.g. vegetable juices, fruit juices, vegetable soups, water, herbal teas, etc.) both help the digestive system to remain efficient and able to deal with most existing deposits of undigested food.

Leaving the dining table while still a little hungry maintains a healthy desire for good, nutritious foods. Completely extinguishing the fire of one's appetite through overeating, on the other hand, leads to intestinal congestion, the proliferation of destructive bacteria and yeast, poor absorption of nutrients, and food cravings.

Food cravings are characterized by a strong, even overwhelming, desire for energy-boosting (which really means energy-depleting)foods and beverages such as sugar, sweets, white flour products, potato chips, coffee, tea, power drinks, and soft drinks. They quickly raise blood sugar to abnormally high levels while stimulating the whole body into overdrive. Once the fuel for generating this *high* experience is used up, the blood sugar drops to an abnormally low level, which creates lethargy, mood swings, anger and frustration, and even depression.

To undo this uncomfortable feeling resulting from such energy-depletion, the now-addict seeks to find comfort provided by these energizing foods and beverages. This effect has earned them the sobriquet *comfort foods*.

Loving a particular food doesn't mean you are craving it. If you truly love to eat a certain food, you can also easily live without it. If you crave it, though, not having it can drive you insane. The bottom line is that whatever foods you crave are also the ones that keep you physically, mentally and emotionally imbalanced. These are also the mostly likely foods and beverages to cause gallstones. Consciously under eating a bit, eating wholesome, nutrient-rich foods, and cleansing the liver/gallbladder and intestinal tract are quick ways to end overeating and food cravings.

10. Maintain Regular Mealtimes

The body is controlled by numerous circadian rhythms, which regulate the most important functions in the body in accordance with preprogrammed time intervals. Sleep, the secretion of hormones and digestive juices, the elimination of waste, and so on, all follow a specific daily routine. If these cyclic activities become disrupted more often than they are adhered to, the body becomes imbalanced and cannot fulfill its essential tasks. All tasks are naturally aligned with and dependent on the schedule dictated by the circadian rhythms.

Having regular mealtimes makes it easy for the body to prepare for the production and secretion of the right amounts of digestive juices for each meal. Irregular eating habits, on the other hand, confuse the body. Furthermore, its digestive power becomes depleted by having to adjust to a different mealtime each time you eat. Skipping meals here and there, eating at different times, or eating between meals especially disrupts the cycles of bile production by the liver cells. The result is the formation of gallstones.

By maintaining a regular eating routine, the body's 60 to 100 trillion cells are able to receive their daily quota of nutrients according to schedule, which helps cell metabolism to be smooth and effective. Many metabolic disorders, such as diabetes or obesity, result from irregular eating habits and can be greatly improved by matching one's eating times with the natural circadian rhythms. It is best to eat the largest meal of the day around midday and only light meals at breakfast (no later than 8:00 a.m.) and dinner (no later than 7:00 p.m.).

11. Ideally, Eat a Balanced Vegetarian/Vegan Diet

Eating a balanced vegetarian/vegan diet is one of the most effective ways to prevent the formation of gallstones, cancer, heart disease, diabetes, osteoporosis, depression, and many other illnesses. If you feel you cannot right away or solely live on foods that are of vegetable origin, then at least try to substitute red meat with free-range chicken, rabbit, or turkey for some time. Eventually, you may be able to go fully vegetarian.

All forms of animal protein decrease the solubility of bile, which is a major risk factor for gallstones.

Aged cheese, commercial yogurt, and highly processed and refined foods create an imbalanced constitution of bile. Moreover, try to avoid fried and deep-fried foods. Consuming the heated oils (packed with harmful trans fatty acids) used by fast food restaurants is an especially quick way to produce gallstones.

You can greatly reduce the risk of developing gallstones by adding more vegetables, salads, fruits, legumes, nuts, seeds and complex carbohydrates to your diet. Drinking 2 to 3 oz. fresh carrot juice daily or once every few days just before the lunch meal prevents stones from being formed.

For complete guidelines on how to eat a healthy, life-sustaining diet according to your body type, see my book *Timeless Secrets of Health and Rejuvenation*.

12. Avoid 'Light Food' Products

Several scientific studies show that eating *light foods* actually encourages appetite and overeating, and does not reduce weight. Before they were introduced into the human food chain, light foods were fed to animals that subsequently began to gain weight faster than normal. The same happened in humans when they started eating these unnatural foods on a regular basis.

The Director of the Framingham Study[220], William Castelli, M.D., published a study about this astonishing discovery in the July 1992 issue of the *Archives of Internal Medicine*: "At Framingham, we found that the people who ate the most saturated fat, the most cholesterol and the most calories weighed the least, were more physically active, and had the lowest serum cholesterol levels."

The more *enzymatic energy* that is contained in food, the faster we feel satisfied, and the more efficiently the food is converted into usable energy and bioavailable nutrients. In contrast, eating low-calorie light foods impairs bile secretion, digestion, and excretory functions. Elevated levels of blood fat indicate that bile secretions are low, blood vessel walls are thickening, and fats are not being adequately digested and absorbed. Hence, a person with high blood fats actually suffers from a fat deficiency. In direct response to an increased demand for fats in the cells and tissues of the body, a low-fat diet may actually raise cholesterol production in the liver. The side effects of this survival maneuver by the body include the development of gallstones, weight gain, and/or wasting.

Low-fat and other low-calorie diets are damaging to one's health and should be prescribed only, if at all, in acute liver and gallbladder disorders where the digestion and absorption of fat are severely disrupted.

After all gallstones are removed and liver functions are normalized, it is necessary to gradually increase fat and calorie consumption to meet the high-energy demands of the human body. The presence of gallstones in the liver and gallbladder impair the body's ability to properly digest fat and other kinds of high-energy food.

Even minimal consumption of useless light foods interferes with the body's most basic metabolic and hormonal processes if these *foods* are

---

[220]The Framingham study is the longest, most expensive, and largest sample-size heart disease study in history

ingested for a period of several years. This can result in metabolic disorders, such as diabetes, obesity, and cancer.

By eating a diet low in protein, as well as cleansing the liver and gallbladder, normal, balanced fat intake will greatly reduce your risk for developing gallbladder or liver problems, including fatty liver and liver cirrhosis.

13. Eat Unrefined Sea Salt

Refined salt has only few benefits for the body. On the contrary, it is responsible for causing numerous health problems, including gallstones. The only salt that the body can digest, assimilate, and utilize properly is unrefined, unprocessed sea salt or rock salt. For salt to be useful to the body, it needs to penetrate foods - that is, the moisture of the vegetables, grains, and legumes must be allowed to dissolve the salt. If salt is used in its dry state, it enters the body in a non-ionized form and creates thirst, which is a sign of being poisoned (see *Hidden Risks of Refined Salt*, Chapter 3).

You may dissolve a pinch of salt in a small amount of water and add that to foods that are not usually cooked. This will aid in the digestion of those items while helping to deacidify the body. Adding a pinch of salt to drinking water generates alkaline properties and provides you with important minerals and trace elements.

It may be worth mentioning that food should taste delicious, but not salty, in and of itself. Pitta and Kapha body types require less salt than the Vata body type[221].

Important Functions of Real Salt in the Body:

- Stabilizes irregular heartbeat and regulates blood pressure - in conjunction with water
- Extracts excess acidity from the cells in the body, particularly the brain cells
- Balances sugar levels in the blood, which is particularly important for diabetics

---

[221] To determine your Ayurvedic body type, refer to my book *Timeless Secrets of Health and Rejuvenation*

- Is essential for the generation of hydroelectric energy in the cells of the body
- Is vital for the absorption of nutrient components through the intestinal tract
- Is needed to clear the lungs of mucus and sticky phlegm, particularly in those suffering from asthma and cystic fibrosis
- Clears up catarrh and congestion in the sinuses
- Is a strong natural antihistamine
- Can prevent muscle cramps
- Helps prevent excess saliva production; saliva that is flowing out of the mouth during sleep may indicate salt deficiency
- Makes bones firm; 27 percent of the body's salt content is located in the bones; salt deficiency and/or eating refined salt versus real salt are major causes of osteoporosis
- Regulates sleep; acts as a natural hypnotic
- Helps prevent gout and gouty arthritis
- Is vital for maintaining sexuality and libido
- Can prevent varicose veins and spider veins on the legs and thighs
- Supplies the body with over 80 essential mineral elements; refined salt, such as the common table salt, has been stripped of all but 2 of these elements. In addition, refined, commercial salt contains harmful additives, including aluminum silicate, a primary cause of Alzheimer's disease.

14. The Importance of Ener-Chi Art

Ener-Chi Art is a unique method of rejuvenation that consists of viewing different energized art pictures which I have created to help restore a balanced flow of chi (vital energy) through the organs and systems in the body. The approach can be likened to acupuncture or acupressure, but without the use of needles or pressure. The benefits occur within less than one minute of viewing the corresponding art pictures. I consider this healing approach to be a profound tool in facilitating a more successful outcome to all other natural healing methods.

When chi flows properly through the cells of the body, the cells can more efficiently remove their metabolic waste products, more readily absorb all the oxygen, water, and nutrients they need, and conduct any necessary repair work more swiftly. The body can restore its health and vitality much more easily when there is constant, unrestricted availability of chi.

Although I consider the liver flush to be one of the most effective tools to help the body return to balanced functioning, by itself it may not be able to restore the body's overall vital energy, as a result of many years of congestion and deterioration. Test results have shown that Ener-Chi Art may very well fill this gap.

The picture on the cover of this book is designed to restore chi in the liver and gallbladder, but because it is a digital print, it is not activated or energized. However, activated prints of these pictures are made available through www.ener-chi.com.

The use of Ener-Chi Ionized Stones is another practical and effective tool to improve one's health and vitality (for more information on Ener-Chi Art and Ionized Stones, see Other Books and Products by Andreas Moritz at the end of this book).

15. Get Enough Sleep

Tiredness precedes any type of disease, whether it is cancer, heart disease, or AIDS. Although impaired liver functions, low immunity, and overeating can also cause fatigue, in most cases it results from a lack of quality sleep, i.e. the sleep before midnight.

Some of the most vital processes of purification and rejuvenation in the body are initiated and carried out during the two hours of sleep before midnight. Physiologically, there are two entirely different types of sleep, as verified by brain wave measurements. These are before-midnight sleep and after-midnight sleep.

Sleep that occurs in the 2 hours before midnight includes deep sleep and it is often referred to as beauty sleep. Deep sleep occurs for about one hour and generally lasts from 11:00 p.m. to midnight. During deep sleep, you are in a dreamless state of consciousness where oxygen consumption in the body drops by about 8 percent. The rest and relaxation that you gain during this hour of dreamless sleep is nearly 3 times as deep as you would get from the same amount of sleep after midnight (when oxygen consumption in the body rises again).

Deep sleep hardly ever occurs after midnight. You experience the necessary amount of deep sleep only if you go to sleep at least 2 hours before midnight. If you regularly miss out on deep sleep, your body and mind become overtired and your stress responses become unnaturally high.

Stress responses include secretions of the stress hormones adrenaline, cortisol, and cholesterol (part of the cholesterol secreted during a stress response may end up as gallstones). To keep these artificially derived energy bursts going or depress them, you may feel the urge to use such nerve stimulants as coffee, tea, candy, and sodas, or sedatives like nicotine and alcohol. When the body's energy reserves are finally exhausted, chronic fatigue results.

When you feel tired, all of your body's cells are tired, not just your mind. In fact, your organs, digestive system, nervous system, and the like, will also suffer from a lack of energy and will not be able to function properly. When you are tired, your brain no longer receives adequate amounts of water, glucose, oxygen, and amino acids, which make up its main food supply. This situation can lead to a whole slew of problems in your mind, body, and behavior.

Doctors at the University of California in San Diego have found that losing a few hours of sleep not only makes you feel tired the next day, but can also affect the immune system, possibly impairing the body's ability to fight infection. Since immunity diminishes with increasing fatigue, your body is unable to defend itself against bacteria, microbes, and viruses, and cannot cope with the buildup of toxic substances in the body. Getting enough sleep, therefore, is the most important prerequisite for restoring health to the body and mind.

Try to go to sleep before 10:00 p.m. and rise between 6:00 and 7:00 a.m., or earlier, depending on your sleep requirements. It is best not to use an alarm clock, to allow for a natural phasing out of your sleeping cycles. Removing all gallstones from the liver and gallbladder and getting enough sleep will reduce any tiredness that you may be experiencing during the day. If this problem continues, you may also need to cleanse your kidneys (to dissolve kidney stones, see *Keep Your Kidneys Clean* in Chapter 5).

16. Avoid Overworking

Working too hard for too many hours overtaxes the body's energy system. Overworking particularly stresses the liver. To meet the excessive demand for energy in the brain or in other parts of the body, the liver tries to convert as much complex sugars into simple sugars (glucose) as possible. If a shortfall of energy occurs, or if energy supplies run out altogether, the body must take recourse to an emergency stress response, which makes extra energy available, but at the same time disrupts circulatory and immune functions.

The continuous secretion of adrenaline and other stress hormones that occur in a person who never stops working can eventually turn him or her into a workaholic. This is a condition in which work becomes the major source of excitement in that person's life. The excitement is provided by the thrill effect brought about by the stress hormones.

To avoid exhausting your liver and damaging your immune system, make enough time for yourself. Try to allocate at least one hour each day for meditation, yoga, exercise, listening to music, artistic activities, or being outdoors enjoying nature. The body is not a machine that can run continuously without a break.

Overworking the body and mind in any way will eventually demand extra recovery time from an illness. In the long run, overworking as a means to get things done faster, or to earn money more quickly, not only cuts years off one's life but also cuts life off one's years, as the old saying goes.

The liver is designed to provide energy for about 100 years, according to research done on aging; overextending this *service* damages or destroys the liver prematurely. Living by a code of moderation with regard to eating, sleeping, and working will enable you to maintain an efficient and vital energy system throughout life.

Another good old saying recommends that we spend one-third of our life sleeping, one-third working, and one-third enjoying recreational pursuits. This wise formula maintains balance on all levels of life: physical, mental, and spiritual. Overworking upsets this much-needed state of equilibrium among our body, mind, and spirit.

17. Exercise Regularly

Our technological and economic advancement has led to an increasingly sedentary lifestyle, which requires additional forms of physical movement to keep our bodies vital and healthy. Regular exercise helps to increase our capacity to digest food, eliminate physical impurities, balance our emotions, promote firmness and suppleness, and strengthen our ability to deal with stressful situations.

When performed in moderation, exercise serves as a great immune stimulant and improves neuromuscular integration in all age groups. Boosting self-confidence and self-esteem are important by-products of exercise that stem from an improved oxygen supply to the cells - not to mention the improvement in self-esteem that comes from losing excess fat, seeing muscle definition, feeling stronger, and generally looking great and vibrant. All this results in greater well-being - physically, mentally and emotionally.

The liver, especially, seems to benefit from aerobic exercise. The increased availability of oxygen during and after exercise greatly improves circulation and enhances the flow of venous blood from the liver toward the heart. A sedentary lifestyle slows this process, causing blood flow in the liver to stagnate. This, in turn, leads to the development of gallstones. For that reason, regular, non-strenuous exercise can prevent new stones from forming.

By contrast, the physical exertion that results from over exercising leads to the secretion of excessive amounts of stress hormones, leaving the body restless and shaky. When the body is depleted of energy, it is unable to do the repair work that arises from a strenuous workout. Thus, the cardiovascular system is left weak and vulnerable to other stress factors as well.

Overexertion can also have a detrimental effect on the thymus gland. This gland, which activates lymphocytes (immune cells that defend us against disease) and controls energy supplies, may actually shrink in size, causing the body to become agitated and vulnerable to all kinds of health problems.

In light of this fact, it is best to choose a form of exercise that gives you a sense of joy and satisfaction. Whenever you exercise, make certain that you always breathe through your nose and keep your mouth closed, in order to avoid the harmful adrenaline breathing. (Rapid mouth breathing usually occurs during a typical fight-or-flight response and can trigger the release of stress hormones; it can do the same even without a stress response) Aerobic exercises are effective and beneficial as long as you maintain nasal breathing (versus mouth breathing).

Typically, it takes about one minute of vigorous exercising to get you to the point of very rapid breathing where you can no longer breathe through your nose without becoming lightheaded. If you run out of breath, slow down or stop exercising. You may resume the exercise once your breathing returns to normal.

By repeating this cycle from as few as 3 to as many as 8 times, you will have practiced what is known as interval training - a safe, effective method of exercising that helps your muscles to become stronger and your weight to normalize for hours and days after the exercise.

This simple advice can also prevent you from potential harm, such as exhaustion or the production of too much lactic acid that can easily occur from over exercising.

Considering how crucial exercise is for a healthy body and mind, try to exercise every day or every other day, even if it is only for 10 minutes. It is important, though, not to exceed 50 percent of your capacity for exercise. The main thing is to avoid becoming fatigued. For example, if you can swim for 30 minutes before getting tired, swim for only 15 minutes. In time, your capacity for exercise will increase.

I have done interval training, yoga, stretching and some weight-lifting exercises now for over 40 years, but about 4 years ago I added a whole body vibration exerciser to my exercising tools and I am as excited about it now as I have been when I first tried it. It is by far the best exercising equipment I have ever used. In just 10 minutes, this vibration exerciser quickly contracts and relaxes all the small and large muscles, organs and systems in your body, including the circulatory and lymphatic systems. It's like having a strenuous whole body workout, but without losing any energy at all. The exercise is actually extremely relaxing and rejuvenating.

Just a few minutes of use each day can help you achieve:

- Weight loss through decreased serum cortisol (stress hormone) and stepped-up fat burning
- Core muscle strengthening and conditioning

- Body reshaping through muscle toning
- Enhanced bone density and bone building
- Improved lymphatic drainage
- Reduced pain caused by muscle strain or osteoarthritis
- Improved mobility (ideal for elderly or rehabilitation patients)
- Improved posture and balance
- Anti-aging benefits: increased production of growth hormones up to 361%

Remember, both excessive exercise and a lack of it weaken the immune system, impair liver functions, and flood the blood with harmful substances.

18. Get Regular Sun Exposure

- The Importance of Vitamin D

Your body is capable of synthesizing vitamin D (which is actually a steroid hormone) through a process whereby the sun's ultraviolet rays interact with a form of cholesterol present in the skin, known as cholesterol sulfate. With regular sun exposure, the skin produces a large amount of cholesterol sulfate in order to protect it against microbial invasion, dehydration, and rapid aging.

Sulfur is a powerful protective agent against UV radiation and radiation damage in general. Together with melanin, produced by skin cells, cholesterol sulfate effectively prevents skin cell damage and skin cancers. This protection is lost when the skin rarely becomes exposed to the sun, hence the well-documented high risk of developing skin cancers among people who spend most of their time indoors or who use protective sun screens. Their skin is often extremely deficient in cholesterol sulfate and highly dehydrated, and therefore burns very quickly when suddenly overexposed to the sun.

Cholesterol sulfate also enters the blood, making it available for all the hundreds and thousands of biochemical processes and functions it is responsible for. In its sulfated form, cholesterol is water soluble and flows freely in the blood, and unlike other forms of cholesterol, it does not require a protein to transport it around the blood.

The sulfur in cholesterol sulfate is extremely important for any repair and healing in the body, including damaged genes. As discovered recently, sulfur holds the key in healing genetic diseases. In particular, the sulfur-containing part of plant cells in broccoli has been demonstrated to be an indirect antioxidant.

According to a 2012 review report published in *Frontiers in Genetics*, the compound sulforaphane[222], found in cruciferous vegetables such as broccoli, cabbage, cauliflower, and leafy green vegetables, has an astonishing ability to get certain enzymes to activate the detoxification and antioxidant process. This healing effect, right down to the genetic level, which has been observed over the past 10 years in humans, has now been attributed to sulfur. Not making enough cholesterol sulfate, may therefore explain why the incidence of degenerative diseases and genetic damage is so high among people who are not regularly exposing their skin to the sun and are therefore deficient in sulfated vitamin D. This includes multiple sclerosis, heart failure, and Alzheimer's disease.

Regular exposure to sunlight has been shown to balance cholesterol levels by decreasing LDL (*bad* cholesterol) and increasing HDL (*good* cholesterol)[223] concentrations. However, unlike cholesterol-lowering drugs (statins), sunlight does not increase cholesterol in the bile. Statins are a major cause of gallstones and liver damage because they force the liver to raise LDL levels in bile. Besides liver damage, statins also cause diabetes and diabetes-related diseases, according to an analysis of 72 trials which together involved close to 160,000 patients[224].

In contrast, sunlight has a holistic effect, which means that all functions in the body benefit at the same time. Ultraviolet light has been proven to lower blood pressure, facilitate cardiac output, increase glycogen (complex sugar) stores in the liver, balance blood sugar, improve the body's resistance to infections (as shown by an increase in the number of lymphocytes and phagocytes), enhance the oxygen-carrying capacity of the blood, and increase the production of sex hormones, among many other health benefits. In fact, women who unsuccessfully tried all available methods to become pregnant succeeded once their vitamin D levels normalized.

---

[222]Sulphate heals genetic diseases, Front Genet. 2012; 3:7. Epub 2012 Jan 24
[223] HDL cholesterol is exactly the same as the cholesterol in LDL particles; the only difference between the two lies in the size and density of the proteins that carry the cholesterol (to and away from the liver). Both are essential for the body.
[224]Adverse Events Associated with Individual Statin Treatments for Cardiovascular Disease: An Indirect Comparison Meta-Analysis, QJM, February 2012: 105(2); 145-57, M. Alberton, et al.

Research from 100 countries proves that sunlight strongly protects against cancer, according to a 2012 paper published in the journal *Anticancer Research*[225]. Researchers found that sunlight can prevent at least 15, and probably closer to 24, different types of cancer.

This review consistently found strong inverse correlations with solar UV B for 15 types of cancer: bladder, breast, cervical, colon, endometrial, esophageal, gastric, lung, ovarian, pancreatic, rectal, renal, and vulvar cancer; and Hodgkin's and non-Hodgkin's lymphoma, according the study abstract. Somewhat weaker evidence exists for 9 other types of cancer: brain, gallbladder, laryngeal, oral/pharyngeal, prostate and thyroid cancer; leukemia; melanoma; and multiple myeloma.

The study concluded: "Evidence for the UV B-Vitamin D-cancer hypothesis is very strong in general and for many types of cancers in particular." Now that we know Vitamin D to be essential for maintaining normal DNA health and cell functions, depleting it by not spending enough time in the sun can have devastating consequences, such as heart failure, arthritis, cancer, multiple sclerosis, diabetes, and Alzheimer's' disease.

Most people don't realize that, just like most other animals, the human body was designed to live outdoors, not indoors. We were meant to only spend the nighttime under a protective shelter and then be out and about to search for foods for our sustenance. Yet, the modern lifestyle and educational system forces us to do the exact opposite to what keeps us healthy.

The majority of people living in modern, fast-paced societies is now vitamin D deficient and suffers from the potentially deadly illnesses this directly contributes to, including obesity and obesity-associated conditions. In a study published in the *Journal of Clinical Endocrinology and Metabolism*, April 2010, a team of researchers found that young women with insufficient levels of vitamin D living in southern California were significantly heavier and had greater body mass than their counterparts with sufficient levels of vitamin D[226]. According to lead author, Dr. Vicente Gilsanz, of Children's Hospital Los Angeles, obesity is influenced by vitamin D insufficiency. "We found that vitamin D

[225]Ecological Studies of the UVB-Vitamin D-Cancer Hypothesis. Anticancer Res. 2012 Jan;32(1):223-36
[226]Vitamin D Status and Its Relation to Muscle Mass and Muscle Fat in Young Women, The Journal of Clinical Endocrinology & Metabolism, *April 1, 2010 vol. 95 no. 4 1595-1601*

insufficiency is associated with increased fat infiltration in muscle in healthy young women," says the study conclusion. Vitamin D insufficiency is now very common in young women living even in sun-rich areas of the United States.

For reasons I have explained in my book *Heal Yourself with Sunlight*, sun exposure may be harmful for those who use sunglasses and sunscreens. Blocking out UV B rays, by whatever means, effectively blocks vitamin D production in the body and suppresses the immune system. Since vitamin D also regulates thousands of genes in the body, an insufficiency or deficiency can generate massive metabolic chaos that affects the functions of all its organs and systems. Having fat invade muscle tissue is a very serious condition that shows the body is fundamentally dysfunctional.

Thankfully, the medical community is increasingly becoming aware that Vitamin D deficiency is one of the most common causes of disease, including skin cancers and other cancers, diabetes, osteoporosis, brain diseases like Alzheimer's disease, Parkinson's disease, autism, and even coronary artery disease.

In fact, the researchers of a recent study, titled "Vitamin D Deficiency And Supplementation & Relation To Cardiovascular Health," boldly stated in the abstract: "Recent evidence supports an association between vitamin D deficiency and hypertension, peripheral vascular disease, diabetes mellitus, metabolic syndrome, coronary artery disease, and heart failure." Blood vessel damage alone can be responsible for hundreds of different disease conditions. The research, published in the *American Journal of Cardiology* in February 2012[227], found that vitamin D deficiency was associated with a 3 times increased risk of cardiovascular disease and survival. In other words, vitamin D deficient people are 3 times more likely to die than people with normal vitamin D levels.

In my book *Heart Disease No More*, I make the point that coronary heart disease cannot be considered a disease, but must be seen as a protective healing mechanism that uses cholesterol to help prevent both a heart attack and heart failure. This healing attempt, which is characterized by cholesterol patches being formed alongside damaged parts of an artery, is undermined by the use of cholesterol-lowering drugs like statins.

---

[227] American Journal of Cardiology Volume 109, Issue 3 , Pages 359-363, 1 February 2012, doi:10.1016/j.amjcard.2011.09.020

I have already documented the research that shows how statin drugs contribute to heart disease (see Chapter 3). Dr. Stephanie Seneff, a senior scientist at MIT and author of hundreds of papers published in the peer-reviewed scientific literature, now sheds further light on the true mechanism of coronary heart disease - the healing mechanism.

Dr. Seneff's research shows that the buildup of plaque in cardiovascular disease is also your body's way to compensate for not having enough cholesterol sulfate, normally produced in large amounts when your skin is exposed to sunshine.

Lack of sun exposure causes a drop in your cholesterol sulfate levels and forces your body to employ another mechanism to increase it. Dr. Seneff explains[228].

"The macrophages in the plaque take up LDL, the small dense LDL particles that have been damaged by sugar... the liver cannot take them back because the receptor can't receive them, because they are gummed with sugar basically. So they're stuck floating in your body... Those macrophages in the plaque do a heroic job in taking that gummed up LDL out of the blood circulation, carefully extracting the cholesterol from it to save it - the cholesterol is important - and then exporting the cholesterol into HDL - HDL A1 in particular... That's the good guy, HDL. The platelets in the plaque take in HDL A1 cholesterol and they won't take anything else... They take in sulfate, and they produce cholesterol sulfate in the plaque. The sulfate actually comes from homocysteine. Elevated homocysteine is another risk factor for heart disease. Homocysteine is a source of sulfate. It also involves hemoglobin. You have to consume energy to produce a sulfate from homocysteine, and the red blood cells actually supply the ATP to the plaque. So everything is there and the intent is to produce cholesterol sulfate, and it's done in the arteries feeding the heart, because it's the heart that needs the cholesterol sulfate. If (cholesterol sulfate is not produced) ...you end up with heart failure."

The solution to this problem is to get appropriate amounts of sunlight exposure on your skin. Dr. Seneff explains: "In this way, your skin will produce cholesterol sulfate, which will then flow freely through the blood - not packaged up inside LDL - and therefore your liver doesn't have to make so much LDL. So the LDL goes down. In fact... there is a complete

---

[228]Could THIS Be the Hidden Factor Behind Obesity, Heart Disease, and Chronic Fatigue? September 17 2011 www.articles.mercola.com

inverse relationship between sunlight and cardiovascular disease - the more sunlight, the less cardiovascular disease."

Of course, this also means that by using a statin drug to artificially lower your cholesterol, you effectively block the body's back-up plan to create the cholesterol sulfate your heart needs in order to function and survive. It's hardly surprising to find that the incidence of heart failure doubled in the first decade when statin drugs were on the market, from 1980 to 1990. Is it a mere coincidence that the rate of heart failure continues to rise with the increased use of statins? "It is very clear to me that statins are causing heart failure," Dr. Seneff says.

Dr. Seneff also published a paper that discloses the detrimental impact of low cholesterol and statin drugs on Alzheimer's disease, and I am in complete agreement with her on that.

That said, sunlight exposure can be risky for those living on a diet rich in highly processed, acid-forming foods and refined fats/oils or the products that contain them. In addition, excessive alcohol consumption, cigarettes, and other mineral- and vitamin-depleting substances, such as prescription medicines and hallucinogenic drugs, can make the skin vulnerable to ultraviolet radiation. After you have cleared your liver and gallbladder from all gallstones, and balanced your diet and lifestyle, regular and moderate sun exposure will cause you no harm; in fact, as shown above, it is essential for good health.

Over 42 percent of Americans suffer from vitamin D deficiency, and 47 percent of pregnant women are severely deficient in this important hormone. Their children tend to have weak bones that break easily, even during their childhood years.

You cannot stop a vitamin D deficiency in the long-term by taking supplements. Whereas too much supplemental vitamin D can actually be life-endangering, taking it ongoing in small dosages can suppress the immune system. Sunlight or use of a UV lamp/vitamin D lamp, on the other hand, is the only real, alternative remedy.

To make sufficient amounts of vitamin D, dark-skinned people need to spend at least two to three times longer in the sun than do Caucasians. Their skin absorbs sun rays less efficiently, hence their need for extended sun exposure. Not being exposed to enough sunlight puts African-American men, for example, at a much higher risk of developing cancer of the prostate than white Americans. The use of sunscreens, including sunglasses, multiplies this risk.

The best way to obtain enough sulfated vitamin D is to expose your skin to the sun between 10:00 a.m. and 3:00 p.m., depending on the time of year and where you live. This is a simple test to determine whether you can make vitamin D from the available sunlight or not. If the shadow your body casts on the ground while standing in direct sunlight is longer than your body height, you are not making vitamin D. This is more likely to happen during the winter, spring, and fall seasons, especially for those living at higher latitudes. So make sure your shadow is at least half the length of your body, or use a UV lamp instead.

For maximum benefits, it is best to take a shower before sunbathing. Contrary to common belief, it is important to avoid sunscreens. Not only do sunscreens fail to prevent cancer, but they can actually *cause* it. Sunscreens successfully cancel out the sun's positive effects and your body quickly absorbs the numerous carcinogenic chemicals they contain[229].

Start your sunlight treatment by exposing your entire body (if possible) to direct sunlight for a few minutes, and then increase your exposure time by a few more minutes each day until you reach 20 to 30 minutes. Alternatively, walking in the sun for an hour, with as much exposed skin as possible, has similar benefits. This will give you enough sunlight to produce sufficient amounts of vitamin D and to keep your body and mind healthy (provided you also incorporate the basic aspects of a balanced diet and lifestyle).

The body can store enough vitamin D during the sunny days of the year to last you through a good part of the winter season, but probably not enough to prevent a cold or the flu in springtime. A winter vacation in a warm and sunny location would be ideal to replenish vitamin D stores. Using a tanning bed that uses electronic ballasts instead of magnetic ballasts is ideal. Many commercial tanning beds use magnetic ballasts to generate the UV light, and these produce harmful electromagnetic fields (EMFs). Most of the newer UV tanning beds and standing lights now come with electronic ballasts. Small UV lamps that use electrical ballasts are fine, too. If you hear a loud buzzing noise while in a tanning bed, it is because it has a magnetic ballast system. These alternatives can replenish your vitamin D reserves enough to get you safely through this more or less sunshine scarce part of the year.

---

[229] To learn more about the beneficial effects of sunlight and the harmful effects of sunscreens, see my books *Heal Yourself with Sunlight* and *Timeless Secrets of Health and Rejuvenation*

Please take notice that a tan does not equate with skin damage, as it is often claimed by those who blame the sun for skin cancer. Tanning is your body's natural protection against sunburn; that's why, for example, we have melanin-producing cells. We were born with built-in mechanisms to produce our own natural sunscreen.

Of course, the use of UV-blocking sunscreens nullifies any benefits you may obtain from sun exposure.

Important note about vitamin D supplements:

Before you decide to take a vitamin D supplement, please be aware of the following points:

1. Synthetic Vitamin D_2, which is the form typically prescribed by doctors to treat vitamin D deficiency, has been shown to not only fail to lower mortality, but actually increase it. This was discovered during a 2011 meta-analysis of 50 clinical trials by the *Cochrane Database* that included a total of 94,000 participants[230]. The analysis shows that participants using synthetic vitamin D_2 experienced a 2 percent relative risk increase, while those taking the natural vitamin D_3 decreased their relative risk by 7 percent.

All synthetic drugs, including vitamin D_2, manipulate and weaken the immune system and it is always wise for patients to do their own homework before taking any prescription medication. Don't take your doctor's word for granted. Medical doctors rarely get their information from medical journals, but rather from pharmaceutical companies whose main objective is to sell drugs, regardless whether they do you any good or not. Synthetic vitamin D certainly doesn't.

2. Unlike the form of vitamin D_3 that the skin produces in response to sun exposure, vitamin D_3 supplements do not contain cholesterol sulfate. According to research published in 2003 in the Journal of Lipid Research[231], "cholesterol sulfate is quantitatively the most important known sterol sulfate in human plasma, where it is present in a concentration that overlaps that of the other abundant circulating steroid

---

[230]1. Vitamin D Supplementation for Prevention of Mortality in Adults, The Cochrane Database of Systematic Reviews, July 6, 2011: (7); CD007470, G. Bjelakovic, et al.

2. Meta-analysis Looks at Efficacy of D_2 vs D_3, Vitamin D Council, November 16, 2011: Dr. John Cannell

3. Vitamin D_3 Is More Potent Than Vitamin D_2 in Humans, The Journal of Clinical Endocrinology and Metabolism, March 1, 2011: 96 (3); E447-E452, Robert P. Heaney, et al.

[231]Cholesterol Sulfate in Human Physiology, JLR Papers in Press, May 14, 2003. DOI 10.1194/jlr.R300005-JLR200

sulfate, dehydroepiandrosterone (DHEA) sulfate." Cholesterol sulfate is an important regulatory molecule and component of cell membranes, without which cells could not survive or divide. In platelet membranes cholesterol sulfate supports platelet adhesion, essential for healthy blood flow and proper blood clotting.

Without enough cholesterol sulfate, the body can cause almost every kind of illness that exists. The supplemental form of vitamin D_3 may therefore fail to protect you against heart failure, heart attack, stroke, brain damage, or other illnesses that often result from a deficiency of sulfated vitamin D which only the skin can form from sun exposure. In my view, it is a very irresponsible practice by medical and alternative health practitioners alike, to recommend a vitamin D supplement without also informing their patients that it cannot serve as a substitute for sulfated vitamin D.

3. Unless you have your blood examined while taking vitamin D_3 on a regular basis, it is important to understand the potential risks. When ingested in excess, vitamin D has shown to cause liver damage and death (see other side effects listed below). Nature has purposefully avoided providing unprocessed foods with vitamin D in order to avoid toxicity; even human mother's milk is extremely low in vitamin D. The reason for this is that nature meant for us to make our own vitamin D by exposing ourselves to the sun, not by adding it to processed cow's milk or going on a salmon hunt (both of which contain vitamin D). If the billions of people on this Earth depended on drinking cow's milk and eating salmon, most of the worlds' population wouldn't even exist today.

While there is no doubt that the use of vitamin D supplements can lead to significant improvements of numerous health conditions, including a reduced risk of developing osteomalacia, rickets, osteoporosis, certain cancers, immune deficiency, and multiple sclerosis, there is no reliable way of testing how well a person can actually digest and metabolize this form of vitamin D.

Because vitamin D is a fat-soluble vitamin, it requires sufficient bile to digest and absorb it. Congestion in the liver bile ducts may make vitamin D supplementation useless. That's why even the beneficial vitamin D_3, regardless of the dosage taken, has shown no benefits at all in so many people who take it every day. Of course, if produced by the skin in response to sunlight, vitamin D_3 doesn't require the digestive process to make it available to the blood.

As always, it is important to understand that the vanishing of one health condition can easily lead to another condition that is equally serious. Just adding to the body one or two elements that are lacking is rarely a good strategy, not much different than what the magic bullets used by our symptom-squashing modern medicine is known for. The body is far too complex and holistic in its makeup and intricacies for these rather simplistic approaches to offer anything better than relief. As always, without addressing the underlying cause of an imbalance, the body cannot truly regain its balance, just the appearance of it.

I have seen numerous cases of diseases where the successful removal of a symptom of the disease, such as a cancerous tumor, led to a fatal heart attack or stroke. The recognition that disease symptoms form an integral part of the body's intricate healing mechanisms, the successful removal of these symptoms may not be in the body's best interest. In fact, as in the case of cancer, if achieved through sudden, drastic measures like chemotherapy and radiation, tumor regression can overwhelm the body with a flood of toxins and billions of corpses of cancer cells which can lead to severe congestion and the development of tumors elsewhere, or quickly overwhelm the heart and shut it down.

There is always a certain risk involved by giving steroids like vitamin D to the body. Steroidal drugs were once hailed as miracle drugs because of the amazing benefits they seemed to produce. Now that we know more about how they actually work and the long-term, serious harm they can cause, their benefits have become questionable. Replacing one serious disease with another cannot be counted as a medical achievement. Like they say, the operation was a success, but the patient died.

When taken in excess, vitamin D supplements have been shown to cause nausea, vomiting, poor appetite, weakness, and weight loss. Supplemental vitamin D can also raise blood levels of calcium, called hypercalcemia, thereby altering mental states and causing confusion. Hypercalcemia can cause abnormal heart rhythm. Calcinosis, which is characterized by a buildup of calcium and phosphate in soft tissues, also results from excessive vitamin D intake. When nutrition guru Gary Null overdosed on vitamin D by taking his own product, 'Ultimate Power Meal', he suffered "excruciating fatigue along with bodily pain," and "began to suffer from extreme cracks and bleeding from within his feet," according to an article in the New York Post (updated Feb 24, 2012). It took Null three months to recover, but he continues to occasionally urinate blood.

Taking too much vitamin D and calcium can lead to an increase in total brain lesion volume. According to Dr. Martha E. Payne of Duke University, Durham, North Carolina, taking these two supplements can increase uptake of calcium into the blood vessel walls, leading to vascular calcification. Dr. Martha E. Payne examined calcium and vitamin D intakes by using food frequency questionnaires and MRI scans of 232 elderly men and women (average age: 71 years). Although all of the subjects displayed some brain lesions of varying sizes, those reporting the highest intakes of calcium and vitamin D were also the most likely to have higher total volume of brain lesions. Dr. Payne reported the study findings at a meeting of the American Society for Nutrition, part of Experimental Biology in May, 2007, in Washington, DC.

To reemphasize, while short-term improvements are common when taking large doses of vitamin D supplements, it is possible to overdose on these supplements especially when your vitamin A (not beta carotene) and vitamin K_2 are not properly balanced. How many people are aware of their vitamins A and K blood levels? In any case, hypercalcemia (high blood calcium) is rarely noticed by patients until it is too late and they have already accumulated large deposits of calcium in their heart, lungs, or kidneys. The damage to these organs can be permanent if your vitamin D levels remain elevated for too long. Sunshine-derived vitamin D, on the other hand, can never do that, even if you spend 8 hours a day in the sun for the rest of your life.

19. Take Liver Herbs

A number of herbs can further improve the performance of the liver and keep this crucial organ nourished and vital. They can be made into a concoction and are best taken as a tea for 7-10 days during each change of season or during times of acute illness. Although many herbs will help liver function and assist in maintaining clean blood, the following are among the most important ones:

Dandelion root	(1 oz. or 28 g)
Comfrey root	(½ oz. or 14 g)*1
Licorice root	(1 oz. or 28 g)
Agrimony	(1 oz. or 28 g)
Wild yam root	(1 oz. or 28 g)
Barberry bark	(1 oz. or 28 g)
Bearsfoot	(1 oz. or 28 g)
Tanners oak bark	(1 oz. or 28 g)
Milk thistle herb	(1 oz. or 28 g)

Note*1. Contrary to the opinion of some natural health practitioners, I have never seen any evidence of comfrey's supposed harmful side effects, only benefits, especially for the liver. For a more detailed explanation, see *What about the claimed 'toxic effects' of Comfrey Root?* in this chapter.

2. For botanical names, see Product Information

For maximum effectiveness, it is best to use all these herbs, in combination, if possible. To do this, mix them together in equal parts (except for comfrey root at half the amount), and add 2 tablespoons of this mixture to about 24 oz. (700 ml) of water. Let it stand for 6 hours or overnight; then bring the mixture to a boil, letting it simmer for 5 to 10 minutes before straining it. If you forget to prepare this tea the night before, bring the mixture to a boil in the morning, let it simmer as indicated above, and strain it. Drink 2 cups of this *herbal tea* per day on an empty stomach, if possible. This tea can be taken ongoing or when you feel your liver is sluggish. Those who cannot do liver flushes for some reason may greatly benefit from it, too.

Taken on its own, tea made from the bark of the red lapacho tree, also known as Pau d'Arco, Ipe Roxa, or Taheebo, has been shown to have excellent effects on the liver and the immune system as well.

20. Daily Oil Swishing or Oil Pulling Therapy

Oil therapy is a simple, yet astoundingly effective, method of cleansing the blood. It is effective for numerous disorders, including blood diseases, lung and liver disorders, tooth and gum diseases, headaches, skin diseases, gastric ulcers, intestinal problems, poor appetite, heart and kidney ailments, encephalitis, nervous conditions, poor memory, female disorders, swollen face, and bags under the eyes. The therapy consists of swishing oil in the mouth.

To apply this therapy you need cold-pressed, unrefined sunflower, sesame, or olive oil. In the morning, preferably after awakening or anytime before breakfast, put 1 tablespoon of oil in your mouth, but do not swallow it. Slowly swish the oil in your mouth, chew it, and draw it through your teeth for 3 to 4 minutes. This action thoroughly mixes the oil with saliva and activates the released enzymes. The enzymes draw toxins out of the blood. For this reason, it is important to spit out the oil after no more than 3 to 4 minutes. You do not want any of the released toxins to be reabsorbed. You will find that the oil takes on a milky white or yellowish color as it becomes saturated with germs and toxins.

For best results, repeat this process two more times. Then rinse out your mouth with ½ teaspoon of baking soda, or ½ teaspoon of unrefined sea salt (take either of these dissolved in a small amount of water). This solution will remove all remnants of the oil and toxins. Additionally, you may want to brush your teeth to make sure your mouth is clean. Tongue scraping is also advised.

Some of the visible effects of oil swishing include the elimination of gum bleeding and the whitening of teeth. During times of illness, this procedure can be repeated 3 times a day, but only on an empty stomach. Oil therapy greatly relieves and supports liver functions, as it takes toxins out of the blood that the liver has not been able to remove or detoxify. This benefits the entire organism. If you feel discomfort, do this only once a day.

Some practitioners recommend oil swishing for a duration of 10-15 minutes, but I found that doing it longer than 3-4 minutes at a time does not offer any additional benefits, such as drawing out more toxins.

21. Replace All Metal Tooth Fillings

Metal dental ware is a constant source of poisoning and, possibly, allergic reaction in the body. All metal corrodes in time, especially in the mouth where high concentrations of air and moisture are always present. Mercury amalgam fillings release their extremely toxic compounds and vapor into the body, a reason why German dentists are prohibited by law from giving them to pregnant women. This product has been banned in a number of European countries.

If mercury is considered dangerous for a mother and a fetus, it must be considered dangerous for everyone. The liver and kidneys, in particular, which have to deal with noxious substances, such as those released by metal fillings, become gradually poisoned. Cadmium, for example, which is used to make the pink color in dentures, is 5 times as toxic as lead. It does not take much of it to raise one's blood pressure to abnormal levels.

Thallium, which is also found in mercury amalgam fillings, causes leg pain and paraplegia. It affects the skin and the nervous and cardiovascular systems. All wheelchair patients who have been tested for metal poisoning tested positive for thallium. Many people who were in a wheelchair several years after they received metal fillings, completely recovered after all metal was removed from their mouths. Thallium is lethal at a dose of 0.5 to 1.0 gram.

Other elements contained in metal fillings are known for their cancer-producing (carcinogenic) effects. These include nickel, (which is used in gold crowns, braces, and children's crowns), and chromium. All metals corrode (including gold, silver, and platinum), and the body absorbs them. Women with breast cancer have often accumulated large amounts of dissolved metals in their breasts. Once the mouth is cleared of all metals, they will also leave the breasts. Likewise, cysts in the breasts and ovaries, which the body creates to store toxic, corrosive metals, will shrink and disappear by themselves.

The body's immune system naturally responds to the presence of toxic metals in the body and, eventually, develops allergic reactions. These allergies may show up as a sinus condition, tinnitus, enlarged neck and glands, bloating, enlarged spleen, arthritic conditions, headaches and migraines, eye diseases, and even more serious complications, such as paralysis or heart attacks.

One obvious way to improve such conditions of metal toxicity is to replace all metal fillings with composite fillings that contain *no* metals[232]. If you need major dental work, such as a crown, bridge, or implant, it is best to seek an alternative dentist who uses the least-harmful dental procedures available. Avoid having titanium implants and chose Zirconium implants instead; they are far superior and non-toxic.

Additionally, cleanse the liver and kidneys, and drink tea made from liver herbs (see above recipe) for 10 days after replacing a filling.

22. Avoid Root Canals

Those who have read my book *Timeless Secrets of Health and Rejuvenation* know why I have been so strongly warning against root canals for so many years now. In the early 1960s, my mother, an outspoken promoter of naturopathic ideas and treatments, told me that root canals were responsible for kidney disease, heart disease, arthritic conditions, autoimmune disorders, and malignant cancers.

Little did we understand back then why a dead tooth in the mouth could be responsible for killing someone, but the tireless work and research by some very brave dentists and scientists has made it possible for us to understand the mechanisms behind this sinister phenomenon.

They are *brave*, because performing root canals is a flourishing business for the dental industry around the world and speaking out against this procedure is perceived as a threat against one of its main sources of income. Many good dentists have already lost their licenses for exposing the toxicity of mercury in amalgam fillings. It infuriates the American Dental Association (ADA) when dentists tell their patients that root canals can be a cause of disease in the body.

For many years now, the ADA has used threats, law suits, and professional humiliation to stop these dentists from standing up for their patients and protecting them from root canal-caused diseases. If the ADA were to admit that root canals are, in fact, responsible for causing degenerative diseases, there would be an endless number of costly lawsuits

---

[232] For details on composite fillings, see my book *Timeless Secrets of Health and Rejuvenation*

that would ruin the entire medical industry. It is obvious that the ADA will fight *tooth and nail* to let this happen.

In 2000, over 30 million root canals were performed on unsuspecting patients in the US, and the number has been increasing ever since. At a cost of at least $750 for a front tooth and $1000 for a molar, root canals earn the industry a staggering $25-40 billion annually.

Most conventional dentists, unlike the biological dentists who are aware of the risks, will tell you that root canals are completely safe. How do they know that? Well, they don't, since a root canal operation is one of the many medical procedures that have never been studied for safety. In fact, there is no data *at all* that substantiates the ADA's claim that root canals are safe. Just because root canals have been performed for more than 100 years doesn't make them safe.

How many cardiologists, oncologists, and neurologists are aware that a dead tooth in their patient's mouth serves as an incubator for anaerobic bacteria that produce some of the most deadly toxins in existence? In 1908, microbiology researchers from Mayo's Clinic and from the dental association at the time discovered that bacteria in dead teeth and the toxins they produce enter the blood stream and travel to any point in the body, thereby afflicting disease to that tissue or organ. Dr. Weston Price, the world's most renowned dentist found that when the bacteria found in root canals were transferred into rabbits, 80 to 100 percent of these animals developed the same diseases the human donors had. Heart disease, for example, could be transferred 100 percent of the time.

By the way, multiple pathological bacteria are not only found within root-canalled teeth, but also in the bone adjacent to the teeth and in 99% of wisdom tooth extraction sites. It can take decades before symptoms of degenerative disease resulting from this form of silent poisoning become apparent. And while many people with root canals will never develop a degenerative illness, not everyone will be that lucky.

Dr. Price's main discovery was that it is not possible to sterilize a root-canalled tooth and to even know whether it is still infected or not. Price's research showed that numerous chronic degenerative diseases originate from bacterial agents hidden inside root-filled teeth - the most frequent being heart and circulatory diseases, and also diseases of the joints, brain, and nervous system.

Price's research revealed that each of our teeth has a complex maze of tiny tubules that, if stretched out, would extend for at least three miles. In addition, he identified as many as 75 separate accessory canals in a single central front tooth.

His documented findings showed that typically harmless, beneficial microscopic organisms regularly move in and around these miniscule tunnels. A problem arises, though, when a dentist performs a root canal, not only is the tooth's blood supply cut off, but also the nutrient supply to these organisms. The starving bacteria now must feed on tooth tissue to survive, which causes infection. To be able to infect dead tooth tissue, though, the formerly harmless oral bacteria must mutate into highly toxic and destructive pathogens. Antibiotics and the body's own immune cells that normally subdue pathogens cannot get to them without blood flowing into the dead tooth.

When examined, just about every single root-canalled tooth has been found colonized by pathogens, possibly spreading the infection around the apex and in the periodontal ligament, and as far as into the jawbone where it can create cavitations that rarely heal on their own. According to Weston Price Foundation, in the records of 5,000 surgical cavitation cleanings, only 2 were found healed.

A healthy immune system that is not weakened by a separate disease process or suppressed by vaccines, radiation, an accident, emotional stress, trauma, poor diet, vitamin D deficiency, or other reasons, can easily deal with any of these germs straying away from the tooth. However, when subdued, these pathogens can enter the blood and be transported to other tissues, organs, or glands.

Price showed that when he implanted fragments from a root-canalled tooth of a person who suffered, for instance, from rheumatoid arthritis, into a rabbit, the rabbit quickly became arthritic, too. Similarly, he showed that root canal fragments taken from a person who had suffered a heart attack would also cause a heart attack in rabbits that received an implant of these fragments. He was able to demonstrate this phenomenon 100 percent of the time. The same principle applied not only to heart disease and arthritis, but to kidney disease, joint disorders, neurological diseases (including ALS and MS), autoimmune diseases such as lupus and more, and even cancers.

The German physician, Josef M. Issels (1907-1998), also known as 'The Father of Integrative Medicine', reported that in his 40 years of treating *terminal* cancer patients, 97 percent of them had root canals. Cancer researcher, Dr. Robert Jones, was also able to establish the relationship between root canals and cancerous growths. In a 5-year long study of 300 breast cancer patients, Jones found that 93 percent of women with breast cancer had root canals and the rest of them had other oral pathology. He showed that in nearly all cases, tumors occurred on the same side of the body as the root canal(s). Jones suggested that toxins from the bacteria in an infected tooth or jawbone must be inhibiting the proteins that suppress cancer cell development.

To confirm Dr Price's original research findings, the Toxic Element Research Foundation (TERF) used DNA analysis to determine whether root-canalled teeth are contaminated with pathogens. This was confirmed in 100 percent of the samples tested. According the test results, there were 42 different species of anaerobic bacteria in 43 root canal samples. Cavitations fared even worse: 67 different anaerobic bacteria were found among the 85 samples tested.

Furthermore, the analysis showed that the blood surrounding the root canal tooth had 400 percent more of these bacteria than the tooth itself, which means they could easily be transferred to other parts of the body when the immune systems was weakened or otherwise overtaxed.

There is a place for bacteria inside the body and in the rest of nature. When bacteria are being caged in and must mutate to survive, they become highly toxic and can cause havoc in the blood, heart, brain, liver, kidneys, and elsewhere in the body, but we certainly cannot blame these organisms for that.

It is highly unnatural to keep anything that is dead in the body. People have died because doctors didn't remove a dead limb that died off because of frostbite or gangrene. A dead baby in a mother's womb, a diseased kidney or damaged piece of splintered bone must all be removed; otherwise an inflammatory immune response combined with destructive bacteria will surely kill the host. Why do doctors remove a burst appendix, but don't do the same for a dead tooth? We cannot have it both ways. What is dead must eventually become infected and decomposed. This is a law of nature.

Even the ADA acknowledges that oral bacteria can travel from your mouth to your heart and cause a life-threatening infection. Their answer to combat the bacteria is a treatment with antibiotics, hoping that this somehow makes these bugs go away. Once again, you are on your on when it comes to protecting your health and that of your family.

Of course, the best way to prevent dental problems is by taking care of your diet, and lifestyle. But if you already have had a root canal or cavitations, I strongly recommend you contact a biological dentist who is aware of the risks I have mentioned here. If it is found that you are not at risk of any significant side effects, by all means, keep the root canal. Otherwise, there is really no good alternative as yet to removing a root-canalled tooth. Your dentist will be able to advice you on having a partial denture, a bridge, or an implant made of nontoxic materials such as Zirconium, and to also ensure that the underlying ligament of the extracted tooth is thoroughly shaved and cleaned.

ToxicTeeth.org is a great resource for more information on this topic and for finding a good biological dentist in your area. See also these reference links for the above research findings[233].

23. Bring Balance to Your Emotional Health

On a deeper level, every physically manifested ailment is an imbalanced emotion. Emotions are signals of comfort or discomfort that our body sends us at every moment of our conscious existence. They contain specific vibrations that serve as a kind of weather report, telling us how we feel about ourselves, about others, and about what is good or bad, right or wrong, both in our lives and in our world. Emotions are like reflections from a mirror that reveal to us everything we need to know to go through the trials and tribulations of life. Our body, which can only be *felt*, is precisely such an emotional mirror or messenger. A dirty mirror reflects only certain parts of us or makes us look distorted. If we are emotionally stuck and unable to understand what is happening to us, it is because we are not open to listen to, understand, and follow the messages that our body is trying to convey to us.

All emotional problems indicate a lack of awareness. If we are not completely aware why these emotions and/or physical challenges are there, we are out of touch with ourselves and, hence, are incapable of making positive changes in our life. Many people are so disconnected from their

---

[233]Weston A. Price Foundation; Price-Pottenger Foundation, Weston A. Price Foundation June 25, 2010; Quantum Cancer Management; American Association of Endodontists; Journal of Clinical Microbiology February 2007; Journal of Clinical Microbiology July 2003; Clinical Infectious Diseases June 1996; Science Daily January 4, 2011; The Wealthy Dentist July 12, 2011

feelings that they do not even know what they feel. Practicing mindfulness brings our attention back to where we are and who we are. By staying with our emotions for as long as they last, we can unleash the tremendous creative powers that lie dormant within us. Emotions are not there to be judged or suppressed; they are there to be understood and accepted. As we learn to observe them, we will begin to understand their true meaning. Instead of unconsciously reacting to a difficult situation or person, we will be able to act consciously out of our own free will.

Emotions want to be acknowledged because they are the only way our body can tell us how we truly feel about others and ourselves. By accepting and honoring all our feelings and emotions, rather than repressing them, we begin to experience a different reality in life, one that offers us freedom from judgment and freedom from pain. We will begin to see a sense and purpose in everything that is happening to us, regardless of whether it is right or wrong, good or bad. This eliminates fear, as well as all the other emotions that arise from fear. Balancing our emotions is one of the most important non-physical ways we have to attain a sound state of health, happiness, and peacefulness.

The approaches, messages, and artwork contained in my book, *Lifting the Veil of Duality,* have been designed to bring balance to your emotional health (see *Other Books and Products by Andreas Moritz*). In fact, your entire perception of problems, limitations, disease, pain, and suffering may become profoundly altered after reading that book. In addition, what formerly may have led you to age faster, or perhaps even experience a physical illness, may rapidly become transmuted into powerful opportunities to generate joy, abundance, vitality, and rejuvenation throughout the rest of your life. My healing system, *Sacred Santémony,* described on my website www.ener-chi.com, is a highly effective method to balance the root causes of emotional imbalances.

Also, you may greatly benefit from following this simple procedure for balancing emotions: Transfer your mind back to a beautiful period in your early childhood, perhaps when you were 3 years old. Remember how very free and joyful you were! You had no preconceived notions of what was right or wrong, good or bad, beautiful or ugly. See yourself as this child interacting with other people with wonder, total ease, and innocent openness. You are interested in all there is, and you feel safe, nurtured, and loved. Now go forward in time to a situation in your life where you no longer felt this way, where you felt a lack of love or were ignored, rebuked, criticized, or abused. Notice the contraction and coldness in your heart. Once again, go back to the innocent spirit of your childlike nature and bring it into that situation that caused you so much pain. Fill yourself with that 3-year-old innocence and untainted joy, and radiate it all around you. See it filling everyone with that same joyful radiance. Now move to another event in your life that caused you unhappiness, and repeat this process. Go through every difficult or negative experience in your life, and heal it with your 3-year-old joyful self.

This exercise is so effective because, in reality, there is no linear time. Time is merely a concept we use to separate events that have already happened, are occurring right now, or may unfold sometime in the future. Thus, in truth, past events have just as powerful an effect on us today as they had then. For this reason, there is so much fear, tension, stress, anger, conflict, and violence in our world. Most people cannot let go of their past experiences and, therefore, re-create similar scenarios to deal with them in one way or another. However, by undoing their negative impact through this simple exercise of self-empowerment, you can literally change your past and, thereby, your present and future realities.

It may take 1-2 weeks (20 to 30 minutes per day) to sift through and heal all your past unbalanced emotions in this way, but it is worthwhile. Whenever you react negatively to something in your life, it is because you have had an unbalanced emotional experience before that. By balancing all the unwanted experiences that have occurred between your early childhood and this moment, you can help remove many of the root causes of any existing emotional, mental, physical, and spiritual problems and can prevent new ones from arising.

Continuous emotional stress is a major reason for making new gallstones, since it alters the bile flora and also prevents proper digestion of food (as well as bile salts). If you have difficulties resolving old emotional conflicts on your own, you may wish to employ the help of a qualified practitioner of German New Medicine (GNM)[234]; these conflicts can be resolved within a matter of an hour or two. GNM shows how profoundly an old unresolved emotional conflict or trauma can affect an organ or system in the body and keep it from functioning properly or recovering. I have seen it work miracles for persistent trauma-caused-conditions like Candida overgrowth, arthritis, and cancer.

---

[234]Dr. Hamer's German New Medicine, www.newmedicine.ca, Ilsedora Laker

Chapter 6

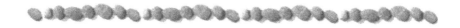

What You Can Expect from the Liver and Gallbladder Flush

A Disease-Free Life

A lthough disease is not part of the body's design, it has built-in and constantly adjusting strategies to heal itself. The word heal is derived from the word *health* or *wholeness*. To heal means to return to wholeness or health. Symptoms of disease merely indicate that the body is already engaged in healing itself to prevent a potentially life-threatening situation from occurring.

Being sick is the indication that the body is doing just that. We *fall ill* when our immune system is down, that is, suppressed and overburdened with accumulated toxic waste. The response of the body to this type of extreme congestion is to clear the toxins in a number of different, and usually unpleasant, ways. These ways are known as symptoms.

The body's methods of cleansing, self-protection and healing often require pain, fever, infection, inflammation, and ulceration[235]. In more serious cases, cancer[236] and a buildup of plaque inside the arterial walls help avert the ill person's imminent demise. Most types of internal suffocation are preceded or accompanied by a blockage of the liver bile ducts. When the liver, which is the main factory and detoxification center of the body, becomes congested with gallstones, disease becomes the much-needed outcome.

When you clear the liver bile ducts of all obstructions and then adopt and maintain a balanced diet and lifestyle, your body naturally returns to a

[235] To learn more about the four major causes of disease, how disease develops, and the true reasons for cancer, heart disease, diabetes, and AIDS, refer to my book *Timeless Secrets of Health and Rejuvenation*

[236] See details in my book *Cancer is not a Disease - It's a Healing Mechanism*

state of balance (homeostasis). This balanced state is what most people call *good health*.

The old saying "An ounce of prevention is worth a pound of cure" applies most appropriately to the liver. If the liver is kept free of gallstones, the body's balanced state is unlikely to be upset. Having a clean liver and keeping it clean almost always means having a clean bill of health.

Health insurance companies and their clients could greatly benefit from the liver and gallbladder flush in several important ways. These companies would be able to lower their premium rates and expenditures considerably, while the insured population would enjoy much better health, fewer sick days from work, and freedom from the fear and pain that typically accompany disease. Older generations would no longer be considered a burden, as they would be able to take care of themselves more and more, rather than less and less. Healthcare costs could be cut drastically, which may be the only way to safeguard continuous progress and prosperity in nations now overwhelmed with debt such as the United States and the United Kingdom.

If the current trend of escalating health expenditures in the United States continues to grow as fast as it has in recent decades, major corporations are likely to end up bankrupt if they continue to offer health insurance as a benefit to their employees. Transferring the burden of employer healthcare to the government or a universal healthcare plan has little if any impact on the massive cost increase caused by symptom-oriented medicine.

In 2001, the cost of healthcare in the United States exceeded the $1 trillion mark, and in 2004, total healthcare spending amounted to $1.9 trillion. That represented 16 percent of the nation's GDP, and there is no end to this trend in sight. Health expenditure in the United States neared $2.6 trillion in 2010 and is estimated to double to over $4 trillion over the next decade.

When healthcare cost grows faster than national income, the survival of a country is at stake. Every person who doesn't take care for his own health contributes to the rise in healthcare spending and the impending national bankruptcy.

Good healthcare cannot be measured by how much money is being spent on treating symptoms of disease. Treating the symptoms of an illness is *sickness care* which inevitably requires further treatments, because the origins of disease are ignored and become only worse if left unattended.

The premise of modern medicine mostly consists of *successfully* treating away symptoms through poisonous drugs, radiation, or surgery. However, this implies suppressing the body's own healing efforts. This means that almost all forms of medical intervention are bound to have harmful side effects, which in turn become the cause of new diseases that require further treatment.

The quick-fix approach of suppressing symptoms of disease is a major cause of chronic illness, premature death, and, of course, spiraling healthcare costs. As mentioned before, over 900,000 people die each year unnecessarily as a direct result of side effects from expensive medical treatments. By comparison, it is very inexpensive to actually cure disease and prevent new diseases from arising.

Conventional healthcare is becoming less and less affordable for most people in the world and is likely to become a rare privilege for a relative few in the future. If the liver and gallbladder flush were to be prescribed by doctors in the United States, even just to patients with gallbladder disease, it could help most of the 31 million gallstone sufferers to live a normal, comfortable life and eliminate or prevent numerous other related illnesses.

I receive about 250 letters/emails from around the world each day. Each of them tells a unique story that speaks volumes in favor of taking active responsibility for one's health. The following testimonial is but a simple example of a turnaround made by a professional musician and music teacher who, at age 24, began to suffer from severe acid reflux disease. Eventually, the pain and reflux were so unbearable that she could no longer sing due to vocal nodes. At age 40 she was plagued by so much pain, insomnia and other health problems that her entire livelihood was threatened.

In her letter to me, she explained, "Acid reflux is death to a vocalist." She continued, "Finally, a HIDA scan was performed which showed that my gallbladder had a 9% ejection rate. I was told it must be removed immediately. When it was taken out, in March 2011, my doctor shared with me that my gallbladder was about to rupture and was 3 times its normal size! He assured me that I would be feeling much better and could eat anything I wanted. Only despite good diet, exercise, abstinence from coffee and alcohol, I experienced only a short-lived relief before I was put back on medication. The proton pump inhibitors (antacids) were no longer providing relief, though. Then, I read your book! My initial liver flush was an amazing experience! Stones passed were quite large and I feel the best I have felt in years (especially since having my gallbladder removed)! My reflux and pain on my right side is improved and I anticipate with joy future cleansing, flushing and return to health. For the first time in many years, I was filled with hope!"

The liver flush does much more than merely restore proper liver and digestive functions; it helps people take active care of their health for the rest of their lives. Taking out an insurance policy against disease cannot guarantee a disease-free life. Good health develops naturally when you keep the body free of gallstones and other toxic waste deposits, and when you fulfill the most basic requirements for maintaining youthfulness and vitality throughout life.

Improved Digestion, Energy, and Vitality

Good digestion comprises three basic processes in the body:

- Ingested food is broken down into its nutrient components
- Nutrients are absorbed and distributed to all the cells and then metabolized efficiently
- The waste products resulting from the breakdown and utilization of food are all eliminated through the excretory organs and systems.

The body requires good digestion in order to guarantee continuous, efficient turnover of its 60 to 100 trillion cells. To sustain homeostasis, the body needs to make 30 billion new cells each day to replace the same number of old, worn-out, or damaged cells. If this process occurs smoothly, day after day and year after year, the new generations of cells in the body will be as effective and healthy as the previous ones. Even if certain cells, such as brain and heart cells, cannot be replaced (although this theory is about to become obsolete, according to new discoveries made in the field of neurogenesis[237]), at least their constituents, such as carbon, oxygen, hydrogen, and nitrogen atoms (all of which make up the

---

[237]Neurogenesis and brain injury: managing a renewable resource for repair

air that we breathe), are nevertheless renewed continuously. In other words, nothing natural in the body can be considered old.

The normal turnover of cells or atoms, however, is no longer complete or efficient in the majority of people who live in a fast-paced world that has little time for a healthy lifestyle and balanced diet. People are unhealthy today because they eat unhealthy foods (and think unhealthy thoughts). In contrast, a nourishing diet consists of natural, unpolluted foods, and fresh, clean water.

Only very few societies have managed to maintain their youth and health at all age levels. Such peoples live in remote and secluded areas, such as the Abkhasian Mountains in Southern Russia; the Himalayan Mountains in India, Tibet, and China; the Andes in South America; the Nicoya region of Costa Rica; and parts of northern Mexico. Their diet consists only of pure, fresh foods.

Thankfully, you don't need to live in remote areas of the world to be healthy. In fact, it is very normal, for example, to have completely clean blood vessels at age 100 or older (see **Figure 14**). The coronary artery in this image came from a 100-year-old American woman who died peacefully in her sleep (not from a disease). Even 1,000 year old trees can still produce healthy leaves and fruits, as a long as sap travels freely to them.

Growing older does not narrow blood vessels and cut off the nutrient supply to the cells of our body (the main cause of turning them old and weak), but an unhealthful diet and lifestyle does.

By cleansing our body and giving it the best possible treatment, we can all raise our quality of life to a high level of energy and vitality, which is the natural state of health that every human being deserves. A well-functioning digestive system and gallstone-free liver provide the main conditions through which the body can regulate the smooth turnover of cells without accumulating toxins. This is perhaps the best antidote to aging and disease any person can have.

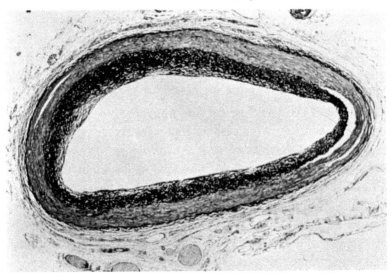

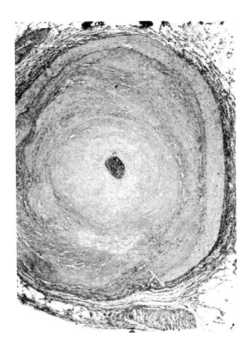

Figure 14: A clear coronary artery of a 100-year-old American woman and a clogged artery of a 50-year old man below that (the red mark in the middle of the second image is a blood clot that caused a fatal heart attack)

Freedom from Pain

Pain is a signal that the body uses to identify and correct certain problems or malfunctioning in the organs, systems, muscles, and joints. Pain is not a disease in itself, but instead is the sign of a proper immune response to an abnormal situation. An abnormal situation could mean congestion of lymph, blood, and waste matter. Any physical congestion leads to a poor supply of oxygen. Oxygen-deprived tissues almost always signal pain. When the pain subsides naturally through cleansing or the body's removing the congestion (without the use of painkillers), it shows that the body has returned to a state of balance. Chronic pain indicates that the immune response and self-cleansing ability of the body are not sufficient and that the cause of the condition is still active and intact.

Cleansing the liver and gallbladder of all gallstones can help to reduce and eliminate pain in the body, regardless of whether it is located in the joints, head, nerves, muscles, or organs. The body is only as healthy as the blood and lymph are. If the blood and lymph contain large amounts of toxins, as occurs when there is congestion in the liver, then irritation, inflammation and infection, or damage to cells and tissues in the weakest parts of body may result. When the functions of digestion, metabolism, and the elimination of waste materials in the body are impaired as a result of poor liver performance, the immune system cannot accomplish its healing work in the body.

The healing response is largely dependent on the efficiency of the immune system, the greatest part of which is located in the intestinal tract. The liver, which is the main organ controlling digestion and cellular metabolism, must be free of all obstructions (gallstones) in order to prevent the immune system from being stressed and overtaxed. When immune power is low in the intestines, it will also be depressed in all other parts of the body.

Pain relief occurs automatically once congestion subsides and the immune system returns to its full power and efficiency. Pain is not something that requires treatment, unless it is unbearable. You would not try fighting the darkness of the night when all you need to do is to switch on the light. It is, in fact, unwise to kill the messenger (pain) that tries to warn you about an approaching enemy. Since chronic pain is caused by chronic congestion, the liver, intestines, kidneys, and lymphatic system should be cleansed before attempting to treat the pain. In almost every case, this approach relieves all pain and restores vibrant health along with proper immune functions.

A More Flexible Body

Physical flexibility is a measure of how well the organs, joints, muscles, connective tissues, and cells are nourished by the food we eat, the water we drink, and the air we breathe. The digestive and metabolic processes that make these nutrients and substances available to the cells need to be in top condition for health to be a real and long-lasting outcome. Stiffness in the joints and muscles indicates the presence of acidic metabolic waste products in these parts of the body owing to poor digestive and eliminative functions.

Anyone who practices yoga, gymnastics, or any other form of exercise and does several liver flushes will notice greatly increased flexibility of the spine, joints, and muscles. Deposits of mineral salts in the neck and shoulder areas begin to lessen, and aches and stiffness disappear. The whole body feels more *connected*, as the connective tissues that keep the cells together become more supple and fluid again.

A river of pure, clean water flows more easily and with less friction than a river that is filled with muck and debris. One of the liver's most important functions is to keep the blood naturally thin so that it can distribute nutrients to the cells, collect waste materials, and carry messenger hormones to their destinations without delay. Keeping your river of life (blood) healthy and clean is of utmost important to your mental and physical health.

Thick blood is a common denominator for most illnesses, and you can recognize it by a lack of flexibility in certain parts of the body, along with other symptoms, including tiredness. If the spine and joints are permanently stiff and painful, this indicates that most of the internal organs are suffering from circulatory problems. Blood circulation greatly improves when gallstones cease to congest the liver. This leads to increased flexibility and mobility throughout the body. A good and regular exercise program helps to support and maintain this newly found flexibility.

A flexible body also suggests that the mind is open and adaptable. A rigid body, by contrast, is a sign of a rigid and fearful mind. As the body is supplied with thinner blood, and as hardened structures begin to soften again, your mental attitude also becomes more expansive and accommodating. This enhances your ability to flow with the opportunities of life in the present moment, adding greater joy and fulfillment to each new day.

Reversal of the Aging Process

Many people view aging as an unavoidable phenomenon that, like a disease, will afflict them eventually. However, this viewpoint applies only to its *negative* consequences. You can just as well see aging as a positive growth process that makes life richer, increases wisdom, and enhances experience and maturity: all assets that are rarely found in one's youth. The negative aspect of the aging process, with which the majority of people identify, is actually a metabolic disorder that develops gradually over a period of time.

The unwanted effects of aging result from malfunctioning that occurs on the cellular level. When the body's cells are unable to remove their daily-generated metabolic waste material fast enough, some of it is deposited in the cell membranes. In fact, the cell membranes become your body's garbage filters. Subsequently, the cells cannot rid themselves of all their own waste because the surrounding connective tissue is congested with other waste material (owing to lymphatic blockage).

In due time, inefficient waste disposal becomes more pronounced and apparent in the body. The withheld waste gradually cuts off the cells' supply of oxygen, nutrients, and water, and increasingly thickens their membranes. The cell membranes of a newborn baby are very thin, nearly colorless, and highly transparent. The average 70-year-old person today has cell membranes that are at least 5 times as thick as those found in a baby's body. The membranes' color is generally brown and, in some cases, even black. This cell-degenerative process is what we generally refer to as *aging*.

During normal aging, which begins right from the beginning of life, all cells in the body are routinely replaced with new cells. On the other hand, during abnormal aging, the newly created cells are not as healthy as the old ones were. The affected tissues or groups of cells have become weaker and suffer malnutrition, thereby giving the new generation of cells a poor start in life. Before long, the membranes of the new cells also become clogged up. They have no chance to develop into healthy young cells.

As more and more of the cells and the surrounding connective tissues become saturated with toxic substances, entire organs in the body begin to age and deteriorate as well.

The skin, which is the largest organ in the body, also begins to suffer from malnourishment. Consequently, it may lose some of its former elasticity, change its natural color, become dry and rough, and develop blemishes that largely consist of metabolic waste products. At this stage, the negative aspect of the aging process becomes visible on the outside. Therefore, it is obvious that external aging of the body, which is a direct result of defective cell metabolism, starts on the inside.

Impaired digestion and liver function are the main causes of inefficient cell metabolism. Both functions improve dramatically when all existing gallstones in the liver and gallbladder are eliminated and other toxic waste materials are removed from the organs, tissues, and cells through simple methods of cleansing (as discussed in this book). As soon as the cells begin to shed their dark skin (a natural result of the cleansing), the absorption of oxygen, nutrients, and water increases, and so does cell vitality.

As digestion and metabolism continue to improve, instead of being old and tired, the cells will become young and dynamic again. Such improvements can easily be seen in an improved skin color and texture, a certain glow in the eyes, and a more positive demeanor. This is the time when the aging process actually reverses, and the positive aspects of aging begin to dominate.

Inner and Outer Beauty

The results of steadily improving cell metabolism will affect the way you feel about your inner self as much as they will show on the outside. Older people look radiant and youthful when they are truly healthy. Young people can look quite old if their bodies are toxic and tired. Naturally, if you want to achieve outer beauty, you must develop inner beauty first.

If your body has accumulated a lot of waste material, it is not capable of imbuing you with a sense of beauty and worthiness. There are still groups of indigenous people living in the most remote parts of the world who enjoy perfect health and vitality. They regularly purge their liver, kidneys, and intestines with oils, herbs, and fluids. These practices have become lost to modern societies, whose main emphasis is on improving the superficial physical appearance and, in the case of an illness, fixing its symptoms rather than removing its cause(s).

Those who have done a series of liver flushes report that they feel much better about their body, their life, and their environment. In many cases, the person's self-esteem and ability to appreciate others improves as the body becomes increasingly purified. The liver cleanse can greatly contribute toward developing vitality and inner beauty. This will not only help to slow or reverse the aging process, but will also make you feel more youthful and attractive, regardless of your age.

Improved Emotional Health

The liver flush has direct implications on how you feel about yourself and others. Under stress, you are likely to become irritable, annoyed, frustrated, and even angry. Most people assume that stress has something to do with the external problems they face in their lives. Yet this is only partially true. Our response to certain issues, situations, or people is only negative because we are not able to cope with them.

The liver, which maintains the nervous system by supplying it with vital nutrients, greatly determines the way we respond to stress. Gallstones impede the proper distribution of nutrients, which forces the body to take recourse to several emergency measures, including the excessive secretion of stress hormones. For a short while, this fast-acting first-aid measure helps to maintain most bodily functions, but eventually the body's equilibrium becomes disturbed and the nervous system is thrown off balance. Given this imbalanced state of internal affairs, any external pressure or demanding situation may trigger an exaggerated stress response that, in turn, may give rise to the feeling of being stressed or overwhelmed.

Our emotional health is intimately linked to our physical health. Cleansing the liver and keeping it clean helps maintain emotional balance. When you remove your gallstones, you also root out any deep-seated anger and resentment that may have been stored there for a long time (the body holds onto various emotions in different body parts[238]). The relief that comes with letting go of past, unresolved issues may create a new sense of being alive. Moreover, the feelings of freedom and euphoria that you commonly experience almost immediately after a liver flush, indicate what can lie in store for you once your liver and gallbladder are completely cleansed. To that effect, I have received countless reports from people around the world who say how cleaning out their liver and gallbladder has helped them end their depression, anxiety, and anger.

A Clearer Mind and Improved Creativity

Clarity of mind, memory recall, creativity, and the ability to concentrate and focus attention all depend on how well the brain and nervous system are nourished. An ineffective circulatory system has a dulling and suppressing effect on all mental processes. This, in turn, stresses and strains the nervous system.

With each new liver flush you undertake, you are likely to notice a further improvement in your mental faculties. Many people report that their mind becomes less turbulent and more relaxed. Others report a sudden influx of expansive thoughts that help to improve their work performance and creative output. Artists generally find an opening of a new dimension to their creative expression, including a more acute perception of colors, shapes, and forms.

Those involved in techniques of spiritual growth or self-improvement will find that the elimination of all gallstones in the liver may help them to gain access to deeper, formerly inaccessible areas within themselves and to use more of their mental potential. The liver flush particularly helps balance the solar plexus chakra, which is considered the body's main emotional center. That's where we experience our *gut feelings*, both negative and positive.

---

[238]See my book *It's Time to Come Alive* for more details.

The solar plexus also represents the energy center in the body responsible for willpower, energy absorption, and distribution; as well as functions of the liver, gallbladder, stomach, pancreas, and spleen. This central switchboard for physical and emotional activities becomes far more comfortable after doing a series of liver flushes.

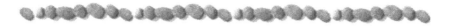

Chapter 7

Ending the Olive Oil Soap Stone Myth

Over the past few years I have been repeatedly asked whether or not the stones passed during the liver flushes are just hardened lumps of olive oil that are somehow manufactured from the cleanse ingredients inside the intestines.

Certain well-known herbalists and doctors, as well as PR-organization arms of the pharma/medical industry, have undertaken great efforts to discredit the beneficial effects of the liver and gallbladder flush. They claim that these gallstones are actually *soap stones* produced in the intestines through saponification of the ingested olive oil.

Some of the most outspoken organizations going after proponents and associations of holistic medicine, such as homeopathic and chiropractic associations, are Quackwatch.com and its sister organization in Europe, EsoWatch.com. While these anti-natural medicine groups claim to be *protectors* of people against quacks and snake oil sellers, they fail to mention anywhere on their extensive web pages the nearly endless cases of medical fraud, medical errors, and often horrific and fatal side effects caused by reckless overuse and abuse of conventional medicine. All their warnings are solely directed against natural medicine, which truly shows where they are coming from.

Quackwatch.com, which is owned by a retired psychiatrist Stephen Barrett, has positioned itself at the top of every search engine on the internet for every keyword related to all the major forms of alternative medical treatments; this is not an easy feat to accomplish without having massive funding from somewhere other than a retirement fund.

This is what medical doctor Ray Sahelian writes in his online Quackwatch.com review "Is Stephen Barrett a Quack?": "I hardly came across reports on his website regarding some of the scams or inaccurate promotion and marketing practices by the pharmaceutical industry. Why is this? Why has Stephen Barrett, M.D. (a retired psychiatrist), focused almost all of his attention on the nutritional industry and has hardly spent time pointing out the billions of dollars wasted each year by consumers on certain prescription and non-prescription pharmaceutical drugs? If he truly claims to be a true consumer advocate, isn't it his responsibility to make sure the big scams are addressed first before focusing on the smaller scams? It's like the government putting all of its efforts going after the poor misusing food stamps while certain big companies cheat billions of dollars from consumers with hardly any governmental oversight."

Dr. Sahelian continues: "Why is there no review of Vioxx (the drug led to more than 27,000 heart attacks and sudden cardiac deaths) on Quackwatch? Why is there no mention on quackwatch.org of the worthless cold and cough medicines sold by pharmaceutical companies and drugstores (which have been shown to cause death in children, according to the CDC's own admission)? Hundreds of millions of dollars are wasted each year by consumers on these worthless and potentially harmful decongestants and cough syrups. Just recently, another 5-year-old child died because she was given just twice the normal dose of cough syrup[239]. Why is there no mention on Quackwatch of the dangers of acetaminophen use, including liver damage? There are probably more people who are injured or die from over-the-counter Tylenol and aspirin use each year than from all the natural supplements people take throughout a year. If Dr. Barrett had focused his career on educating people in reducing the use of useless and dangerous prescription and nonprescription drugs (even just one, acetaminophen) he would have helped many more people than attempting to scare people from the use of supplements."

"Another point I would like to make regarding Quackwatch is that Dr. Barrett often, if not the majority of the time, seems to point out the negative outcome of studies with supplements (you can sense his glee and relish when he points out these negative outcomes), and rarely mentions the benefits they provide. A true scientist takes a fair approach, and I don't see this in my review of the Quackwatch website," says Dr. Sahelian.

I may add to this, that Quackwatch.com fails to mention the now proven fact that 92 percent of all peer-reviewed scientific studies done on pharmaceutical drugs are fraudulent, that over 900,000 people die each year in the US alone as a result of medical treatments and medical errors, and that at least half of all new cancers are caused by mammography, CT scans, and cancer treatments. So far, no person who has done a liver and gallbladder flush has died from it, but millions of people who didn't

---

[239] Five-year-old girl dies after being given just twice the normal dose of over-the-counter cough medicine, NaturalNews.com, April 27, 2012

cleanse their liver and gallbladder have. In fact, liver and gallbladder congestion is a leading cause of death.

Even some of the mass media have joined the witch-hunt and contributed to disseminating fear-inducing information that may sound logical to a layperson, but makes no sense to the true experts and well-informed doctors and scientists familiar with human physiology, basic chemistry, and liver health. Although colon hydrotherapy used to be standard medical practice in most hospitals until the 1920s (before antibiotics became popular), today colon hydrotherapists are also harassed and their licenses taken away on flimsy grounds.

The individuals behind the anti-liver flush movement, which was created *"to protect the health of the people against quacks and charlatans like Andreas Moritz,"* have their own reasons for lodging such statements. They obviously have never done a liver flush themselves or cleaned out their colon and merely repeat what Quackwatch.com, EsoWatch.com, Wikipedia, and other organizations known for targeting holistic medicine and its practitioners have said about it.

Many doctors have become angered over the fact that their patients, by doing a series of liver and gallbladder flushes, were able to avoid gallbladder surgery after they were told (by them) that they *absolutely needed* it. Droves of patients have left their doctors because they were feeling so much better, simply by doing liver flushes, than they had ever felt under their physicians' care.

On the other hand, an increasing number of medical practitioners now offer the liver flush regimen to their patients, with such high success rates across a large number of health conditions, including diseases of the liver and gallbladder, that patients just flock to them, more than ever. Doctors whose principle goal is to help their patients heal themselves are becoming increasingly popular, and they are a lot less stressed than mainstream doctors. They are well aware of their patients' improved conditions following the liver flushes and are not easily deceived by anti-liver flush television documentaries or magazine articles paid for by pharmaceutical companies, medical associations, or resentful physicians.

The following facts prove why the stones passed during liver and gallbladder flushes cannot be olive oil stones, as claimed by some:

1. When combined with citrus juice, olive oil cannot congeal into such relatively hard, dense, waxy stones, as are eliminated during liver flushes. You can easily determine this when you combine the two ingredients as part of the liver flush protocol. A saponification of olive inside the body is not possible, given the short time frame that the olive oil has to travel through the GI tract, and the absence of any saponifying chemicals or hardening agents. The small amount of hydrochloric acid found in an empty stomach has no influence on thickening oils or fats. Proteins are digested by gastric juice. Fats and oils are digested by bile and bile salts.

To saponify fats or oils and turn them into solid soap, you need to use lye. Lye is a corrosive alkaline substance, commonly known as sodium hydroxide ($NaOH$, also known as caustic soda) or, historically, potassium hydroxide (KOH, from hydrated potash). Lye is a highly toxic chemical that can cause serious injury and death. Since you need lye to saponify fats, and lye is not ingested during a liver flush, the body has no capacity whatsoever to manufacture olive oil stones, and certainly not green, beige, yellow, brown, black, or red stones, all of which have been found to be released during the liver cleansing process.

In a Quackwatch.com publication[240], author Peter Moran quoted from a letter of opinion published in the medical journal *Lancet,* after the *Lancet* published an article in favor of liver flushes (which infuriated liver flush opponents). The counter-article written by some group of obscure *scientists* attempted to make doctors and patients believe that the results of an alleged experimentation (no reference given, unheard of for bona fide scientists) were identical to the outcome of a liver flush.

These pseudo-scientists claim: "Experiments revealed that mixing equal volumes of oleic acid (the major component of olive oil) and lemon juice produced several semisolid white balls after the addition of a small volume of a potassium hydroxide solution. On air drying at room temperature, these balls became quite solid and hard. We conclude, therefore, that these green 'stones' (passed during liver flushes) resulted from the action of gastric lipases on the simple and mixed triacylglycerols that make up olive oil, yielding long chain carboxylic acids (mainly oleic

---

[240] The Truth about Gallbladder and Liver "Flushes", Quackwatch.com

acid). This process was followed by saponification into large insoluble micelles of potassium carboxylates (lemon juice contains a high concentration of potassium) or 'soap stones'."

Of course, these so-called *scientists* failed to mention that potassium hydroxide readily turns into white balls or pellets[241] as this picture in Wikipedia shows (see **Figure 15**). There is no need to add olive oil or lemon juice to create these pellets or lumps of corrosive powder. Regardless, potassium hydroxide, which is very corrosive, has a high reactivity toward acids like lemon's citric acid and fatty acids. Surely, almost everyone has seen potassium hydroxide solution leaking from an alkaline battery, as shown in the picture next to it.

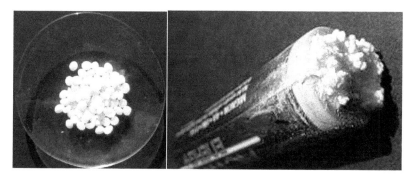

Figure 15: Potassium hydroxide pellets and powder

To then go on and draw the conclusion that these same lab-produced, hard white pellets, somehow created inside the body, magically turn into soft, waxy, bright green colored cholesterol stones, is simply ridiculous. If this weren't such a serious issue with incredibly serious implications, I would think it was a fabulous joke.

According to standard product analysis[242], virgin olive oil has a free acidity (expressed as oleic acid) of no more than 0.8 grams per 100 grams (0.8 percent). Higher concentrations make the olive oil inedible. Doing a laboratory experiment with 100 percent oleic acid does not even remotely resemble what is happening when one ingests the barely 1 percent of free oleic acid found in ½ cup of olive oil. Turning this tiny amount of oleic acid into hundreds of green olive oil *soap stones* requires a miracle. It is certainly anything but science.

---

[241] Potassium Hydroxide Pellets, en.wikipedia.org
[242] Olive Oil Standard Product Analysis, www.oliveoilsource.com

As far as I know, nobody has ever done a liver flush using inedible olive oil composed of free acid of at least over 80 percent, necessary to make soap in a laboratory setting. What this means is that even if, in fact, the olive oil ingested during a regular liver flush could be made into soap stones, there is just not enough free acid available to form even pinhead size soap stones, not to mention the hundreds, and possibly thousands, of lentil-to-chickpea size stones passed during most liver flushes.

These *scientists*, as well as Quackwatch.com, EsoWatch.com and Wikipedia, have also omitted to mention that the body does not produce the caustic, toxic chemical potassium hydroxide that they used in their experiment (if they ever did perform such an experiment, or just read up on it on Wikipedia). Therefore, comparing a chemical reaction using a highly reactive toxic chemical with what is naturally occurring in the human digestive system is not only indicative of pseudoscience, but also highly deceptive and downright irresponsible.

I can only assume that this comparison, using clever scientific jargon that most people cannot understand, or don't know how to verify, was intentional. Real scientists would not be making up such fictitious stories and presenting them as scientific fact. To sum it up, the toxic lye potassium hydroxide is not part of the liver and gallbladder flush and, therefore, saponification of olive oil cannot take place inside the human body.

The statement, "On air drying at room temperature, these balls became quite solid and hard," made by these authors in the Lancet letter refers only to potassium hydroxide which, of course, plays no role in the liver flush. Besides, the gallstones passed during the liver flushes do not dry in the air - they enter the toilet water right away. Again, the comparison does not compute.

The most presumptuous statement made in the *Lancet* letter is the following: "This regime consisted of free intake of apple and vegetable juice until 1800 h, but no food, followed by the consumption of 600 ml of olive oil and 300 ml of lemon juice over several hours." I have worked with the liver flush process for over 15 years, but have never heard of any sane person drinking 600 ml of the mixture, which is over 20 oz. of olive oil, plus 10 oz. of lemon juice! Anyone who tries to do that will vomit like there is no tomorrow!

The correct liver flush regime uses 4 oz. (118 ml) of olive oil, which is merely 20 percent the amount the 40-year-old woman mentioned in the article allegedly ingested. I am extremely doubtful that there is anyone who could drink this much olive oil and not faint. I know that those who have tried drinking 4 oz. of olive oil twice within an hour or two became violently ill. I also doubt that there could be any herbalist that would prescribe this much olive oil and lemon juice to a patient without having homicidal intentions.

2. True medical science as taught, for instance, at Johns Hopkins University, of course, does not share the same views as the pseudo scientists or medical doctors who claim that liver stones don't exist. Under the subject of 'Cholangiocarcinoma' in its online department of Gastroenterology & Hematology, Johns Hopkins describes the existence of intrahepatic biliary gallstones in the following way: "Gallstones vary in size, shape and number, and may be found throughout the biliary tract. The link between cholangiocarcinoma and gallstones is unclear. Intrahepatic gallstones may cause chronic obstruction to bile flow, promote micro injury of the bile ducts, and are associated with a 2-10% risk of the development of cholangiocarcinoma (see **Figure 1a** in Chapter 1).

Congenital cystic dilation of intrahepatic biliary ducts (Caroli's disease), and choledochus cysts have also been closely associated with development of cholangiocarcinoma (bile duct cancer)[243].

Therefore, to ignore, deny, or ridicule the existence of intrahepatic biliary gallstones is a foolish and inexcusable mistake that can have serious consequences for millions of people. Although liver cancer has been an extremely rare disease just half a century ago, this is no longer the case today. An average man's lifetime risk of getting liver or bile duct cancer is now about 1 in 94, while an average woman's risk is about 1 in 212, according to 2012 statistics published by the American Cancer Society[244].

By comparison, according the recently released 2008 statistics on autism rates, 1 in 88 children will develop autism. Even if only 2-10 percent of all liver cancers are caused by liver bile duct congestion (due to biliary stones), the number of cancers is still extremely high. Regardless, liver cancer is only one of the many extremely serious consequences of liver bile duct obstruction, as you can derive from Chapter 1 of this book.

---

[243]Intrahepatic Biliary Gallstones, Johns Hopkins University, Gastroenterology & Hematology, Cholangiocarcinoma: Causes; http://www.hopkins-gi.org
[244]Liver cancer statistics, American Cancer Society http://www.cancer.org

3. Many laboratories have confirmed that the stones passed during liver and gallbladder flushes consist of mostly cholesterol and bile salts (see example in Figure 1b of Chapter 1). This means, the released stones must have originated in the liver or gallbladder. This is a link to a "Thesis on the liver cleanse" by Cristina Carugati, School of Naturopathy, Bissone, Switzerland, which contains verifiable laboratory reports as well[245].

4. Millions of people all over the world have reported success with the liver flush. If it were useless, it would not have spread through word of mouth like it has. An ongoing liver flush survey on CureZone.com has shown that about 75 percent of the people who have done a liver flush have benefited from it[246] (please note that for lasting improvements, one must ensure that all the stones are removed from the liver and gallbladder; doing just one liver flush alone is not sufficient).

World renowned Dr. Thomas Rau, of the Biological Medicine Network and Medical Director of the 50-year-old Paracelsus Clinic in Switzerland, who has used my liver flush protocol for over a decade now, confirms that it has greatly benefited thousands of his patients. He says it is very easy to prove the effects of the liver and gallbladder flushes through ultrasound. In every case where ultrasounds showed dilated bile ducts before doing liver flushes (because of their congestion with gallstones), they showed complete normalization after liver flushing.

Author and naturopathic physician Alan Baklayan has also been using the liver and gallbladder protocol to help his patients effectively normalize their cholesterol levels. And I have received letters/emails from hundreds of physicians stating that they, too, found the liver and gallbladder flush to be their most effective method of helping their patients heal from a multiple range of disorders.

5. Olive oil does not assume the putrid smell that emanates from most intrahepatic and extrahepatic gallstones that are released. The smell is unlike that produced by any type of fecal matter. Laboratory-produced soap stones do not emit this putrid smell.

---

[245] Thesis on the Liver Cleanse by Cristina Carugati, School of Naturopathy, Bissone, Switzerland, ener-chi.com (Resources > Links to Helpful websites)
[246] CureZone Liver Flush Survey, Curezone.com

6. Analysis of released gallstones reveals that the majority of them contain all of the basic ingredients that make up bile fluid. Organic matter may also be present. Many of these stones consist of layers and layers of old, dark-green bile, something that does not happen overnight. The rest of the stones are the typical, rock-hard mineral stones found in the gallbladder. The red or black bilirubin stones some people pass during their flushes certainly cannot pass off as olive oil *soap stones*.

7. During the liver flush, the olive oil mixture does not pass into the liver, as it would if it were eaten with food. Its only action is to prompt a powerful discharge of bile from the liver and gallbladder, thereby removing stones via their respective pathways. Neither the liver nor the gallbladder can therefore act as a soap stone factory.

8. Once the liver and gallbladder are completely clean, no more gallstones are released after ingesting the oil/citrus juice mixture. If these stones were indeed made from olive oil, they would continue to be produced during liver flushes performed after the liver has been completely cleansed and all bile ducts clear and open. However, this is not the case. The liver flush produces no more stones once the liver is clean, regardless of how much olive oil one ingests.

Besides, the olive oil consumed during liver flushes does not always produce the same results. During one flush, only 50 stones may come out, whereas during the next one, as many as 1,000 may be expelled. Sometimes, no stones come out at all when a large clogged biliary duct in the liver just hasn't opened up yet. During the following flush, however, there may be hundreds of stones coming out. If the olive oil mixture alone were to turn into olive oil stones, as claimed, the same number of stones and types of stones would have to be made each time.

9. Because of intolerance to olive oil, some people have used, for example, pure macadamia nut oil (which is colorless) during their flushes and produced precisely the same green-colored stones. Cholesterol stones that exactly match these green stones can be found in the bile ducts of dissected livers (see **Figure 3b**). Some people have used golden-colored olive oil for the liver flushes, but obtained the same results when they used a slightly green-colored olive oil.

10. If stones were just blobs of olive oil, why do so many people get cured from chronic illnesses, such as asthma, allergies, cancer, heart disease, diabetes, and even paralysis, after passing numerous stones during their liver flushes?

11. Many people have released stones of different colors: black, red, green, white, yellow, and tan. Olive oil does not have coloring agents in it to produce stones of different hues, much less of such a colorful variety.

12. People who have sent their stones in for chemical analysis have received reports that almost all the stones were made from cholesterol and salts. These constituents are identical to those in the cholesterol stones found in gallbladders that have been removed. A very small number of stones contained organic matter of unknown origin. Organic matter can easily become trapped in bile sludge that turns into stones inside the liver's bile ducts.

13. Quite a few individuals, including myself, have sometimes passed green cholesterol stones on the evening of the flush, even before taking the olive oil mixture. Others, who had already done several liver flushes, have reported stones coming out during the apple juice phase, all without the help of any olive oil. The stones that come out on their own display no different shape, color, or smell than the ones released during the actual flushes.

14. It is conventional medicine that has actually proved the existence of gallstones in the bile ducts of the liver (see *Diseases of the Gallbladder and Bile Ducts,* in Chapter 1). The medical term for these stones is *intrahepatic stones,* or *biliary stones.* These green stones, made of cholesterol and some bile constituents, are, in fact, oily and, therefore, melt and decompose when exposed to warmer air temperatures, oxygen, and airborne bacteria. Cholesterol itself consists of about 96 percent water. While these cholesterol stones are easily broken down when released into the environment, this does not occur when they remain trapped in the bile ducts of the liver. Cholesterol stones in the gallbladder tend to become hardened and calcified over several months and years.

Plenty of photographs have been taken of dissected livers and are in the medical archives of university clinics that show the presence of these stones in the bile ducts of the liver (see **Figure 3b**, as well as **Figure 1a** from Johns Hopkins University). The research cited and referenced in this book is further proof of their existence.

15. It is a medically proven fact that millions of people regularly pass green sludge, sometimes consisting of dozens of green cholesterol stones, in response to eating a very fatty meal. These stones are *not* composed of the oils or fats that were ingested. They are forced out of the liver and gallbladder along with the expelled bile. Unfortunately, unlike during liver flushing, some of the stones get caught in the common bile duct or even in the pancreatic duct. There is no difference between such stones that are released involuntarily and those passed voluntarily (and intentionally) during a liver flush.

Anyone who drinks half a cup of olive oil on an empty stomach (without taking citrus juice and Epsom salt) will also release the same types of stones as passed during the liver flushes. This will make it very clear to them that these stones are not a product of citrus juice and Epsom salt acting on the olive oil and making *soap stones*. However, unlike during a proper liver flush, they may also suffer a gallstone attack or pancreatitis as a result of some of the released stones getting stuck in the common bile or pancreatic duct because they did not use the bile duct-relaxing Epsom salt.

16. Someone recently asked me the following question: "I found a rather credible argument against the stones hypothesis, basically claiming that at least some of the stones we see after the flush are amalgamations of bile formed in the intestines. He describes an experimental sequence with dyes[247]. I'd love to know what you think of it."

The experiment itself actually explains what happens when we ingest such toxic substances as dye, especially on an empty stomach. The person who wrote this post, first tried natural dyes, such as beetroot juice and activated charcoal, neither of which are treated as toxins by the body. If stones passed during a liver flush were indeed formed as a result of olive oil, juice, and bile combining to form stones, these natural dyes would have had to have red or black dye in them, just like they would color stools red or black.

---

[247]The Liver flush dye experiment: http://www.curezone.com/forums/fm.asp?i=67726#i

The synthetic dyes used in the experiment, E124 (Ponceau 4R) and E102 (Tartrazine), on the other hand, are highly toxic for the body. Their toxicity is multiplied manifold when ingested without solid food. When ingested in liquids, these dyes are immediately carried to the liver for detoxification, where they enter bile ducts and combine with bile. Bile can coagulate and clump together, forming bile stones just as quickly as an egg that is being boiled can become hard within minutes. When discharged during the liver flush these stones may have dye in them.

However, this may not be the main reason for the coloration of stones, as observed by this person. The first batch of stones discharged from the liver or gallbladder can easily absorb synthetic dye color which has a particularly small molecular structure. Synthetic dyes can even stain the hardest quartz crystals.

In the above experiment, the dye entered the stones via lesser dense structures/pathways where the stones were more porous. That's why the stones are not uniformly red, but contain just streaks of red color. Again, most bile stones are not solid at all and absorb dye quite readily, almost like a sponge. After all, most cholesterol is water-soluble; only parts of the stones contain densely packed cholesterol crystals that reject water, and dye.

The vast majority of stones released during liver and gallbladder flushes are greasy, fatty, waxy stones that consist of mostly cholesterol fats (as well as other bile constituents and organic materials), which makes them lighter than water (hence they float in water). They may contain a large amount of bacteria which produce toxic, smelly gases. When placed outdoors, especially in the sun, airborne bacteria will quickly decompose them, and the cholesterol fats will melt like butter. If kept in the refrigerator, this will not happen. When saturated with synthetic dyes, the dyes will remain behind. Bacteria simply cannot decompose synthetic chemicals.

I receive thousands of emails each year from people who have regained their health doing liver flushes. Some of them report they already release stones during the preparation phase, before ingesting any oil or Epsom salt. Malic acid and apple juice have been shown to release stones in some individuals, and so has Epsom salt. If synthetic dye were to be added to Epsom salt or apple juice, these same individuals would also pass stones that are stained red. In truth, though, the stones are the same green cholesterol stones that show up in dissected livers.

Ultimately, if olive oil were turned into stones, a person would produce the same amount of stones each time, given that the same method of cleansing is used. However, this is clearly not the case. Different people pass different amounts and types of stones each time they perform a liver flush.

I have not passed any stones in many years although I still do one liver flush each year, using the exact same formula. I am not the only one. Over the years, I have received reports from thousands of people from around the world who have cleaned out their livers and no longer pass any stones, or just very few, during their maintenance cleanses. If the oil mixture were in fact responsible for causing these stones, the oil would produce about the same amount of stones each time.

My bile secretion and digestion are excellent. I used to suffer one gallstone attack once every 2 months, for many years (over 40 attacks). Not passing any stones anymore is therefore not due to a dysfunctional liver and gallbladder.

17. Some critics (M.D.s) claim that the results from the liver flush are just due to the placebo effect, and nothing else. I am not sure how the liver flush could possibly be the result of a placebo effect. The calcified stones released by the gallbladder, usually after 5 to 8 liver flushes, but as early as the first liver flush, are identical to those found in dissected gallbladders. They do not disintegrate and remain stone hard. Only semi-calcified stones may shrink in time; yet the calcified shell remains intact.

I am also not sure how wishful thinking and positive expectation can cause the liver and gallbladder to release hundreds and thousands of stones over a series of liver flushes, and then no longer have the same result (once the liver is clean). Since the person does not really know if and when his or her liver is actually clean, shouldn't the placebo bear the same results *every time* a person does a liver flush? I wish it were this easy.

I personally suffered over 40 gallbladder attacks during a period of more than 10 years, and my gallbladder was packed with stones, causing a painful, short spinal scoliosis. Since my first liver flush, I never suffered another attack. The scoliosis, among other health problems, vanished after my twelfth flush. After that, none of my annual flushes has produced any stones, although I used exactly the same procedure. My gallbladder is completely clean and efficient now.

If the placebo effect can accomplish all that, then by all means, why not promote it as an effective treatment? However, I have never heard of anyone who passed gallstones and became healthier afterwards just by having hopeful expectations. Every person who does a liver flush expects to pass stones but, sometimes, no stones come out at all. Others who suspect that they do not have any stones at all, or not anymore, may still pass many of them. The placebo has, therefore, very little, if any, influence on the outcome or liver flushes.

Thousands of people from all over the world have saved their gallbladders through liver flushing. Others have fully regained their health and even saved their own lives by doing this flush. Those who intentionally promote or spread the strange and unsubstantiated claim that gallstone-flushing is a placebo and somehow produces olive oil *soap stones*, rob their compatriots and themselves of the opportunity to benefit their own health. This is something they will have to live with.

Ignorance cannot be cured. It needs to be replaced with knowledge.

The following is an unedited, unabbreviated experience report I have received from someone who started off with skepticism, and it sums up this chapter very well:

"For years I've been having pains in my lower-right abdomen. I thought it was my appendix. So I got tested. My appendix was removed yet I still had the pains. Next a couple doctors (I've seen dozens for different reasons) suggested I get an ultrasound. So I did. Turned out my gallbladder was packed with stones. Very interesting to see one of my organs filled to the rim. The surgery was expensive and I wasn't too hot on the idea of having a second surgery in less than two months. Eventually, I ran into someone who told me all about the liver flush. I was like, "What the hell did you say?" Sounded like bull to me, and I was almost sure it was, but what did I have to lose? Well, a few stones, I guess. I took Epson salts and the olive oil drink, and the next morning I saw green balls in the toilet, some floating, others on the bottom of the toilet. It was cool but I figured it had to be the olive oil or some other food residue. So I took it to the labs of the University of Chicago. I have a friend who knows someone who offered to help me out and run the tests on a couple of the stones – yes, I fished them out of the toilet!! Sick!!!!! Then, I told my doctor about it. He said not to expect anything. I was way ahead of him. I was psyching myself up for another surgery, trying to prove to myself it was the only thing I can do. Then I received the lab results. The test explained the stones were made of bile salts, parasitic infestation of some kind and one was calcified, in which case the technician explained to me that's why it sank. I went back to my doctor and told him. He didn't believe it, and, frankly, neither did I. Then I got another ultrasound; and the result? My gallbladder was less than half-full of stones unlike before when it was completely filled up. Since then I've done slightly more than ten flushes and, eventually, another ultrasound detected a clear gallbladder. As for the pain? Well, that went away at flush number four or five. And my complexion has dramatically improved, which I noticed had changed after the third flush. I had acne for fourteen years. I think it's safe to say that not only is America a young country, naive politically and socially, but we've also gone way off base in the field of medicine. In particular, doctors here, for the most part seem to be great at relaying long-held information, but in the world-wide picture, they can learn a lot from more 'open-minded' parts of the world. No offense, docs. It's not just you. It's time to rid ourselves of pride and admit that we, as a nation, can use some guidance. Since my gallbladder ordeal, I've learned of more than a dozen people who've naturally cured themselves of the 'incurable'. A few from cancer and another one from arteriosclerosis; and then, AIDS. Crazy, I know. His doctors didn't believe it either, all fourteen of them who each did a blood work-up. Cheers."

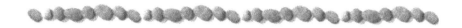

Chapter 8

Summing Up

C leansing the liver is not something that was invented recently. All ancient cultures and civilizations knew of the necessity to keep the liver clean. Plenty of useful cleansing formulas still exist that were handed down through the generations, either by ancestral education or by traditional healers. Although the exact mechanisms of these time-tested cleansing procedures were not as well understood then as they are today (through methods of scientific understanding and investigation), they are no less valid, scientific, and effective than any recently developed therapy.

Medical science has yet to come to terms with the fact that numerous useful methods of healing have worked for millions of people throughout the ages and can make all the difference in the treatment of the most threatening diseases that plague modern societies.

Every house and appliance requires some form of maintenance or repair work from time to time; otherwise, it will lose its ability to carry out the true purpose for which it was designed. The same principle applies to the liver. No other organ in the body besides the brain is as complex and has as many vital functions as the liver.

We clean our teeth and wash our skin every day because we know that exposure to food, air, chemicals, and normal metabolic processes tends to leave residues that can make us feel unclean and uncomfortable. Not many people, however, think that the same principle of cleaning also applies to the inner parts of the body. The lungs, skin, intestines, kidneys, and liver deal with a tremendous amount of internally produced waste, which is a necessary by-product of breathing, digestion, and metabolism.

Under normal circumstances, the body can properly deal with the metabolic waste products that accumulate daily by eliminating them safely from the system. These normal circumstances include eating nutritious and organic foods, living in a pollution-free environment, having plenty of physical movement and exercise, and living a balanced, joyful lifestyle. Yet how many of us can claim to live such natural, fulfilling lives? What happens when our diet, lifestyle, and environment are no longer balanced enough to suit the body's requirements for energy, nourishment, and frictionless circulation? One organ that suffers the most from an overload of toxic chemicals, poor quality of food, and lack of exercise is the liver. Hence, it is of utmost importance for everyone who is concerned about their health to ensure that their liver is cleansed and remains free of any unnecessary obstructions.

Cleansing the liver is not something someone else can do for you. Rather, it is a self-help method that requires a profound sense of self-responsibility and trust in the natural, innate wisdom of the body. You will only feel drawn toward liver flushing when you know deep within yourself that this is something you absolutely have to do. Liver flushing requires a certain amount of commitment and discipline because once you have begun the process you don't want to stop doing it until your liver is completely clean. If you do not feel you are ready to make that commitment, it may be best to put this book aside for the time being and wait. When the time is right, you will feel the definite impulse or desire to improve your liver's functioning and pick up the book and read it again.

Although the liver flush is not a cure for diseases, it sets the precondition for the body to heal itself. In fact, it is rare for an ailment not to improve by increasing liver performance. To understand the great significance of the liver flush, one needs to personally experience how it feels to have a liver that has been relieved of two handfuls of gallstones. For millions of people, the liver flush has been an "amazing" experience, which is reason enough for me to share it with those willing to help themselves.

The doctor of the future will give no medicine
but will interest his patients in the care of the human frame,
in diet, and in the cause and prevention of disease.
~ Thomas Edison ~

Product Information

All website addresses are for countries in North America, unless otherwise specified.

Colema Boards
Wellness Products
www.ener-chi.com

Colema Boards for Europe (in France):
Bernard CLAVIERE
www.colon-net.com
bernardgironde@yahoo.com

Enema bags
www.enemasupply.com
www.healthandyoga.com
www.therawfoodworld.com/index.php

Squatty Potty Toilet Stool
www.ener-chi.com

Organic Sulfur Crystals
Wellness Products
www.ener-chi.com

Ener-Chi Art by Andreas Moritz
www.ener-chi.com

Ener-Chi Ionized Stones
www.ener-chi.com

Unrefined Salts
www.saltworks.us
www.celtic-seasalt.com
www.realsalt.com
www.himalayancrystalsalt.com

Herbs for the Kidney Cleanse and Liver Tea
www.presentmoment.com (based in Minneapolis, Minnesota)
Mail Order: 1-800-378-3245 or 1-612-824-3157
herbshop@presentmoment.com
Note: Herbs are very fresh and potent and available as a pre-mix.
For European countries visit: www.andreas-moritz.eu

Magnetic Clay (to remove heavy metals from the body)
Magnesium oil (to end or prevent magnesium deficiency)
See *Ancient Minerals* under "Wellness Products"
Zeolite (to remove toxins/heavy metals and balance pH)
Under "Wellness Products":www.ener-chi.com

Products for Alternative Versions of the Liver Flush

In North America:

- **Gold Coin Grass, Chinese Gentian and Bupleurum**
  Prime Health Products (Toronto, Canada)
  www.sensiblehealth.com
  Tel: 416-248-2930, 416-248-0415
  jchang@sensiblehealth.com

- **Chanca Piedra Extract (Raintree Nutrition)**
  www.herbspro.com/ChancaPiedra

- **L-Malic Acid Powder, Food Grade**
  http://purebulk.com/l-malic-acid

- **Colosan**
  Family Health News
  Tel: 1-800-284-6263 or 1-305-759-9500
  www.familyhealthnews.com
  www.prana-luz.com (Spain, Europe)

In Europe:
- Organic cranberry juice
- Organic Aloe Vera Juice
- Malic acid
- Gold coin grass,

- Chanca Piedra
- Enzian and Bupleurum tinctures
- Andreas Moritz Kidney Cleanse Tea
- Andreas Moritz Liver Cleanse Tea

www.andreas-moritz.eu

Water Purification

- **LIFE Water Ionizers**

www.ener-chi.com

- **Adya Ceramic Water Filtration System**

www.amazon.com
www.adyawatereurope.eu (Netherlands, Europe)

- **Aqua Lyros - Structured Water (Germany)**

www.ener-gie.com

- **Prill Beads for Water Improvement**

www.Global-Light-Network.com
www.prana-luz.com (Spain)

Botanical Names for Kidney Cleanse Herbs

Marjoram	*Origanum majorana*
Cat's claw	*Uncaria tomentosa*
Comfrey root	*Symphytum officinale*
Fennel seed	*Foeniculum vulgare*
Chicory herb	*Chichorium intybus*
Uva ursi or bearberry	*Arctostaphylos*
Hydrangea root	*Hydrangea arborescens*
Gravel root	*Eupatorium purpureum*
Marshmallow root	*Althaea officinalis*
Golden rod herb	*Solidago virgaurea*

Botanical Names for Liver Tea Herbs

Dandelion root	*Taraxacum officinale*
Comfrey root	*Symphytum officinale*
Licorice root	*Glycyrrhiza glabra*
Agrimony	*Agrimonia eupatoria*
Wild yam root	*Dioscorea villosa*
Barberry bark	*Berberis vulgaris*
Bearsfoot	*Polymnia uvedalia*
Tanners oak bark	*Quercus robur*
Milk thistle herb	*Silybum marianum*

To order books, Ener-Chi Art pictures, Ionized Stones and some other products mentioned in this book, contact:

Ener-Chi Wellness Center, LLC
Website: www.ener-chi.com
Toll free: 1-866-258-4006 (USA)
Local (709) 570-7401 (Canada)

For selected products in Europe visit
www.andreas-moritz.eu
(see more details below)

To purchase Ener-Chi Art pictures in Europe, visit:
www.buchshop-fiedler.de

For other books by Andreas Moritz in German, visit:
http://shop.unitedbookgroup.com
(select Andreas Moritz - Bücher)

Other Books and Products by Andreas Moritz

Timeless Secrets of Health and Rejuvenation
Breakthrough Medicine for the 21st Century
(550 pages, 8 ½ x 11 inches)

This book meets the increasing demand for a clear and comprehensive guide that can help people to become self-sufficient regarding their health and well-being. It answers some of the most pressing questions of our time: How does illness arise? Who heals, and who doesn't? Are we destined to be sick? What causes aging? Is it reversible? What are the major causes of disease, and how can we eliminate them? What simple and effective practices can I incorporate into my daily routine that will dramatically improve my health?

Topics include: The placebo effect and the mind/body mystery; the laws of illness and health; the four most common risk factors for disease; digestive disorders and their effects on the rest of the body; the wonders of our biological rhythms and how to restore them if disrupted; how to create a life of balance; why to choose a vegetarian diet; cleansing the liver, gallbladder, kidneys, and colon; removing allergies; giving up smoking, naturally; using sunlight as medicine; the new causes of heart disease, cancer, diabetes, and AIDS; and a scrutinizing look at antibiotics, blood transfusions, ultrasound scans, and immunization programs.

Timeless Secrets of Health and Rejuvenation sheds light on all major issues of healthcare and reveals that most medical treatments, including surgery, blood transfusions, and pharmaceutical drugs, are avoidable when certain key functions in the body are restored through the natural methods described in the book. The reader also learns about the potential dangers of medical diagnosis and treatment, as well as the reasons why vitamin supplements, *health foods*, low-fat products, *wholesome* breakfast cereals, diet foods, and diet programs may have contributed to the current health crisis rather than helped to resolve it. The book includes a complete program of healthcare, which is primarily based on the ancient medical system of Ayurveda and the vast amount of experience Andreas Moritz has gained in the field of health restoration during the past 30 years.

Cancer is Not a Disease! It's A Healing Mechanism
Discover Cancer's Hidden Purpose, Heal its Root Causes, and be Healthier Than Ever!

In this expanded, 2012 edition of *Cancer is Not a Disease,* Andreas Moritz proves the point that cancer is the physical symptom that reflects our body's final attempt to deal with life-threatening cell congestion and toxins. He claims that removing the underlying conditions that force the body to produce cancerous cells, sets the preconditions for complete healing of our body, mind, and emotions.

This book confronts you with a radically new understanding of cancer - one that revolutionized the current cancer model. On the average, today's conventional *treatments* of killing, cutting out, or burning cancerous cells offer most patients a remission rate of a mere 7 percent, and the majority of these survivors are *cured* for not more than just 5 years. Prominent cancer researcher and professor at the University of California at Berkeley, Dr. Hardin Jones, stated: "Patients are as well, or better off, untreated..." Any published success figures in cancer survival statistics are offset by equal or better scores among those receiving no treatment at all. More people are killed by cancer treatments than are saved by them.

Cancer is Not a Disease shows you why traditional cancer treatments and even cancer diagnoses are often fatal, what actually causes cancer, and how you can remove the obstacles that prevent the body from healing itself. Cancer is not an attempt on your life; on the contrary, this *terrible disease* is the body's final, desperate effort to save your life. Unless we change our perception of what cancer really is, it will continue to threaten the life of nearly 1 out of every 2 people. This book opens a door for those who wish to turn feelings of victimhood into empowerment and self-mastery, and disease into health.

Topics of the book include:
- Reasons the body is forced to develop cancer cells
- How to identify and remove the causes of cancer
- Why most cancers disappear by themselves, without medical intervention
- Why radiation, chemotherapy, and surgery never cure cancer
- Why some people survive cancer despite undergoing dangerously radical treatments

- The roles of fear, frustration, low self-worth, and repressed anger in the origination of cancer
- How to turn self-destructive emotions into energies that promote health and vitality
- Spiritual lessons behind cancer

Lifting the Veil of Duality
Your Guide to Living without Judgment

"Do you know that there is a place inside you - hidden beneath the appearance of thoughts, feelings, and emotions - that does not know the difference between good and evil, right and wrong, light and dark? From that place you embrace the opposite values of life as One. In this sacred place you are at peace with yourself and at peace with your world." - Andreas Moritz

In *Lifting the Veil of Duality*, Andreas Moritz poignantly exposes the illusion of duality. He outlines a simple way to remove every limitation that you have imposed upon yourself during the course of living in the realm of duality. You will be prompted to see yourself and the world through a new lens: the lens of clarity, discernment, and non-judgment. You will also discover that mistakes, accidents, coincidences, negativity, deception, injustice, wars, crime, and terrorism all have a deeper purpose and meaning in the larger scheme of things. So naturally, much of what you will read may conflict with the beliefs you currently hold. Yet you are not asked to change your beliefs or opinions. Instead, you are asked to have an *open mind*, for only an open mind can enjoy freedom from judgment.

Our personal views and world views are currently challenged by a crisis of identity. Some are being shattered altogether. The collapse of our current world order forces humanity to deal with the most basic issues of existence. You can no longer avoid taking responsibility for the things that happen to you. When you *do* accept responsibility, you also empower and heal yourself.

Lifting the Veil of Duality shows how you create or subdue your ability to fulfill your desires. Furthermore, you will find intriguing explanations about the mystery of time, the truth and illusion of reincarnation, the oftentimes misunderstood value of prayer, what makes relationships work and why so often they don't. Find out why injustice is an illusion that has managed to haunt us throughout the ages. Learn about our original separation from the Source of life and what this means with regard to the current waves of instability and fear that so many of us are experiencing.

Discover how to identify the angels living amongst us and why we all have light-bodies. You will have the opportunity to find the ultimate God within you and discover why a God seen as separate from yourself keeps you from being in your Divine Power and happiness. In addition, you can find out how to heal yourself at a moment's notice. Read all about the *New Medicine* and the destiny of the old medicine, the old economy, the old religion, and the old world.

It's Time to Come Alive!
Start Using the Amazing Healing Powers of Your Body, Mind, and Spirit Today!

In this book, Andreas Moritz brings to light man's deep inner need for spiritual wisdom in life and helps the reader develop a new sense of reality that is based on love, power, and compassion. He describes our relationship with the natural world in detail and discusses how we can harness its tremendous powers for our personal and humanity's benefit. *It's Time to Come Alive* challenges some of our most commonly held beliefs and offers a way out of the emotional restrictions and physical limitations we have created in our lives.

Topics include: What shapes our destiny, using the power of intention, secrets of defying the aging process, doubting - the cause of failure, opening the heart, material wealth and spiritual wealth, fatigue - the major cause of stress, methods of emotional transformation, techniques of primordial healing, how to increase the health of the five senses, developing spiritual wisdom, the major causes of today's earth changes, entry into the new world, the 12 gateways to heaven on earth, and much more.

Simple Steps to Total Health!
Andreas Moritz with co-author John Hornecker

By nature, your physical body is designed to be healthy and vital throughout life. Unhealthy eating habits and lifestyle choices, however, lead to numerous health conditions that prevent you from enjoying life to the fullest. In *Simple Steps to Total Health*, the authors bring to light the most common cause of disease, which is the buildup of toxins and residues from improperly digested foods that inhibit various organs and systems from performing their normal functions. This guidebook for total health provides you with simple but highly effective approaches for internal cleansing, hydration, nutrition, and living habits.

The book's 3 parts cover the essentials of total health: Good Internal Hygiene, Healthy Nutrition, and Balanced Lifestyle. Learn about the most common disease-causing foods, dietary habits and influences responsible for the occurrence of chronic illnesses, including those affecting the blood vessels, heart, liver, intestinal organs, lungs, kidneys, joints, bones, nervous system, and sense organs.

To be able to live a healthy life, you must align your internal biological rhythms with the larger rhythms of nature. Find out more about this and many other important topics in *Simple Steps to Total Health*. This is a must-have book for anyone who is interested in using a natural, drug-free approach to restore total health.

Heart Disease No More!
(Excerpted from *Timeless Secrets of Health and Rejuvenation*)

Less than one hundred years ago, heart disease was an extremely rare illness. Today it kills more people in the developed world than all other causes of death combined. Despite the vast quantity of financial resources spent on finding a cure for heart disease, the current medical approaches remain mainly symptom-oriented and do not address the underlying causes.

Even worse, overwhelming evidence shows that the treatment of heart disease or its presumed precursors, such as high blood pressure, hardening of the arteries, and high cholesterol, not only prevents a real cure, but also can easily lead to chronic heart failure. The patient's heart may still beat, but not strongly enough for him to feel vital and alive.

Without removing the underlying causes of heart disease and its precursors, the average person has little, if any, protection against it. Heart attacks can strike whether you have undergone a coronary bypass or have had stents placed inside your arteries. According to research, these procedures fail to prevent heart attacks and do nothing to reduce mortality rates.

Heart Disease No More, excerpted from the author's bestselling book, *Timeless Secrets of Health and Rejuvenation*, puts the responsibility for healing where it belongs: on the heart, mind, and body of each individual.

It provides the reader with practical insights about the development and causes of heart disease. Even better, it explains simple steps you can take to prevent and reverse heart disease for good, regardless of a possible genetic predisposition.

Diabetes - No More!
Discover and Heal Its True Causes
(Excerpted from *Timeless Secrets of Health and Rejuvenation*)

According to bestselling author Andreas Moritz, diabetes is not a disease; in the vast majority of cases, it is a complex mechanism of protection or survival that the body chooses in order to avoid the possibly fatal consequences of an unhealthy diet and lifestyle.

Despite the body's ceaseless self-preservation efforts (which we call *diseases*), millions of people suffer or die unnecessarily from these consequences. The imbalanced blood sugar level in diabetes is but a symptom of illness, and not the illness itself. By developing diabetes, the body is neither doing something wrong, nor is it trying to commit suicide. The current diabetes epidemic is man-made, or rather, factory-made, and, therefore, can be halted and reversed through simple but effective changes in diet and lifestyle. *Diabetes - No More!* provides you with essential information on the various causes of diabetes and how anyone can avoid them.

To stop the diabetes epidemic you need to create the right circumstances that allow your body to heal. Just as there is a mechanism to becoming diabetic, there is also a mechanism to reverse it. Find out how!

This book is excerpted from the author's bestselling book, *Timeless Secrets of Health and Rejuvenation*.

Ending The AIDS Myth
It's Time to Heal the TRUE Causes!
(Excerpted from *Timeless Secrets of Health and Rejuvenation*)

Contrary to common belief, no scientific evidence exists to this day to prove that AIDS is a contagious disease. The current AIDS theory falls short in predicting the kind of AIDS disease an infected person may be manifesting, and no accurate system is in place to determine how long it will take for the disease to develop. In addition, the current HIV/AIDS theory contains no reliable information that can help identify those who are at risk for developing AIDS.

On the other hand, published research actually proves that HIV only spreads heterosexually in extremely rare cases and cannot be responsible for an epidemic that involves millions of AIDS victims around the world. Furthermore, it is an established fact that the retrovirus HIV, which is composed of human gene fragments, is incapable of destroying human cells. However, cell destruction is the main characteristic of every AIDS disease.

Even the principal discoverer of HIV, Luc Montagnier, no longer believes that HIV is solely responsible for causing AIDS. In fact, he showed that HIV alone could not cause AIDS. Increasing evidence indicates that AIDS may be a toxicity syndrome or metabolic disorder that is caused by immunity risk factors, including heroin, sex-enhancement drugs, antibiotics, commonly prescribed AIDS drugs, rectal intercourse, starvation, malnutrition, and dehydration.

Dozens of prominent scientists working at the forefront of AIDS research now openly question the virus hypothesis of AIDS. Find out why! *Ending the AIDS Myth* also shows you what really causes the shutdown of the immune system and what you can do to avoid this.

Heal Yourself with Sunlight
Use Its Secret Medicinal Powers to Help Cure Cancer, Heart Disease, Hypertension, Diabetes Arthritis, Infectious Diseases, and much more.

This book by Andreas Moritz provides scientific evidence that sunlight is essential for good health, and that a lack of sun exposure can be held responsible for many of today's diseases.

Ironically, most people now believe that the sun is the main culprit for causing skin cancer, certain cataracts leading to blindness, and aging. Only those who take the *risk* of exposing themselves to sunlight find that the sun makes them feel and look better, provided they don't use sunscreens or burn their skin. The UV rays in sunlight actually stimulate the thyroid gland to increase hormone production, which in turn, increases the body's basal metabolic rate. This assists both in weight loss and improved muscle development.

It has been known for several decades that those living mostly in the outdoors, at high altitudes, or near the equator, have the lowest incidence of skin cancers. In addition, studies have revealed that exposing patients to controlled amounts of sunlight dramatically lowered elevated blood pressure (up to 40 mm Hg drop), decreased cholesterol in the blood stream, lowered abnormally high blood sugars among diabetics, and increased the number of white blood cells which we need to help resist disease. Patients suffering from gout, rheumatoid arthritis, colitis, arteriosclerosis, anemia, cystitis, eczema, acne, psoriasis, herpes, lupus, sciatica, kidney problems, asthma, as well as burns, have all shown to receive great benefit from the healing rays of the sun.

There is ample scientific evidence to show that vitamin D deficiency due to lack of regular sun exposure is responsible for most diseases prevalent in modern societies where most people spend most of their time indoors. In addition, the use of sunscreens often leads to a life-threatening vitamin D deficiency.

This book reveals the true reasons the masses are fed the misinformation that the sun is harmful to our health.

Hear the Whispers, Live Your Dream
A Fanfare of Inspiration

Listening to the whispers of your heart will set you free. The beauty and bliss of your knowingness and love center are what we are here to capture, take in, and swim with. You are like a dolphin sailing in a sea of joy. Allow yourself to open to the wondrous fullness of your selfhood, without reservation and without judgment.

Judgment stands in the way, like a boulder trespassing on your journey to the higher reaches of your destiny. Push these boulders aside and feel the joy of your inner truth sprout forth. Do not allow another's thoughts or directions for you to supersede your inner knowingness, for you relinquish being the full, radiant star that you are.

It is with an open heart, a receptive mind, and a reaching for the stars of wisdom that lie within you, that you reap the bountiful goodness of Mother Earth and the universal I AM. For you are a benevolent being of light and there is no course that can truly stop you, except your own thoughts, or allowing another's beliefs to override your own.

May these expressions of love, joy and wisdom inspire you to be the wondrous being that you were born to be!

Feel Great, Lose Weight
Stop Dieting and Start Living

No rigorous workouts. No surgery. In this book, celebrated author Andreas Moritz suggests a gentle - and permanent - route to losing weight. In this ground-breaking book, he says that once we stop blaming our genes and take control of our own life, weight loss is a natural consequence.

"You need to make that critical mental shift. You need to experience the willingness to shed your physical and emotional baggage, not by counting calories but by embracing your mind, body and spirit. Once you start looking at yourself differently, 80 percent of the work is done."

In Feel Great, Lose Weight, Andreas Moritz tells us why conventional weight loss programs don't work and how weight loss experts make sure we keep going back. He also tells us why food manufacturers, pharmaceutical companies, and health regulators conspire to keep America toxically overweight.

But we can refuse to buy into the Big Fat Lie. Choosing the mind-body approach triggers powerful biochemical changes that set us on a safe and irreversible path to losing weight, without resorting to crash diets, heavy workouts, or dangerous surgical procedures.

Vaccine-nation
Poisoning the Population, One Shot at a Time!

Andreas Moritz takes on yet another controversial subject, this time to expose the Vaccine Myth. In *Vaccine-nation*, Moritz unravels the mother of all vaccine lies - that vaccines are safe and they prevent disease. Furthermore, he reveals undeniable scientific proof that vaccines are actually implicated in most diseases today.

This book reveals:

- Statistical evidence that vaccines never actually eradicated infectious diseases, including polio
- How childhood vaccines, flu shots, and other kinds of inoculations systemically destroy the body's immune system
- The massive increase of allergies, eczema, arthritis, asthma, autism, acid reflux, cancer, diabetes (infant and childhood), kidney disease, miscarriages, many neurological and autoimmune diseases, and Sudden Infant Death Syndrome (SIDS) is largely due to vaccines

- Why vaccinated children have 120 percent more asthma, 317 percent more ADHD, 185 percent more neurologic disorders, and 146 percent more autism than those not vaccinated
- The shocking fact that most outbreaks of infectious diseases occur largely among those who are fully vaccinated
- Vaccines lack long-term safety testing and most vaccine side effects are never reported in order to protect vaccine-makers from liability suits.

To this day, national health agencies still refuse to conduct long-term double blind control studies to prove vaccines are both safe and work better than the placebo effect. The Centers for Disease Control (CDC) say that we shouldn't test such drugs (vaccines) on human beings because that would be *"unethical"*. However, pumping little children with 35 vaccine shots that are loaded with dangerous toxins and proclaiming that this would cause *no* harm can hardly be considered safe and ethical. We are asked to just trust them on this, in the complete absence of proof that vaccines are safe and effective to prevent disease. Avoiding comparison studies is not really a reasonable excuse today, as many parents *have already* opted out of at least some, if not all, vaccines for their children anyway. So there are many children available for such kind of research.

In *Vaccine-nation*, Moritz minces no words while unraveling these and other skeletons in Big Pharma's closet and cautions you not to buy into the hollow claims of vaccine makers. In his characteristic style, Moritz offers a gentle and practical approach to a disease-free life, which rests on the fulcrum of the mind-body connection, cleansing of the body, and naturally healthy living.

Art of Self Healing (book)
Collection of all Ener-Chi Art healing pictures (oil on canvas by Andreas Moritz). Size 12 x 14 inches; contains 32 high-quality art prints.

Andreas Moritz has developed a new system of healing and rejuvenation designed to restore the basic life energy (chi) of an organ or a system in the body within a matter of seconds. Simultaneously, it also helps balance the emotional causes of illness.

Eastern approaches to healing, such as acupuncture and shiatsu, are intended to enhance well-being by stimulating and balancing the flow of chi to the various organs and systems of the body. In a similar manner, the energetics of Ener-Chi Art is designed to restore a balanced flow of chi throughout the body.

According to most ancient systems of health and healing, the balanced flow of chi is the key determinant for a healthy body and mind. When chi flows through the body unhindered, health and vitality are maintained. By contrast, if the flow of chi is disrupted or reduced, health and vitality tend to decline.

A person can determine the degree to which the flow of chi is balanced in the body's organs and systems by using a simple muscle testing procedure. To reveal the effectiveness of Ener-Chi Art, it is important to apply this test both before and after viewing each Ener-Chi Art picture.

To allow for easy application of this system, Andreas has created a number of healing paintings that have been *activated* through a unique procedure that imbues each work of art with specific color rays (derived from the higher dimensions). To receive the full benefit of an Ener-Chi Art picture, all it requires is to look at it for less than a minute. During this time, the flow of chi within the organ or system becomes fully restored. When applied to all the organs and systems of the body, Ener-Chi Art sets the precondition for the whole body to heal and rejuvenate itself.

Alzheimer's - No More!
Discover the True Causes and Immediate Remedies
(expected publication date December 2012)

All books are available as paperback and electronic books through the Ener-Chi Wellness Center.

Ener-Chi Ionized Stones

Ener-Chi Ionized Stones are stones and crystals that have been energized, activated, and imbued with life force through a special process introduced by Andreas Moritz, the creator of Ener-Chi Art.

Stone ionization has not been attempted before because stones and rocks have rarely been considered useful in the field of healing. Yet, stones have the inherent power to hold and release vast amounts of information and energy. Once ionized, they exert a balancing influence on everything with which they come into contact. The ionization of stones may be one of our keys to survival in a world that is experiencing high-level pollution and destruction of its eco-balancing systems.

In the early evolutionary stages of Earth, every particle of matter on the planet contained within it the blueprint of the entire planet, just as every cell of our body contains within its DNA structure the blueprint of our entire body. The blueprint information within every particle of matter is still there - it has simply fallen into a dormant state. The ionization process *reawakens* this original blueprint information and enables the associated energies to be released. In this sense, Ener-Chi Ionized Stones are alive and conscious, and are able to energize, purify, and balance any natural substance with which they come into contact.

Ener-Chi Ionized Stones
Instructions for use

■ Drinking Ionized Water
Placing an Ionized Stone next to a glass of water for about half a minute ionizes the water. Ionized water is a powerful cleanser that aids digestion and metabolism, and energizes the entire body.
■ Eating Ionized Foods
Placing an Ionized Stone next to your food for about half a minute ionizes and balances it. Due to the pollution in our atmosphere and soil, even natural organic foods are usually somewhat polluted. Such foods are also impacted by ozone depletion and exposure to electro-magnetic radiation in our planetary environment. These negative effects tend to be neutralized through the specified use of Ionized Stones.
■ Ionized Foot Bath

By placing Ionized Stones (preferably pebbles with rounded surfaces) under the soles of the feet, while the feet are immersed in water, the body begins to break down toxins and waste materials into harmless organic substances.

■ Enhancing Healing Therapies

Ionized Stones are ideal for enhancing the effects of any healing therapy. For example, "LaStone Therapy" is a popular new therapy that is offered in some innovative health spas. This involves placing warm stones on key energy points of the body. If these stones were ionized prior to being placed on the body, the healing effects would be enhanced. In fact, placing Ionized Stones on any weak or painful part of the body, including the corresponding chakra, has healthful benefits. If crystals play a role in the therapy, ionizing them first greatly amplifies their positive effects

■ Aura and Chakra Balancing

Holding an Ionized Stone or Ionized Crystal in the middle section of the spinal column for about 30 seconds balances all of the chakras, or energy centers, and tends to keep them in balance for several weeks or even months. Since energy imbalances in the chakras and auric field are one of the major causes of health problems, this balancing procedure is a powerful way to enhance health and well-being.

■ Attached to Main Water Pipe of Home

Attaching a stone to the main water pipe will ionize your water and make it more absorbable and energized.

■ Placed in or near the Electrical Fuse Box

By placing a larger Ionized Stone in, above, or below the fuse box in your house, the harmful effects of electromagnetic radiation become nullified. You can verify this by doing the muscle test (as shown on the instruction sheet for Ener-Chi Art) in front of a TV or computer, both before and after placing the stone on the fuse box. If you don't have a fuse box that is readily accessible, you can place a stone next to the electrical cable of your appliances or near their power sockets.

■ Used in Conjunction with Ener-Chi Art

Ionized Stones may be used to enhance the effects of Ener-Chi Art pictures. Simply place an Ionized Stone over the related area of the body while viewing an Ener-Chi Art picture. For example, if you are viewing the Ener-Chi Art picture related to the heart, hold an ionized stone over the heart area while viewing the picture. The nature of the energies involved in the pictures and the stones is similar. Accordingly, if the stones are used in combination with the pictures, a resonance is created which greatly enhances the overall effect.

■ Creating an Enhanced Environment

Placing an Ionized Stone near the various items that surround you for about half a minute helps to create a more energized and balanced environment. The Ionized Stones affect virtually all natural materials, such as wood floors, wood or metal furniture, stone walls, and brick or stone fireplaces. In work areas, especially near computers, it is a good idea to place one or more Ionized Stones at strategic locations. The same applies to sleeping areas, such as putting stones under your bed or pillow.

■ Improving Plant Growth

Placing Ionized Stones next to a plant or flowerpot may increase their health and beauty. This automatically ionizes the water they receive, whether they are indoor or outdoor plants. The same applies to vegetable plants and organic gardens.

■ Creating More Ionized Stones

Make any number of ionized stones simply by holding your seed stone against any other stones or crystals for 40-50 seconds. Your new stones will have the same effect as the seed stone.

To order Books, Ener-Chi Art and Ener-Chi Ionized Stones please contact:

Ener-Chi Wellness Center, LLC
Website: http://www.ener-chi.com
Toll free: 1(866) 258-4006 (USA)
Local (709) 570-7401 (Canada)

About Andreas Moritz

Andreas Moritz is a medical intuitive; a practitioner of Ayurveda, iridology, shiatsu, and vibrational medicine; a writer; and an artist. Born in southwest Germany in 1954, Moritz had to deal with several severe illnesses from an early age, which compelled him to study diet, nutrition, and various methods of natural healing while still a child.

By age 20, he had completed his training in both iridology (the diagnostic science of eye interpretation) and dietetics. In 1981, he began studying Ayurvedic medicine in India and finished his training as a qualified practitioner of Ayurveda in New Zealand in 1991. Rather than being satisfied with merely treating the symptoms of illness, Moritz has dedicated his life's work to understanding and treating the root causes of illness. Because of this holistic approach, he has had great success with cases of terminal disease where conventional methods of healing have proved futile.

Since 1988, he has practiced the Japanese healing art of shiatsu, which has given him insights into the energy system of the body. In addition, he has devoted 8 years of research into consciousness and its important role in the field of mind/body medicine.

Andreas Moritz is the author of the following books on health and spirituality:
- Timeless Secrets of Health and Rejuvenation
- Cancer is Not a Disease
- The Amazing Liver and Gallbladder Flush
- Lifting the Veil of Duality
- It's Time to Come Alive
- Heart Disease - No More!
- Simple Steps to Total Health
- Diabetes - No More!
- Ending the AIDS Myth
- Heal Yourself with Sunlight
- Feel Great, Lose Weight
- Vaccine-nation: Poisoning the Population, One Shot at a Time
- Alzheimer's No More!
- Art of Self-Healing
- Hear the Whispers, Live Your Dream

During his extensive travels throughout the world, Andreas has consulted with heads of state and members of government in Europe, Asia, and Africa, and has lectured widely on the subjects of health, mind/body medicine, and spirituality. Moritz has a free forum, "Ask Andreas Moritz," on the large health website CureZone.com (5 million readers and increasing). Although he recently stopped writing for the forum, it contains an extensive archive of his answers to thousands of questions on a variety of health topics.

Since taking up residence in the United States in 1998, Moritz has been involved in developing a new and innovative system of healing called *Ener-Chi Art* that targets the root causes of many chronic illnesses. Ener-Chi Art consists of a series of light ray-encoded oil paintings that can instantly restore vital energy flow (chi) in the organs and systems of the body. Moritz is also the creator of *Sacred Santémony - Divine Chanting for Every Occasion,* a powerful system of specially generated frequencies of sound that can transform deep-seated fears, allergies, traumas, and mental or emotional blocks into useful opportunities for growth and inspiration within a matter of moments.

INDEX

Additional scientific references about intrahepatic gallstones

1. Best, R. R.: The Incidence of Liver Stones Associated with Cholelithiasis and Its Clinical Significance. Surg. Gynecol. Obstet., 78:425, 1944.

2. Chiam, H. K., Unni, P. N. and Hwang, W. S.: Cholelithiasis in Singapore. Part II. A Clinical Study. Gut, 11:148, 1970.

3. Cobo, A., Hall, R. C., Torres, E. and Cuello, C. J.: Intrahepatic Calculi. Arch. Surg., 89:936, 1964.

4. Cook, J., Hou, P. C., Ho, H. C. and McFadzean, A. J. S.: Recurrent Pyogenic Cholangitis. Brit. J. Surg., 42:188, 1954.

5. Digby, K. H.: Common Duct Stones of Liver Origin. Brit. J. Surg., 17:578, 1930.

6. Glenn, F. and Moody, F. G.: Intrahepatic Calculi. Ann. Surg., 153:711, 1961.

7. Glenn, F.: Christopher's Textbook of Surgery (Ed. 7). Philadelphia, W. B. Saunders, 1960, 778.

8. Harrison-Levy, A.: The Biliary Obstruction Syndrome of the Chinese. Brit. J. Surg., 49:674, 1962.

9. Jones, S. A., Steedman, R. A., Keller, T. B. and Smith, L. L.: Transduodenal Sphincteroplasty (Not Sphincterotomy) for Biliary and Pancreatic Disease. Amer. J. Surg., 118:292, 1969.

10. Maki, T.: Cholelithiasis in the Japanese. Arch. Surg., 82:599, 1961.

11. Maki, T., Sato, T., Yamaguchi, I. and Sato, T.: Treatment of Intrahepatic Gallstones. Arch. Surg., 88:260, 1964.

12. Miyake, H.: Gallstone in Kyushu, Japan. Arch. Surg., 85:425, 1962.

13. Palmer, R. H.: Gallstones Produced Experimentally by Litho-cholic Acid in Rats. Science, 148:1339, 1965.

14. Palmer, R. H.: Production of Bile Duct Hyperplasia and Gallstones by Lithocholic Acid. J. Clin. Invest., 45:1255, 1966.

15. Rufanov, I. G.: Liver Stones. Ann. Surg., 103:321, 580, 1936.

16. Stock, P. E. and Tinckler, L. F.: Choledochoduodenostomy in the Treatment of Cholangiohepatitis. Surg. Gynecol. Obstet., 101:599, 1955.

17. Stock, F. E. and Fung, J. H. Y.: Oriental Cholangiohepatitis. Surgery, 84:409, 1962.

18. Walters, W.: Cholangiohcpatitis or Recurrent Pyogenic Cholangitis with Intrahepatic and Extrahepatic Bile-pigment Stones. Editorial, JAMA, 178:934, 1961.

Notes

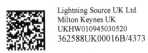

Lightning Source UK Ltd.
Milton Keynes UK
UKHW010945030520
362588UK00016B/4373

9 780984 595440